CASE STUDIES

Stahl's Essential Psychopharmacology

CASE STUDIES Stahl's Essential Psychopharmacology

Stephen M. Stahl
University of California at San Diego
University of Cambridge, UK

Debbi A. Morrissette
Editorial Assistant

with illustrations by
Nancy Muntner

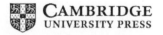
CAMBRIDGE
UNIVERSITY PRESS

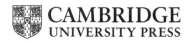

Shaftesbury Road, Cambridge CB2 8EA, United Kingdom

One Liberty Plaza, 20th Floor, New York, NY 10006, USA

477 Williamstown Road, Port Melbourne, VIC 3207, Australia

314–321, 3rd Floor, Plot 3, Splendor Forum, Jasola District Centre, New Delhi – 110025, India

103 Penang Road, #05–06/07, Visioncrest Commercial, Singapore 238467

Cambridge University Press is part of Cambridge University Press & Assessment, a department of the University of Cambridge.

We share the University's mission to contribute to society through the pursuit of education, learning and research at the highest international levels of excellence.

www.cambridge.org
Information on this title: www.cambridge.org/9780521182089

First published 2011
8th printing 2023

Printed in Great Britain by CPI Group (UK) Ltd, Croydon CRO 4YY

A catalogue record for this publication is available from the British Library

ISBN   978-0-521-18208-9   Paperback

Contents

= designates a "Lighting Round," a short case without a tutorial

Contents

Introduction

Joining the *Essential Psychopharmacology* series here is a new idea –
namely, a case book. *Essential Psychopharmacology* started in 1996 as a
textbook (currently in its third edition) on *how psychotropic drugs work*. It
then expanded to a companion *Prescriber's Guide* in 2005 (currently in its
fourth edition) on *how to prescribe psychotropic drugs*. In 2008, a website
was added (*stahlonline.org*) with both of these books available online in
combination with several more, including an *Illustrated* series of several books
covering specialty topics in psychopharmacology. Now comes a *Case Book*,
showing *how to apply the concepts* presented in these previous books *to real
patients in a clinical practice setting*.

Why a case book? For practitioners, it is necessary to know the science of
psychopharmacology – namely, both the mechanism of action of psychotropic
drugs and the evidence-based data on how to prescribe them – but this is
not sufficient to become a master clinician. Many patients are beyond the
data and are excluded from randomized controlled trials. Thus, a true clinical
expert also needs to develop the art of psychopharmacology: namely, how to
listen, educate, destigmatize, mix psychotherapy with medications and use
intuition to select and combine medications. The art of psychopharmacology
is especially important when confronting the frequent situations where there is
no evidence on which to base a clinical decision.

What do you do when there is no evidence? The short answer is to combine
the science with the art of psychopharmacology. The best way to learn this
is probably by seeing individual patients. Here I hope you will join me and
peer over my shoulder to observe 40 complex cases from my own clinical
practice. Each case is anonymized in identifying details, but incorporates real
case outcomes that are not fictionalized. Sometimes more than one case
is combined into a single case. Hopefully, you will recognize many of these
patients as the same as those you have seen in your own practice (although
they will not be the exact same patient, as the identifying historical details are
changed here to comply with disclosure standards and many patients can look
very much like many other patients you know, which is why you may find this
teaching approach effective for your clinical practice).

I have presented cases from my clinical practice for many years online (e.g.,
in the master psychopharmacology program of the Neuroscience Education
Institute (NEI) at neiglobal.com) and in live courses (especially at the annual
NEI Psychopharmacology Congress). Over the years, I have been fortunate to
have many young psychiatrists from my university and indeed from all over

the world, sit in on my practice to observe these cases, and now I attempt to bring this information to you in the form of a case book.

The cases are presented in a novel written format in order to follow consultations over time, with different categories of information designated by different background colors and explanatory icons. For those of you familiar with *Essential Psychopharmacology: The Prescribers Guide*, this layout will look quite familiar. Included in the case book, however, are many unique sections as well; for example, presenting what was on the author's mind at various points during the management of the case, and also questions along the way for you to ask yourself in order to develop an action plan. Also, these cases incorporate ideas from the recent changes in maintenance of certification standards by the American Board of Psychiatry and Neurology for those of you interested in recertification in psychiatry. Thus, there is a section on Performance in Practice (called here "confessions of a psychopharmacologist"). This is a short section at the end of every case, looking back and seeing what could have been done better in retrospect. Another section of most cases is a short psychopharmacology lesson or tutorial, called the "Two Minute Tute," with background information, tables and figures from literature relevant to the case on hand. Shorter cases of only a few pages do not contain the Tutes, but get directly to the point, and are called "Lightning Rounds." Drugs are listed by their generic name, and often have a brand name mentioned the first time they appear in a case. A generic and brand name index is included at the back of the book for your convenience. Lists of icons and abbreviations are provided in the front of the book.

The case-based approach is how this book attempts to complement "evidence based prescribing" from other books in the *Essential Psychopharmacology* series, plus the literature, with "prescribing based evidence" derived from empiric experience. It is certainly important to know the data from randomized controlled trials, but after knowing all this information, case based clinical experience supplements that data. The old saying that applies here is that wisdom is what you learn AFTER you know it all. And so, too, for studying cases after seeing the data.

A note of caution. I am not so naive as to think that there are not potential pitfalls to the centuries-old tradition of case-based teaching. Thus, I think it is a good idea to point some of them out here in order to try to avoid these traps.

Do not ignore the "law of small numbers" by basing broad predictions on narrow samples or even a single case.

Do not ignore the fact that if something is easy to recall, particularly when associated with a significant emotional event, we tend to think it happens more often than it does.

Do not forget the recency effect, namely, the tendency to think that something that has just been observed happens more often than it does.

According to editorialists (1), when moving away from evidence-based medicine to case-based medicine it is also important to avoid:
- Eloquence- or elegance-based medicine
- Vehemence-based medicine
- Providence-based medicine
- Diffidence-based medicine
- Nervousness-based medicine
- Confidence-based medicine

I have been counseled by colleagues and trainees that perhaps the most important pitfall for me to try to avoid in this book is "eminence-based medicine," and to remember specifically that:
- Radiance of gray hair is not proportional to an understanding of the facts
- Eloquence, smoothness of the tongue and sartorial elegance cannot change reality
- Qualifications and past accomplishments do not signify a privileged access to the truth
- Experts almost always have conflicts of interest
- Clinical acumen is not measured in frequent flier miles

So, it is with all humility as a practicing psychiatrist that I invite you to walk a mile in my shoes, experience the fascination, the disappointments, the thrills and the learnings that result from observing cases in the real world.

Stephen M. Stahl, M.D, Ph.D.

(1) Isaccs D and Fitzgerald D, Seven alternatives to evidence based medicine, British Medical Journal 1999, 319:7225

In memory of Daniel X. Freedman, mentor, colleague, and scientific father.

To all the courageous patients and their families that have been part of my practice of psychiatry over the years

To Cindy, my wife, best friend, and tireless supporter.

To Jennifer and Victoria, my daughters, for their patience and understanding of the demands of authorship.

List of Icons

	Pre and Posttest Assessment Question
	Lightning Round
	Patient Intake
	Psychiatric History
	Social and Personal History
	Medical History
	Family History
	Medication History
	Current Medications

	Psychotherapy History
	Mechanism of Action Moment
	Attending Physician's Mental Notes
	Further Investigation
	Case Outcome
	Case Debrief
	Take-Home Points
	Performance in Practice: Confessions of a Psychopharmacologist
	Tips and Pearls
	Two-Minute Tute

Abbreviations used in this book

ACE	angiotensin converting enzyme	MSLT	multiple sleep latency test
ADHD	attention deficit hyperactivity disorder	MTHFR	methylene tetrahydrofolate reductase
BMI	body mass index	NE	norepinephrine
BP	blood pressure	NIMH	National Institute of Mental Health
BUN	blood urea nitrogen		
CBT	cognitive behavioral therapy	NMDA	N-methyl-d-aspartate
CD	conduct disorder	NOS	not otherwise specified
COMT	catechol O methyl transferase	NRI	norepinephrine reuptake inhibition
CSF	cerebrospinal fluid	OCD	obsessive compulsive disorder
CT	computerized tomography	ODD	oppositional defiant disorder
DA	dopamine	PFC	prefrontal cortex
DBS	deep brain stimulation	PET	positron emission tomography
DKA	diabetic ketoacidosis	prn	as needed (Latin)
DLPFC	dorsolateral prefrontal cortex	PSG	polysomnogram
ECT	electroconvulsive therapy	PTSD	post traumatic stress disorder
EEG	electroencephalogram	qhs	at bedtime (Latin)
EMDR	eye movement desensitization and reprocessing	REM	rapid eye movements
EPS	extrapyramidal symptoms	RLS	restless legs syndrome
ESS	Epworth sleepiness scale	SAMe	S-adenosyl-methionine
fMRI	functional magnetic resonance imaging	SERT	serotonin transporter
		SNRI	serotonin norepinephrine reuptake inhibitor
GAD	generalized anxiety disorder		
HHS	hyperglycemic hyperosmolar syndrome	SOREMP	sleep onset rapid eye movement periods
HMO	health maintenance organization	SSRI	serotonin selective reuptake inhibitor
ICU	intensive care unit		
IM	intramuscular	TBI	traumatic brain injury
MAOI	monoamine oxidase inhibitor	TCA	tricyclic antidepressant
MDD	major depression disorder	TMS	transcrancial magnetic stimulation
MDE	major depressive episode		
MRI	magnetic resonance imaging	VNS	vagal nerve stimulation

The Case: The man whose antidepressants stopped working

The Question: Do depressive episodes become more difficult to treat and more recurrent over time?

The Dilemma: When can you stop antidepressant treatment and what do you do if medications that worked in the past no longer work?

Pretest Self Assessment Question (answer at the end of the case)

When should antidepressant maintenance become indefinite?

A. Following remission from one episode of major depression
B. Following remission from two episodes of major depression
C. If there is a particularly severe episode or one with suicidality, especially if a positive family history for depression
D. Following remission from three episodes of major depression
E. On a case by case basis

Patient Intake

- 63-year-old man with the worst depression and anxiety he has ever felt

Psychiatric History: First Episode

- Age 42, became depressed and anxious after his episode of atrial fibrillation
- Felt vulnerable and afraid of death
- After his hospitalization for atrial fibrillation, which resolved with medications, he felt depression, anxiety, "butterflies in his stomach" and felt like his whole body was "plugged into an electrical circuit"
- Began having suicidal thoughts
- This episode also coincided with the death of his mother
- Treatment with alprazolam (Xanax) and clonazepam (Klonopin): no improvement
- Sertraline (Zoloft) treatment 100 mg/day and he was much improved within 2–3 months, functioning normally at work but had sexual side effects
- Felt totally normal after 6 months and discontinued sertraline

Social and Personal History

- Married 33 years, 3 children
- Non smoker
- No drug or alcohol abuse

Medical History

- Atrial fibrillation age 42, resolved with medication
- Hypercholesterolemia
- BP normal
- BMI normal
- Normal fasting glucose and triglycerides

Family History

- Mother: depression and alcohol abuse
- Maternal uncle: alcohol abuse
- Son: depression
- Daughters: one with mild depression, one with postpartum depression

Medications One Year Following the First Episode of Depression

- Antiarrhythmic
- Statin for cholesterol
- Antihypertensive
- Aspirin

Psychiatric History: Second Episode

- Relapsed into his second episode of major depression at age 52, 10 years after his first episode and 9 ½ years after stopping sertraline
- Symptoms same as last time
- Fear, anxiety, depression, "plugged into a circuit"
- Suicidal thoughts
- Symptoms worse in the morning
- Unable to function and wife had to drive him to work for 3 months
- Depression could have been triggered in part by his taking partial early retirement just before this episode, and feeling vulnerable again and worried about whether this meant his life was over
- For some reason, not given sertraline again at first, but paroxetine (Paxil) which showed no benefit
- Switched to sertraline 150 mg/day with supplemental clonazepam (Klonopin) prn anxiety, and symptoms resolved within 2–3 months but with recurrent sexual dysfunction, same as the first time
- Discontinued sertraline after 1 year

Psychiatric History: Third Episode

- Relapsed into a third episode of major depression at age 58, 6 years after his last episode, and 5 years after stopping sertraline the second time

- Symptoms exactly the same again, with fear, anxiety, suicidal thoughts, unable to function, symptoms worse in the morning
- Was not started on sertraline again because of prior sexual dysfunction, but given bupropinon SR (Wellbutrin SR), but no improvement after 8 weeks
- Added sertraline again, and helped after 8 weeks (completely normal) and stopped bupropion but continued sertraline for a year and then discontinued it

Psychiatric History: Fourth Episode

- Relapsed into a fourth episode of major depression at age 61, 3 years after his last episode and 2 years after discontinuing sertraline for the 3rd time
- The patient had gone back to work, had been very successful again, and retired again
- Brought up worries about his mortality again
- However, doing volunteer work and this helps a bit
- This time, given venlafaxine XR (Effexor XR) and this worked even faster than before and he did not have sexual dysfunction, but discontinued it after less than a year

Based on just what you have been told so far about this patient's history and recurrent episodes of depression, do you think it was a mistake to allow him to discontinue his antidepressant after

- *this last fourth episode?*
- *after his third episode?*
- *after his second episode?*

Psychiatric History: Fifth Episode

- Patient has been suffering with fifth episode for 15 months
- New psychosocial factors from marital difficulties seem to have triggered this episode
- Same symptoms as before
- The referring psychiatrist has given venlafaxine 75–150 mg, which worked for his last (fourth) episode, but no response this time to 8 weeks of treatment at this dose, plus another 8 weeks at 375 mg/day (4 months total treatment)
- This is very atypical for him, where antidepressants worked quickly and robustly in the past
- Has severe psychomotor retardation and strong thoughts but no active plans for suicide
- For months 5 through 11, venlafaxine was augmented with
  - Dextroamphetamine (Dexedrine) 20 mg/day

- Buspirone (Buspar) 30 mg/day
- Clonazepam 2 mg in the morning and 2 mg at night
- Lorazepam (Ativan) 2 mg in the morning and 2 mg at night
• This treatment regimen associated with only a partial response, and continuing depression, anxiety, guilt, hopelessness and suicidal ideation
• Switched the venlafaxine back to sertraline 200 mg/day which had worked in the past, along with continuing the same augmentation medications above, but no response for months 12 through 15 of treatment of this fifth episode
• He seems to have developed treatment resistant depression
• Would this have happened in any event, or could this have been prevented by earlier maintenance treatment?
• He now presents to you 15 months into his fifth episode of major depression, not responding to standard treatments

Attending Physician's Mental Notes: Initial Psychiatric Evaluation

• Patient has been suffering through fifth episode of depression for 15 months
• Here is a case that indeed is linked to psychosocial stressors, but seems to have new episodes of depression coming closer and closer together following discontinuation of his antidepressant
• First recurrence 9½ years after stopping sertraline the first time
• Second recurrence 5 years after stopping sertraline the second time
• Third recurrence 2 years after stopping sertraline the third time
• He is now here only a year after stopping his venlafaxine following his fourth episode of depression
• Treatment guidelines are consistent with discontinuing antidepressants 9 to 12 months after remission from a first episode of depression, with long term maintenance after the second episode reserved perhaps for very severe cases. Clearly the third episode of major depression should be treated indefinitely with antidepressant maintenance, and no doubt, after a fourth episode, indefinite antidepressant maintenance is indicated
• One wonders if the fourth episode and the current fifth episode could have been prevented if he had been treated in maintenance after his third episode
• Now, attending physician is a bit worried that the medications will not work as well this time
• Perhaps changes have occurred in the brain, with shrinkage of the hippocampus and/or prefrontal cortex due to 4 previous and now a fifth episode of depression, and that might make the current fifth episode very difficult to treat

- Is this the natural history of treatment resistant depression in the making?

How would you treat him?

- Increase the dose of dextroamphetamine
- Increase the dose of buspirone
- Augment with bupropion
- Augment with L-methylfolate (Deplin), or thyroid or SAMe
- Augment with an atypical antipsychotic, especially aripiprazole or quetiapine
- Refer for TMS
- Refer for ECT
- Augment with mirtazapine (Remeron)
- Switch to an MAOI

Attending Physician's Mental Notes: Initial Psychiatric Evaluation, Continued

- Has not responded to bupropion in the past, and not clear his buspirone or amphetamine is helpful, and he does not need two different benzodiazepines
- Maybe too treatment resistant for a natural product
- He has anxiety and is quite depressed, so suggest an anxiolytic/ sedating/sleep inducing antidepressant like mirtazapine, while discontinuing his dextroamphetamine, buspirone, and consolidating his two benzodiazepines into one
- Could have added an atypical antipsychotic, but because of his cardiovascular status, patient wished to try mirtazapine first
- Patient willing to do all of this but discontinue his amphetamine, although he does agree to reduce the dose
- Mirtazapine 15 mg/day added and given at night
- Lorazepam discontinued and clonazepam increased to 2.5 mg in the morning and 1 mg at night
- Buspirone discontinued
- Dextroamphetamine decreased to 10 mg/day in the morning

Attending Physician's Mental Notes: First Interim Followup, Month 18 (3 months after initial psychiatric evaluation)

- Referring psychiatrist maintained the above medication treatment, and patient finally started feeling better at month 18, which the patient attributed to sertraline
- Far from well yet
- Feels worst in the morning, his usual pattern (disorganized, lacking energy, anxious)

- Suggested his mirtazpine dose be increased and to add quetiapine (Seroquel)
- Maintained sertraline 200 mg/day
- Increased mirtazapine to 30 mg/day at night
- Maintained dextroamphetamine 10 mg in the morning
- Maintained clonazapem 2.5 mg in the morning and 1 mg at night
- Added quetiapine, tapered up to 300 mg/day

Attending Physician's Mental Notes: 2nd Interim Followup, Month 22

- Referring psychiatrist maintained the above medication treatment, but no improvement
- Still very depressed in the morning
- Recommended starting MAOI
- Washed out of sertraline, mirtazapine, dextroamphetamine
- Continued clonazapam, quetiapine
- MAOI started in 7 days (equals 7 half lives of sertraline, mirtazapine; only 5 half life washout of these is required before starting an MAOI)
- Transdermal selegilene 6 mg/24 hours prescribed

Attending Physician's Mental Notes: 3rd Interim Followup, Month 24

- Referring psychiatrist made the changes suggested above, but discontinued quetiapine because of excessive daytime sedation and some initial worsening of psychomotor retardation
- No side effects attributable to transdermal selegilene
- 4–5 weeks after starting MAOI, began to feel better
- Now he looks, if anything, a bit hypomanic, but upon close examination, patient is somewhat exhuberant about getting well, having waited 2 years to respond from this fifth episode
- Let's hope he does not stop his antidepressant this time

Case Debrief

- The patient has a 13 year history of recurrent unipolar major depressive episodes
- His first 4 episodes were readily treated to full remission and he discontinued treatment each time several months to a year after remitting
- His subsequent episodes came in an ever escalating pattern, with less and less time between them
- By the time of his fifth episode, he had become treatment resistant, and took two years to get better
- He responded to a single action agent several times (SSRI), then a dual action agent the fourth time (SNRI) and finally, after failing SSRI and SNRI

treatment plus multiple augmentation strategies the fifth time, required an MAOI

Take-Home Points

- Major depression can be recurrent, and recurrences can possibly indicate disease progression potentially manifested as shorter and shorter periods of wellness between subsequent episodes, with eventually poor interepisode recovery, and ultimately, treatment resistance
- This may be linked to changes in brain structure and neurotrophic factors
- Patients with 3 or more episodes of depression should be treated indefinitely with antidepressant maintenance
- Antidepressant-induced sexual dysfunction can be a powerful reason to discontinue antidepressants, despite the risks of recurrence and treatment resistance

Performance in Practice: Confessions of a Psychopharmacologist

- What could have been done better here?
  - There is no question the patient should have been treated with maintenance antidepressants after his third episode of depression, possibly preventing his fourth and fifth episodes, and possibly preventing the development of treatment resistance
  - The patient was very religious and did not believe in psychotherapy, but perhaps more efforts should have been made to get him into psychotherapy to deal with his issues about his own mortality and his reactions to psychosocial stressors
- Possible action item for improvement in practice
  - Make a concerted effort to see that patients with recurrent episodes of major depression and who need maintenance treatment are not lost to followup

Tips and Pearls

- MAO inhibitors have fallen out of favor in the United States and are not used at all in many countries
- These agents remain powerful alternatives for cases like this one, with treatment resistance
- Some myths about dangers, side effects, diet and drug interactions regarding MAOIs can be dispelled with re-study of the facts about these agents, such as those shown below

Two-Minute Tute: A brief lesson and psychopharmacology tutorial (tute) with relevant background material for this case
- **How MAOIs work**
- **Tips on how to use MAOIs**
- **Brain changes in recurrent depression**
- **See also Case 10, Two Minute Tute, p 113**

Table 1: Currently approved MAO inhibitors

Name (trade name)	Inhibition of MAO- A	Inhibition of MAO-B	Amphetamine properties
phenelzine (Nardil)	+	+	
tranylcypromine (Parnate)	+	+	+
isocarboxazid (Marplan)	+	+	
amphetamines (at high doses)	+	+	+
selegiline transdermal system (Emsam)			
brain	+	+	+
gut	+/-	+	+
selegiline low dose oral (Deprenyl, Eldepryl)	-	+	+
rasaligine (Agilect/Azilect)	-	+	-
moclobemide (Aurorix, Manerix)	+	-	-

Table 2: MAO inhibitors with amphetamine actions or amphetamines with MAO inhibitions

Drug	Comment
amphetamine	MAOI at high doses
tranylcypromine (Parnate)	also called phenylcyclopropylamine, structurally related to amphetamine
Selegiline	metabolized to L-methamphetamine
	metabolized to L-amphetamine
	less amphetamine formed transdermally

Table 3: MAO enzymes

	MAO-A	MAO-B
Substrates	5-HT	Phenylethylamine
	NE	DA
	DA	Tyramine
	Tyramine	
Tissue distribution	Brain, gut, liver, placenta, skin	Brain, platelets, lymphocytes

Table 4: Suggested tyramine dietary modifications for MAO inhibitors*

Food to avoid	Food allowed
Dried, aged, smoked, fermented, spoiled, or improperly stored meat, poultry, and fish	Fresh or processed meat, poultry, and fish
Broad bean pods	All other vegetables
Aged cheeses	Processed and cottage cheese, ricotta
cheese, yogurt	
Tap and nonpasteurized beers	Canned or bottled beers and alcohol (have little tyramine)
Marmite, sauerkraut	Brewer's and baker's yeast
Soy products/tofu	

*No dietary modifications needed for low doses of transdermal selegiline or for low oral doses of selective MAO-B inhibitors.

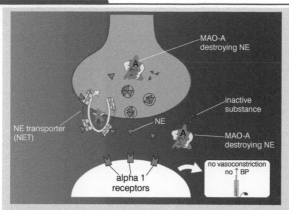

Figure 1: Normal NE Destruction

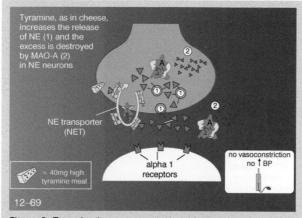

Figure 2: Tyramine increases norepinephine release

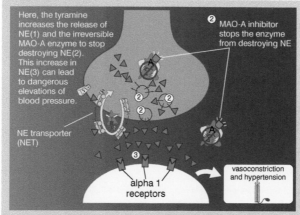

Figure 3: Inhibition of MAO-A and tyramine

Table 5: Potentially dangerous hypertensive combos: agents when combined with MAOIs that can cause hypertension (theoretically via adrenergic stimulation)

Decongestants
phenylephrine (alpha 1 selective agonist)
ephedrine* (ma huang, ephedra) (alpha and beta agonist; central NE and DA releaser)
pseudoephedrine* (active stereoisomer of ephedrine – same mechanism as ephedrine)
phenylpropanolamine* (alpha 1 agonist; less effective central NE/DA releaser than ephedrine)
Stimulants
amphetamines
methylphenidate
Antidepressants with NRI (norepinephrine reuptake inhibition)
TCAs
NRIs
SNRIs
NDRIs
Appetite suppressants with NRI
sibutramine*
phentermine

*withdrawn from markets in the United States and some other countries

Table 6: Potentially lethal combos: agents when combined with MAOIs that can cause hyperthermia/serotonin syndrome (theoretically via SERT inhibition)

Antidepressants
SSRIs
SNRIs
TCAs (especially clomipramine)
Other TCA structures
cyclobenzaprine
carbamazepine
Appetite suppressants with SERT inhibition
sibutramine*
Opioids
dextromethorphan
meperidine
tramadol
methadone
propoxyphene

*withdrawn from markets in the United States and some other countries

Table 7: Tyramine content of cheese

Cheese		mg per 15g serving
English STILTON		17.3
Kraft® grated PARMESAN		0.2
Philadelphia® CREAM CHEESE		0

Table 8: Tyramine content of commercial chain pizza

Serving		mg per serving
1/2 medium double cheese, double pepperoni		1.378
1/2 medium double cheese, double pepperoni		0.063
1/2 medium double cheese, double pepperoni		0

Table 9: Tyramine content of wine

Wine		mg per 4-oz serving
Ruffino CHIANTI		0.36
Blue Nun® WHITE		0.32
Cinzano VERMOUTH		0

Table 10: Are brain changes progressive in depression?

- A frontal-limbic function disconnection is present in depression and correlates with the duration of the current depressive episode
- Hippocampal volume loss is greater with longer periods of untreated depression
- The likelihood that a life stress precipitates a depressive episode is greatest for the first episode of depression and declines with each subsequent episode, although the risk of subsequent episodes increases as though prior episodes of depression as well as life stressors are causing subsequent episodes
- More episodes as well as residual symptoms both predict poorer outcome in terms of more relapses
- Antidepressants may boost trophic factors, normalize brain activity, suggesting that successful and early treatment may attenuate progressive maladaptive brain changes and improve the clinical course of the illness
- Symptomatic remission may be the clinician's benchmark for enhancing the probability of arresting disease progression
- Sustained remission may be a clinician's benchmark for reversing the underlying pathophysiology of major depression

Posttest Self Assessment Question: Answer

When should antidepressant maintenance become indefinite?

A. Following remission from one episode of major depression
   - Guidelines suggest this is not necessary unless particularly severe and other risk factors such as suicidality and a highly positive family history
B. Following remission from two episodes of major depression
   - This is ambiguous, with non complicated cases not requiring indefinite maintenance but complex, severe or suicidal cases probably needing maintenance
C. If there is a particularly severe episode or one with suicidality, especially if a positive family history for depression
   - Yes
D. Following remission from three episodes of major depression
   - Definitely yes
E. On a case by case basis
   - No, should be more systematic than this as shown in the answers above

Answer: C and D

References

1. Stahl SM, Mood Disorders, in Stahl's Essential Psychopharmacology, 3rd edition, Cambridge University Press, New York, 2008, pp 453–510
2. Stahl SM, Antidepressants, in Stahl's Essential Psychopharmacology, 3rd edition, Cambridge University Press, New York, 2008, pp 511–666
3. Stahl SM, Selegilene, in Stahl's Essential Psychopharmacology The Prescriber's Guide, 3rd edition, Cambridge University Press, New York, 2009, pp 489–96
4. Stahl SM, Sertraline, in Stahl's Essential Psychopharmacology The Prescriber's Guide, 3rd edition, Cambridge University Press, New York, 2009, pp 497–502
5. Stahl SM, Venlafaxine, in Stahl's Essential Psychopharmacology The Prescriber's Guide, 3rd edition, Cambridge University Press, New York, 2009, pp 579–584
6. Trivedi MH, Rush AJ, Wisniewski SR et al. Evaluation of outcomes with citalopram for depression using measurement-based care in STAR*D: implications for clinical practice. Am J Psychiatry 2006; 163: 28–40
7. Rush AJ, Trivedi MH, Wisniewski SR et al. Bupropion-SR, sertraline, or venlafaxine-XR after failure of SSRIs for depression. N Engl J Med 2006; 354(12): 1231–42
8. Rush AJ, Trivedi MH, Wisniewski SR et al. Acute and longer-term outcomes in depressed outpatients requiring one or several treatment steps: a STAR*D report. Am J Psychiatry 2006; 163: 1905–17
9. Warden D, Rush AJ, Trivedi MH et al. The STAR*D Project results: a comprehensive review of findings. Curr Psychiatry Rep 2007; 9(6): 449–59
10. Judd LL, Akiskal HS, Maser JD et al. Major depressive disorder: a prospective study of residual subthreshold depressive symptoms as predictor of rapid relapse. J Affect Disord. 1998; 50(2–3): 97–108
11. Kendler KS, Thornton LM, Gardner CO Stressful life events and previous episodes in the etiology of major depression in women: an evaluation of the "kindling" hypothesis. Am J Psychiatry 2000; 157: 1243–51

The Case: The son who would not take a shower

The Question: Will a 32-year-old with an 18-year history of psychotic disorder ever be able to live on his own?

The Dilemma: How can aging parents no longer with the health or the means to support an adult patient with a serious mental illness move their son towards independence without decompensating his psychotic illness or making him homeless?

Pretest Self Assessment Question (answer at the end of the case)

Patients who have shown only partial response on valproate can benefit from augmentation with lamotrigine. If valproate affects the plasma levels of lamotrigine, which would be the proper titration schedule to follow for lamotrigine?

A. Valproate does not affect the plasma levels of lamotrigine, and thus no adjustments in the titration schedule are required
B. Valproate increases the plasma levels of lamotrigine, and thus the titration schedule should be halved
C. Valproate decreases the plasma levels of lamotrigine, and thus the titration schedule should be doubled
D. Valproate should never be given in the presence of lamotrigine

Patient Intake

- 32-year-old man
- Chief complaint by the patient: parents will not leave him alone
- Chief complaint by the parents: son will not take care of his hygiene or his room, and is not on a trajectory towards ever living on his own

Psychiatric History

- Onset of illness age 18 characterized, at times, as schizophrenia, and at times as an affective state, of depressive but not manic in nature
- Most likely schizoaffective disorder with prodromal onset, perhaps at the age of 14 and with full onset at age 16 or 17, with a final diagnosis and hospitalization first at age 18
- Has had multiple hospitalizations, last one being 1 ½ years ago
- Has had four suicide attempts
- Has taken numerous medications over the years with variable results

Social and Personal History

- Lives in a home that was built for him at the back of his parents' property
- Parents now retired and concerned about their need to support him on a reduced income, and what will happen to him after they can no longer care for him
- Has accumulated some college credits, is artistic, reads books, and has a high IQ
- Has poor general hygiene, including rare brushing of teeth, sleeping in his clothes, not taking showers, and getting skin infections from poor hygiene
- Has poor habits, is difficult and obstructionist to changing habits
- Parents have never had him evaluated for social security disability

Medical History

- Obese
- Dyslipidemia with moderately elevated fasting triglycerides
- Normal fasting glucose

Family History

- Maternal great-grandfather: depression, received ECT, committed suicide at age 72
- Maternal aunt: bipolar disorder

Patient Intake

- Patient arrived on time at appointment and was accompanied by parents
- Patient is a tall, huge, overweight man
- He comes into the office with a wide brimmed leather Australian style bush hat, and when he takes it off reveals a shaved head
- He also has a large, poorly kempt and scraggly brown beard
- Altogether he has a very scary somewhat bizarre appearance and demeanor
- He initially eyed the physician with suspicion
- When the mother began the interview by speaking about herself, he would frequently interrupt and very fluently and forcibly voice objections to most of what she said
- When directly prompted by physician to explain what was wrong with him, he had a great deal of thought blocking and silence, and was unable to respond in a coherent manner

- Patient is quite guarded about his delusions and hallucinations in the presence of physician, but experiences both according to his past history
- Patient has persistent delusions of thinking that he should die
- Is tormented by thoughts telling him that he is a vile and despicable person who needs to die
- Receives messages that he is "one of them"; that is, one of the people who prey on the weak
- Patient believes his problems are due to events in his childhood related to his memory, whether actual or not, that he was molested by boys at a military school when he was in 7th or 8th grade
- When around children, he believes he could harm them, and voices tell him he could harm them telepathically, especially by molesting them telepathically
- Believes he can telepathically hurt his sister's dog
- Believes God speaks to him, and no one can convince him that God does not think that he is a vile person

Current Medications

- Ziprasidone (Geodon): 80 mg in the morning; 160 mg at night
- Sertraline (Zoloft): 200 mg in the morning
- Valproate ER (Depakote ER): 1500 mg at night

Attending Physician's Mental Notes: Initial Psychiatric Evaluation

- This patient is severely ill
- It is not clear whether the parents are providing helpful support or are fostering dependency
- The key is to urgently help the family make progress towards the goal of having the patient develop long-term independence, or at least behavior and skills consistent with another living arrangement such as a group home or board and care facility rather than homelessness

Further Investigation

Is there anything else you would like to know about this patient?

- What about substance abuse?
  - Upon inquiry, the patient states he smokes marijuana most days
  - No alcohol
  - The parents seem unaware that this might be contributing in a major way to the patient's overall disability and personal hygiene

Of the following choices, what would you do?
- Increase the dose of ziprasidone (Geodon)
- Add a mood stabilizer
- Switch to another atypical antipsychotic

If you would switch to another atypical antipsychotic, which one would you choose?
- Aripiprazole (Abilify)
- Clozapine (Clozaril)
- Olanzapine (Zyprexa)
- Quetiapine (Seroquel)
- Risperidone (Risperdal)

Case Outcome: First and Second Interim Followup Visits Over 3 Months

- Patient was titrated to 400 mg clozapine at night
- A few months later, parents are still concerned that he is not on track to living independently
- They complain he is not able to do the simplest of things such as getting up on time, taking his medications, eating regularly, and scheduling his own rides with a community transport service
- Mother believes that clozapine has some effect, in that it keeps him from becoming actually suicidal although he continues to have suicidal thoughts
- Mostly she believes clozapine keeps him out of the hospital
- Patient agrees that clozapine helps him remain out of hospital, but wants to stop his medications as he feels marijuana is the best treatment, and wants to only take medical marijuana

What would you do next?
- Augment with carbamazepine
- Augment with lamotrigine
- Augment with lithium
- Add a second antipsychotic to clozapine
- Suggest cognitive behavioral therapy
- Suggest drug dependence therapy

Case Outcome: Third and Subsequent Followup Visits Over Months 3 to 6

- Patient was augmented with lamotrigine, as this mood stabilizer was shown to be useful in treatment-resistant cases even with partial response only to clozapine

- As patient is on valproate, he should be given half of the normal titration schedule for lamotrigine:
  - For the first two weeks: 25 mg every other day
  - Week three: increase to 25 mg per day
  - Week five: increase to 50 mg per day
  - Week six: increase to 100 mg per day
- Patient was open to a cognitive behavioral therapy as an approach to his lack of insight into his delusions and hallucinations, and his problems with his hygiene
- Patient appears to emotionally blackmail his parents into not setting limits for him; he knows there will be no consequences for him not taking care of himself
- Parents are encouraged to look for a placement outside of the home, and to state that if patient does not follow certain rules such as taking care of getting up at the right time, taking his medications, taking care of his hygiene, and taking care of arranging his own transportation, he would have to go to an alternative home
- Patient needs to show willingness to change to avoid certain penalties
- Family referred to social services for an assessment, for possible social security disability evaluation, and evaluation of alternative living arrangements
- Family also referred to patient and family support groups for information and support

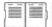

Case Debrief

- Parents of children with mental disorders are often confronted with difficult choices that may involve the placement of their child
- When these children grow up, they may sometimes, intentionally or not, keep their parents "hostage" of their disorder
- Comorbid substance abuse is common and patients often lack the motivation to stop this. Drug abuse may also contribute to lack of motivation to develop social skills for independent living, as being dependent and abusing drugs is too often seen as an easier path and a better life
- Physicians and mental health professionals of all types can help the entire family get through these difficult choices, and may be able to guide the parents as well as the children to a common path of understanding
- There is no easy road in the treatment of a family member with a mental disorder. . . .

Performance in Practice: Confessions of a Psychopharmacologist

- What could have been done better here?
  - Should referral to social security have been done years earlier?
  - Should family therapy have been done years earlier or started immediately at the time of the first evaluation when giving clozapine and then lamotrigine, and not 6 months later?
  - Is this a medication issue of treatment resistance, or a family issue?
  - Do the parents need better skills in dealing with the patient?
- Possible action items for improvement in practice
  - Serve as better liaison with local patient and family support groups

Two-Minute Tute: A brief lesson and psychopharmacology tutorial (tute) with relevant background material for this case
– Negative symptom description
– Role of marijuana in schizophrenia

Table 1: What are negative symptoms?

Domain	National Institute of Mental Health (NIMH) Term*	Translation
Dysfunction of communication	Alogia	Poverty of speech, e.g. talks little, uses few words
Dysfunction of affect	Blunted affect	Reduced range of emotions (perception, experience, and expression), e.g. feels numb or empty inside, recalls few emotional experiences, good or bad
Dysfunction of socialization	Asociality	Reduced social drive and interaction, e.g. little sexual interest, few friends, little interest in spending time with (or little time spent with) friends
Dysfunction of capacity for pleasure	Anhedonia	Reduced ability to experience pleasure, e.g. finds previous hobbies or interests unpleasurable
Dysfunction of motivation	Avolition	Reduced desire, motivation, persistence, e.g. reduced ability to undertake and complete everyday tasks; may have poor personal hygiene

*These terms were agreed to represent domains of negative symptoms during an NIMH-supported consensus conference of experts

Table 2: What do negative symptoms predict?

Worse quality of life
Worse social functioning
Worse interpersonal relationships
Worse work performance
Worse overall outcome

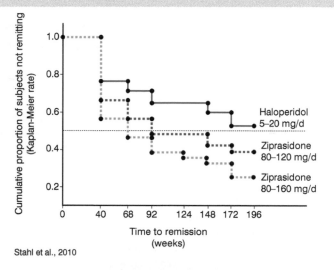

Stahl et al., 2010

Figure 1: Negative symptom remission after very long term treatment.

Standard doses of an atypical antipsychotic ziprasidone were superior to low doses of ziprasidone and to the conventional antipsychotic haloperidol in enhancing the number of patients with remission of their negative symptoms.

Cannabis and Psychosis

- Cannabis increases the risk of psychotic symptoms in individuals from the general population
- In patients with an established psychotic disorder, cannabis
  - Has a negative effect on illness course
  - Causes more and earlier relapses
  - Causes more frequent hospitalization
  - Causes poorer psychosocial functioning
  - Causes loss of brain tissue at twice the rate of patients with schizophrenia who do not use cannabis

So Why Do Patients with Psychosis Use Cannabis?
- Principal motives may be
  - Enhancement of positive affect
  - Social acceptance
  - Coping with negative affect/negative symptoms
- Studies suggest patients with psychosis
  - Are more sensitive to the mood enhancing effects of cannabis
  - But are also more sensitive to the psychosis inducing effects of cannabis
  - Since the rewards are immediate and the adverse consequences are delayed, this can set up a vicious cycle of deleterious use of cannabis in patients with schizophrenia

Posttest Self Assessment Question: Answer

Patients who have shown only partial response on valproate can benefit from augmentation with lamotrigine. If valproate affects the plasma levels of lamotrigine, which would be the proper titration schedule to follow for lamotrigine?

A. Valproate does not affect the plasma levels of lamotrigine, and thus no adjustments in the titration schedule are required
B. Valproate increases the plasma levels of lamotrigine, and thus the titration schedule should be halved
C. Valproate decreases the plasma levels of lamotrigine, and thus the titration schedule should be doubled
D. Valproate should never be given in the presence of lamotrigine

Answer: B

References

1. Stahl SM, Clozapine, in Stahl's Essential Psychopharmacology The Prescriber's Guide, 3rd edition, Cambridge University Press, New York, 2009, pp 113–8
2. Stahl SM, Lamotrigine, in Stahl's Essential Psychopharmacology The Prescriber's Guide, 3rd edition, Cambridge University Press, New York, 2009, pp 259–65
3. Stahl SM, Valproate, in Stahl's Essential Psychopharmacology The Prescriber's Guide, 3rd edition, Cambridge University Press, New York, 2009, pp 569–74
4. Goff DC, Keefe R, Citrome L, et al. Lamotrigine as add-on therapy in schizophrenia. J Clin Psychopharmacol 2007; 27: 582–9
5. Stahl SM, Halla A, Newcomer JW, et al. A post hoc analysis of negative symptoms and psychosocial function in patients with

schizophrenia: a 40-week randomized double-blind study of ziprasidone versus haloperidol followed by a 3-year double-blind extension trial. J Clin Psychopharmacol 2010; 30: 425–430

6. Harrow M, Hansford BG, Astrachan-Fletcher EB, Locus of control: relation to schizophrenia, to recovery, and to depression and psychosis – a 15-year longitudinal study. Psychiatry Research 2009, 168: 186–192

7. Harvey PD, Bellack AS, Toward a terminology for functional recovery in schizophrenia: is functional remission a viable concept. Schiz Bull 2009; 35: 300–306

8. Roder V, Brenner HD, Muller D, et al. Development of specific social skills training programmes for schizophrenia patients: results of a multicentre study. Acta Psychiatrica Scand 2008; 105: 262–71

9. Stahl SM and Buckley PF, Negative symptoms of schizophrenia: a problem that will not go away. Acta Scandinavia Psychiatrica 2007, 115: 4–11

10. Buckley PF and Stahl SM, Pharmacological treatment of negative symptoms of schizophrenia: therapeutic opportunity or Cul-de-Sac? Acta Scandinavia Psychiatrica 2007; 115: 93–200

11. Murray RM, Morrison PD, Henquet C et al. Cannabis, the mind and society: the hash realities. Nat Rev Neurosci 2007; 8: 885–95

12. Grech A, Van Os J, Jones PB et al. Cannabis use and outcome of recent onset psychosis. Eur Psychiatry 2005; 20: 349–53

13. Henquet C, Van Os J, Kuepper R et al. Psychosis reactivity to cannabis use in daily life: an experience sampling study. Br J Psychiatry 2010; 196: 447–453

Lightning Round

The Case: The man who kept hitting his wife over the head with a frying pan

The Question: How do you treat aggressive behavior in a patient with early Alzheimer's Disease?

The Dilemma: Can Alzheimer patients ever be treated with black box antipsychotics?

Pretest Self Assessment Question (answer at the end of the case)

An elderly patient presents with memory and cognitive problems as well as behavioral issues. Based on the reports of family members and various neuropsychological tests, you diagnose your patient with probable Alzheimer's disease. All of the following statements are true about using atypical antipsychotic in the treatment of Alzheimer's disease, except one. Which one is false?

A. Evidence-based treatments of the behavioral symptoms of dementia are pointing to risks but not benefits of atypical antipsychotics.

B. The CATIE-AD study shows no convincing evidence of efficacy of atypical antipsychotics for behavioral symptoms of dementia.

C. Black box warnings of increased incidence of death appearing on all antipsychotics have increased the perception of risk for these agents.

D. Because of poor evidence for their efficacy in treating behavioral symptoms, atypical antipsychotics should rarely, if ever, be given to elderly Alzheimer's patients.

Patient Intake

- 83-year-old-man
- Chief complaint: none
- Patient is brought in by his wife saying she has noticed changes in her husband's memory and behavior for the past year

Psychiatric History

- Patient's wife is known to you as a previous patient with recurrent episodes of major depression, now resolved
- Wife comes to you now with her husband designated as the patient because of his temper, shouting and irritability
- Patient used to attend sessions with his wife, so is known to the attending physician over many years
- She wants an evaluation and treatment of his behavior
- Husband is not aware of changes in his memory but does know that he has been evaluated by several doctors over the past year and that his wife is concerned about his memory

25

- Wife says that for the last year, the patient loses temper and shouts readily, out of character for him
- He is increasingly obsessive about money
- He admits that these observations are true
- Certain behaviors are perseverative and make no sense
- He is irritable, impulsive, and shows signs of poor judgment
- The patient's driver's license has been suspended and he is not permitted to drive as he has failed his written test on three occasions
- When provoked, the patient likes to take an iron frying pan and hit his wife on the head with it; she has been bruised but not knocked unconscious; he is remorseful but keeps doing it
- Wife is afraid he will hurt her and does not want to have to place him outside of the home as he refuses to go at this time
- However, he will soon be placed in a nursing home if this behavior is not controlled and if the danger of injury to the wife is not removed
- Initially placed on donepezil (Aricept)
- No improvement after two months
- Switched to galantamine (Razadyne)
- No improvement after two more months
- Trial of citalopram (Celexa)
- No improvement after two more months and in fact the patient is deteriorating
- Patient's wife asks for an antipsychotic but neither the family physician nor the neurologist will prescribe one because of the black box warning of increased risk of cardiovascular events and death if these medications are used in elderly Alzheimer patients plus little evidence-based proof that they work for agitation in Alzheimer's disease from controlled clinical trials

Patient Intake

- Patient arrives with his wife and he is dressed in a tennis outfit having just played tennis and looks younger than his stated age
- Cooperative at the time of the interview
- Unable to remember three objects at three minutes
- Euthymic, willing to cooperate with transferring financial guardianship of his considerable assets to his wife with the consulting advice of a daughter by a previous marriage and a local stock broker, who will be an advisor but not have signature authority; he is judged not competent to handle his funds

Social and Personal History

- Patient is a wealthy retired entrepreneur
- Hobby is tennis

- Married 33 years, no children from this marriage
- Previous marriage 19 years, one daughter
- Non smoker
- No drug or alcohol abuse

Medical History

- Patient has been evaluated by 2 neurologists and a psychologist
- CT and MRI brain scans show moderately severe cortical atrophy
- Patient received a clinical diagnosis of probable Alzheimer's disease

Medications

- Lanoxin for mild congestive heart failure
- Imuran prophylaxis for myasthenia gravis, which occurred seven years ago but is now in remission
- Diovan for hypertension
- Doxazosin for urinary frequency
- Coumadin for phlebitis and pulmonary emboliu, past 25 years

Family History

- Two brothers: Alzheimer's disease

Of the following choices, what would you do?

Add antipsychotic

Add antidepressant

Add divalproex (Depakote)

Add gabapentin (Neurontin)

Add selegilene (Eldepryl)

Use behavioral interventions

Other

Case Outcome

- Discussed options, including behavioral and environmental interventions, which the patient and his wife feel are not applicable
- Discussed the controversies about using antipsychotics for the behavioral symptoms of dementia, including increased risk of cardiovascular events and even death
- Suggested trying first another selective serotonin reuptake inhibitor (SSRI)
- Both patient and his wife refuse – they have already wasted 6 months on ineffective treatments
- Patient states that he is not depressed and won't take an antidepressant
- Wife wants something that will work on aggressive symptoms

immediately or she fears that he will have to be placed soon in a nursing home
- After explaining risks, benefits, and alternatives, they agree to a trial of risperidone
- Excellent response, patient's behavior improves and no longer gets provoked or tries to assault wife with the frying pan

Case Debrief

- This high functioning patient with early Alzheimer's disease is beginning to deteriorate behaviorally
- Empiric trials of two acetylcholinesterase inhibitors were not effective for either memory or for behavioral symptoms, although sometimes these agents can work for both types of symptoms
- Empiric trial of an SSRI was not effective and behavioral interventions for this higher functioning patient were not deemed appropriate
- Although many would believe the risks outweigh the benefits, with informed consent a trial of low dose risperidone (Risperdal) stopped the aggressive behavior, reduced the risk of injury to the wife, and prolonged the time to admission to a nursing home, showing that in this case, at least short term the benefits outweighed the risks for administering an atypical antipsychotic
- Despite evidence-based large trials, sometimes you only need a trial of a drug in one patient to make the case that a treatment works

Take-Home Points: General

- It has been very difficult to prove in randomized controlled trials that antipsychotics are effective for the behavioral symptoms of dementia
- So-called evidence-based studies of treatments of the behavioral symptoms of dementia are pointing to risks but not benefits of atypical antipsychotics
- In particular, the well known CATIE-AD study shows no convincing evidence of efficacy of atypical antipsychotics for behavioral symptoms of dementia, reducing the perception of efficacy of these agents
- Black box warnings of increased incidence of death, now for all antipsychotics, have increased the perception of risk for these agents

Take-Home Points: So What To Do?

- When appropriate, first-line treatment should be considered as interventions to identify and manage reversible precipitants of behavioral symptoms of dementia
- These include treating causes of behavior symptoms of dementia whenever possible such as

- Pain
- Nicotine withdrawal
- Medication side effects
- Undiagnosed medical, neurological, and psychiatric conditions
- Provocative environments that are either too stimulating or not stimulating enough

• When considering medications for the behavioral symptoms of dementia, there is little evidence for efficacy of anything but much better understanding of the risks of medication

• Thus, many experts now advocate a first-line treatment of agitation and aggression in dementia with an SSRI, e.g., citalopram

• If that fails, there is some rationale and some open label and anecdotal evidence for the efficacy of beta blockers, valproate, gabapentin, and selegilene

• All of these agents have a better risk profile than atypical antipsychotics even if they do not have any better evidence of efficacy

Take-Home Points: Whither the Antipsychotic in Alzheimer's Disease?

• If an antipsychotic is considered, especially if an SSRI fails, empiric trials of an atypical antipsychotic, such as risperidone, can be done if risk benefit assessment is consistent with the trial and with documentation of informed consent and documentation of efficacy if the treatment is to be continued

• Be wary, however, of mistaking Alzheimer dementia for Lewy Body dementia as these patients should generally not receive antipsychotics even though they may have prominent behavioral symptoms, due to the risk of increasing parkinsonian symptoms and complications from that; in such cases quetiapine or clozapine could be considered if any agent at all in this class

• Guidelines for treating the behavioral symptoms of dementia remain unclear and controversial with insufficient studies of this increasingly common problem as the number of patients with dementia continues to increase

Tips and Pearls

• This patient was somewhat aware of his behavioral symptoms but, if you believe him, unaware of his memory problems

• He illustrates an old adage for how to differentiate whether memory problems in the elderly are due to depression or to dementia; namely, if you complain about your memory you are more likely to be depressed

• However, if your spouse complains about your memory, you more likely have dementia

Posttest Self Assessment Question: Answer

An elderly patient presents with memory and cognitive problems as well as behavioral issues. Based on the reports of family members and various neuropsychological tests, you diagnose your patient with probable Alzheimer's disease. All of the following statements are true about using atypical antipsychotic in the treatment of Alzheimer's disease, except one. Which one is false?

A. Evidence-based treatments of the behavioral symptoms of dementia are pointing to risks but not benefits of atypical antipsychotics

B. The CATIE-AD study shows no convincing evidence of efficacy of atypical antipsychotics for behavioral symptoms of dementia

C. Black box warnings of increased incidence of death appearing on all antipsychotics have increased the perception of risk for these agents

D. Because of poor evidence for their efficacy in treating behavioral symptoms, atypical antipsychotics should rarely if ever be given to elderly Alzheimer's patients

– This is an overinterpretation of the black boxed warning and the decision to prescribe an antipsychotic in a patient with behavioral symptoms in dementia should be an individual one based upon the unique set of risks and benefits in a given situation

Answer: D

References

1. Sultzer DL, Davis SM, Tariot PN et al. Clinical symptom responses to atypical antipsychotic medications in Alzheimer's disease: phase 1 outcomes from the CATIE-AD effectiveness. Am J Psychiatry 2008; 165: 844–54

2. Rosenheck RA, Leslie DL, Sindelar JL et al. Cost-benefit analysis of second-generation antipsychotics and placebo in a randomized trial of the treatment of psychosis and aggression in Alzheimer disease. Arch Gen Psychiatry 2007; 64(11): 1259–68

3. Liperoti R, Onder G, Landi F et al. All-cause mortality associated with atypical and conventional antipsychotics among nursing home residents with dementia: a retrospective cohort study. J Clin Psychiatry 2009; 70(10): 1340–7

4. Ballard C, Corbett A, Chitramohan R et al. Management of agitation and aggression associated with Alzheimer's disease: controversies and possible solutions. Curr Opin Psychiatry 2009; 22: 532–40

5. Burke AD and Tariot PN. Atypical antipsychotics in the elderly: a review of therapeutic trends and clinical outcomes. Expert Opin Pharmacother 2009; 10(15): 2407–14

6. Suh GH. The use of atypical antipsychotics in dementia: rethinking Simpson's paradox. Int Psychogeriatr 2009; 21(4): 616–21

7. Barak Y, Baruch Y, Mazeb D et al. Cardiac and cerebrovascular morbidity and mortality associated with antipsychotic medications in elderly psychiatric inpatients. Am J Geriart Psychiatry 2007; 15(4): 354–6

8. Finkel S, Kozma C, Long S et al. Risperidone treatment in elderly patients with dementia: relative risk of cerebrovascular events versus other antipsychotics. Int Psychogeriatr 2005; 17(4): 617–29

9. Meeks TW and Jeste DV. Beyond the black box: what is the role for antipsychotics in dementia. Curr Psychiatr 2008; 7(6): 50–65

10. Dorsey ER, Rabbani A, Gallagher SA et al. Impact of FDA black box advisory on antipsychotic medication use. Arch Intern Med 2010; 170(1): 96–103

11. Salzman C, Jeste DV, Meyer RE et al. Elderly patients with dementia-related symptoms of severe agitation and aggression: consensus statement on treatment options, clinical trials methodology, and policy. J Clin Psychiatry 2008; 69(6): 889–98

12. Stahl SM, Dementia and Its Treatment in Stahl's Essential Psychopharmacology, 3rd edition, Cambridge University Press, New York, 2008, pp 899–942

13. Stahl SM, Risperidone, in Stahl's Essential Psychopharmacology The Prescriber's Guide, 3rd edition, Cambridge University Press, New York, 2009, pp 475–81

The Case: The son who would not go to bed

The Question: What do you do when SSRIs and behavioral therapy fail to reverse disability in OCD for more than 19 years?

The Dilemma: How to improve quality of life for a patient with treatment-resistant OCD

Pretest Self Assessment Question (answer at the end of the case)

Which of the following are evidence-based treatments for obsessive compulsive disorder?

A. High dose paroxetine (Paxil) (>40 mg)
B. High dose sertraline (Zoloft) (>200 mg)
C. SNRIs (serotonin norepinephrine reuptake inhibitors)
D. Atypical antipsychotic augmentation of SSRIs (serotonin selective reuptake inhibitors)

Patient Intake

- 34-year-old man with a chief complaint of "paranoia"
- Parents, who asked for the appointment and with whom the patient lives, are approaching their own retirement and concerned about the patient's ability to ever live on his own and what will happen to all of them after their money runs out, or to him, after their deaths

Psychiatric History

- The patient has had obsessive compulsive symptoms since kindergarten and has been under psychiatric care since he was 15
- As a child he had problems relating with other children at least in part due to early symptoms (e.g., they could not touch his books without washing their hands)
- He has been totally disabled and receiving social security income since he was 21, with symptoms including obsessions, compulsions, general anxiety, paranoia, and depression
- He currently has many rituals that occupy all his waking hours
- For example, his nighttime rituals include turning off the light, thinking of Jesus while not thinking of the devil, swallowing three times, thinking of a girl, going to his bed, blinking three times, and thinking of Jesus again – if he does this perfectly he can then go to sleep; if not, he repeats it over and over until he does it perfectly and is able to go to bed
- Additionally, he has problems standing in crowds or being with other people as he feels they are clearly thinking of him and are out to get him

- He states that he no longer wants to go through the hassle of being out with other people because it makes him uncomfortable
- Thus, he has withdrawn into himself; he currently lives with his parents, stays home, naps during the day, and has very little interaction with other people
- He has no friends, no girlfriends, relates mostly to his family, and is mostly alone
- He is not unhappy about this arrangement, is mostly comfortable with his life, and has given up on plans to change his life

Medication History

- Numerous psychotropic drugs especially over the past 20 years, including several different selective serotonin reuptake inhibitors (SSRIs) and augmentation strategies
- At first, perhaps 25% improvement in intensity and duration of symptoms, but no longer clear whether medications are doing any good whatsoever

Psychotherapy History

- Has had several years of outpatient behavioral therapy and cognitive behavioral therapy with numerous therapists over the past 20 years
- Basically, about every 5 years they try again with new therapists and new psychiatrists to see if any new medications or any new psychotherapy will be effective
- Little to no response to these psychotherapeutic interventions, but it has been 5 years since making a serious effort at psychotherapy or trying new medications, so wanting to try something again

Social and Personal History

- He graduated high school and held a job for one year prior to getting full disability (social security disability plus Medicare)
- He was able to go to college for ten years and get an associate degree in art
- He has worked intermittently for a few days or weeks for cash but otherwise has had nothing in the way of employment since age 21

Medical History

- Overweight
- BMI 29
- Type II diabetes
- Hypertension

- BP 145/88 on treatment
- Fasting glucose and trigylcerides elevated

Family History

- Maternal grandparents: depression
- Maternal aunts: anxiety and depression

Patient Intake

- Extremely severe, relatively treatment-resistant, and fully disabling OCD
- He understands a great deal about the sophisticated issues regarding his illness, but also lacks a great deal of insight into how his habits are sabotaging any chance of a meaningful life and also how this is making family members suffer
- However, he was responsive to preliminary discussion of this and appears motivated to get better
- He has no current suicidal ideation, delusions, hallucinations, or thought disorder
- He reports no bad side effects

Current medications

- Paroxetine (Paxil; Seroxat) 40 mg twice per day
- Quetiapine (Seroquel)100 mg three times per day
- Risperidone (Risperdal) 3 mg twice per day
- Trihexyphenidyl (Artane) and benztropine (Cogentin) 2 mg three times per day
- Gabapentin (Neurontin) 3000 mg twice per day
- Bupropion (Wellbutrin) XL 300 mg + bupropion SR 150 mg once per day
- Lamotrigine (Lamictal) 100 mg once per day
- Rosiglitazone maleate and metformin for diabetes
- Lisinopril for blood pressure

In your clinical experience, would you expect a patient such as this to respond to any medication regimen alone?

- Yes
- No

Attending Physician's Mental Notes: Initial Psychiatric Evaluation

- OCD is a difficult disorder to treat and often requires both medication and cognitive behavioral therapy (CBT)
- Response to medication alone may be particularly unlikely for a patient with this history of treatment resistance and maladaptive behaviors

Despite taking several psychotropic medications at high doses, the patient does not appear to have robust efficacy nor does he report bad side effects. Which of the following would be your next step?

- Take plasma drug levels
- Adjust medications
- Recommend restarting CBT with a new therapist
- Recommend alternative therapy such as deep brain stimulation (DBS)

Attending Physician's Mental Notes: Initial Psychiatric Evaluation, Continued

- As mentioned, some form of treatment in addition to medication is likely to be necessary for this patient; however, it may also be beneficial to adjust his current medication regimen
- The patient is taking very high doses of paroxetine and gabapentin without apparent intolerance
- This could be because he has taken these medications for so long and has become tolerant to them
- It is also possible that he is not absorbing the medications; he also may not be taking the medications as reported and be partially noncompliant; thus, before adjusting any medications it may be best to obtain plasma drug levels
- He and his parents say he is taking the gabapentin for general anxiety symptoms, which they say are severe, and he is taking bupropion and lamotrigine for depression, but they say he has more of an "I don't care" attitude than real depression or sadness

Further investigation

Is there anything else you would especially like to know about this patient?

- What about details concerning his past medication treatments and his past behavioral therapy?
  - Has taken fluoxetine (Prozac) up to 80 mg, citalopram (Celexa) up to 60 mg, no response but well tolerated
  - Has taken clomipramine (Anafranil) up to 150 mg, no response, poorly tolerated

- Each for over 12 weeks
- Has tried brief augmentation with buspirone (Buspar), lithium, and benzodiazepines without further improvement
- CBT (cognitive behavioral therapy) with more than 3 therapists over 20 years, at least 6 months each, with little or no response to weekly sessions

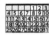

Case Outcome: First Interim Followup, Week 3

- Blood work confirms that despite high doses, the plasma levels of paroxetine and gabapentin are only moderate, assuming he takes the medication as reported
- Plasma levels are low for risperidone, quetiapine, bupropion, and lamotrigine
- Because SSRIs are the best-evidenced treatments for OCD, even though there is limited documentation of high dose utility of SSRIs in OCD, the paroxetine dose is nevertheless raised to 60 mg twice a day to achieve higher plasma levels
- Although gabapentin plasma levels are only moderate, the daytime dose (currently 3000 mg) is actually decreased (to 2000 mg)
- Although gabapentin can improve anxiety it is not specifically approved in OCD and could be contributing to the patient's need to take daytime naps, although the naps are not really due to fatigue or sleepiness, but to boredom and lack of stimulating daytime activities

Would you continue his atypical antipsychotics?
- Yes, continue both risperidone and quetiapine
- Continue risperidone but discontinue quetiapine
- Continue quetiapine but discontinue risperidone
- No, discontinue both risperidone and quetiapine

Would you continue his bupropion and lamotrigine?
- Yes, continue both bupropion and lamotrigine
- Continue bupropion but discontinue lamotrigine
- Continue lamotrigine but discontinue bupropion
- No, discontinue both bupropion and lamotrigine

Case Outcome: First Interim Followup, Week 3, Continued

- It may be preferable to use one rather than two atypical antipsychotics, particularly as plasma levels of both are currently low and thus neither one has necessarily been given an adequate trial
- The dose of quetiapine is increased to 800 mg/day while risperidone and trihexyphenidyl are discontinued
- There is no evidence of efficacy for either bupropion or lamotrigine

in OCD and since he has not clearly experienced problems with depression both of these medications are discontinued
- Adjusted medication regimen
  - Paroxetine 60 mg twice per day
  - Gabapentin 2000 mg in the morning and 3000 mg at night
  - Quetiapine 800 mg once per day
- Rosiglitazone maleate and metformin for diabetes, lisinopril for blood pressure

In addition to the adjustments to medications, which of the following would you be most likely to recommend to this patient?
- CBT (cognitive behavioral therapy)
- DBS (deep brain stimulation)
- Cingulotomy
- Gamma knife surgery
- Both CBT and DBS
- Both CBT and cingulotomy
- Both CBT and gamma knife surgery
- None of the above

Attending Physician's Mental Notes: First Interim Followup, Week 3

- CBT is likely a necessary component of treatment for many patients with OCD, particularly when there are multiple maladaptive behaviors as with this patient
- DBS is approved for treatment-resistant OCD
- Involves two surgical procedures, one to implant electrodes in the brain and a second to implant a neurostimulator in the chest
- Stimulation is generally constant but can be temporarily turned off by holding a hand-held magnetic device over the area of the chest where the neurostimulator is located
- DBS may be preferable to cingulotomy or gamma knife surgery, both of which are permanent and reserved as a last resort

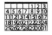

Case Outcome: First Interim Followup Visit, Week 3, Continued

- Information about nonmedication options was discussed, with the assignment of the patient and his parents to read about DBS
- Parents also assigned to investigate 1 to 3 month residential CBT treatment programs at two academic medical centers specializing in OCD

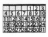

Case Outcome: Second Interim Followup Visit, Week 7

- No change in status, no side effects including no weight gain
- No increase in fasting triglycerides or glucose
- Not interested in DBS
- Residential CBT treatment programs for OCD not covered by insurance or Medicare, and cost tens of thousands of dollars

How long does it take someone with OCD to respond to initiation of an SSRI or to change from one SSRI to another?

- 1 month
- 2 months
- 3 months
- 6 months

Attending Physician's Mental Notes: Second Interim Followup, Week 7

- Initiation of treatment with an SSRI can take up to 12 weeks to see notable changes, although some patients respond faster
- Thus, it may take another month or two to determine whether the increase in paroxetine and quetiapine (and discontinuation of risperidone, lamotrigine and bupropion) will have any additional therapeutic actions
- No changes in medications or dosage recommended for another 2 months
- There is a reality TV show in Southern California on OCD, and part of the production is to pay for residential CBT treatment and the parents were encouraged to contact the show's producers to see if their son would be eligible
- Parents also told to investigate a third academic medical center's 3 week day treatment program about 100 miles from their home which would be less expensive than a longer program that is residential

Case Outcome: Third Interim Followup Visit, Week 15

- No change in status, no side effects, no weight gain, no change in fasting triglycerides or glucose
- TV show not interested in their case
- The day treatment program is several thousand dollars but the parents will pay for it with savings, and move him to an apartment near the medical center for 21 days
- Can enroll in the next month
- Decide to leave medications the same as a stable platform for new cognitive behavioral treatment

Case Outcome: Fourth Interim Followup Visit, Week 21

- Patient completed 3 week day treatment program, with rituals reduced, but obsessions not really changed
- Now at home and reverting to old rituals and habits
- Patient resigned to his situation
- Parents, mother now in her late 60s and father in his early 70s, both retired, very discouraged and worried about their future and his
- Discussed various medical treatment options and told about DBS once again

What would you do now?
- Try additional evidence based medication treatment strategies for resistant OCD
- Refer to DBS center
- Investigate family dynamics, dependency issues
- Let well enough alone

Case Debrief

- Many patients with OCD experience resistance to medication treatment and maladaptive behaviors that require multimodal treatment approaches
- Adjustments to this patient's medications simplified his regimen but did not result in significant improvement in efficacy
- In order to experience improvement in symptoms and higher quality of life this patient will likely require ongoing medication treatment with trials of medication doses and combinations that have been effective in resistant cases coupled with residential treatment for behavioral therapy
- DBS remains an option if he does not experience sufficient improvement with medication and CBT

Take-Home Points

- Many patients with OCD either do not respond to SSRIs or do not respond sufficiently to achieve functional independence, a vocation or a social life
- Many patients with OCD also do not respond to available CBT, especially nonresidential treatment if the OCD is severe
- Practical considerations and cost mean that residential CBT is out of reach for most patients with OCD, as is DBS
- Nevertheless, some patients can improve with pharmacologic approaches that have not been exhausted in this patient even if the prognosis for independent living remains poor

Performance in Practice: Confessions of a Psychopharmacologist

- What could have been done better here?
  - Since this case is obviously refractory to both medications and to CBT, should referral to DBS have been done earlier and more aggressively?
  - Should dependency issues and family dynamics have been investigated earlier when therapeutic optimism for everyone was higher?
  - Should more aggressive augmentation strategies been initiated earlier?
- Possible action items for improvement in practice
  - Research better links with residential CBT programs for OCD and alternative forms of financing
  - Research better links with DBS centers, including information on whether as experimental protocol, medical expenses such as surgery and stimulator are covered by research grants or by Medicare

Tips and Pearls

- It appears that there are some pharmacokinetic or compliance issues here that may be interfering with drug absorption
- Plasma drug levels are often neglected in treatment resistant cases, but may open the door to rational uses of high or even heroic dosing
- This suggests also that the patient may be a good candidate for a trial of intravenous clomipramine, to bypass pharmacokinetic problems

Mechanism of Action Moment

- Only serotonergic antidepressants seem to work in OCD whereas serotonergic, noradrenergic and/or dopaminergic antidepressants seem to work in depression
- Serotonergic agents must block the serotonin transporter by 80% or more for them to work in depression (Figure 1)
- Serotonergic agents are often dosed similarly in OCD, but anecdotes suggest that higher doses may work better in some OCD patients
- This could be due to the fact that occupancy of serotonin transporter between 80% and 100% occurs at higher drug doses, and results in higher serotonin levels in the synapse and greater OCD efficacy
- Alternatively, since intravenous serotonergic agents such as clomipramine are also effective in some patients who do not respond to seemingly adequate doses of oral agents, it may be that high oral doses or intravenous administration is required in some OCD patients to even attain the critical level of 80% occupancy of serotonin transporters

PATIENT FILE

Two-Minute Tute: A brief lesson and psychopharmacology tutorial (tute) with relevant background material for this case
- Pharmacologic treatments of OCD
- Relationships between SSRI dose and SERT occupancy
- Improvement of OCD by DBS

Table 1: Recommendations for the Pharmacologic Treatment of OCD

Treatment type	Agent	Examples	Recommended Dose for Adults (mg/day)
Standard Treatments	SSRI	Citalopram Escitalopram Fluoxetine Fluvoxamine Paroxetine Sertraline	20–60 10–20 20–60 100–300 40–60 50–200
	TCA	Clomipramine	75–300
Alternative Treatments	High dose SSRI	Citalopram Escitalopram Fluoxetine Fluvoxamine Paroxetine Sertraline	60–120 20–60 60–160 300–450 60–120 200–400
	Intravenous	Clomipramine	
	non SSRIs	Mirtazapine Phenelzine Venlafaxine	
Augmentation	SSRI + Clomipramine	Citalopram + clomipramine Fluvoxamine + clomipramine Fluoxetine + clomipramine	
	Atypical antipsychotics	Olanzapine Risperidone Quctiapine others	
	Pindolol Buspirone Clonazepam Riluzole Topiramate N-acetylcysteine		

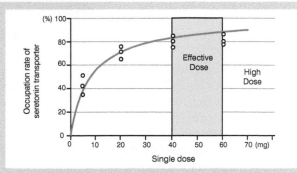

Figure 1: Relationship between SSRI dose and SERT (Serotonin Transporter) occupation

80% SERT occupancy is the level at which clinical efficacy can be expected. This is achievable by administration of most SSRIs, at standard doses. Higher doses, achieving higher SERT occupancy, may be effective in some OCD patients.

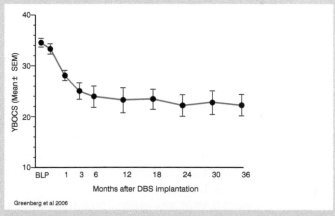

Greenberg et al 2006

Figure 2: OCD Severity improvement during long term DBS, n=10
YBOCS = Yale Brown Obsessive Compulsive Scale

Posttest Self Assessment Question: Answer

Which of the following are evidence-based treatments for obsessive compulsive disorder?

A. High dose paroxetine (>40 mg)
    – Although many SSRIs have been reported in small studies at high doses, there is little if anything on paroxetine in the literature
B. High dose sertaline (>200 mg)
    – Probably the largest and best designed study has been comparing 200 mg to 400 mg of sertraline, with good therapeutic effects of the high dose but more side effects
C. SNRIs (serotonin norepinephrine reuptake inhibitors
    – A few case series have been reported of effective treatment by venlafaxine in OCD
D. Atypical antipsychotic augmentation of SSRIs
    – Many small studies and a few literature reviews, some patients benefit but others do not

Answer: B, C and D

References

1. Skapinakis P, Papatheodorou T, Mavreas V, Antipsychotic augmentation of serotonergic antidepressants in treatment-resistant obsessive compulsive disorder: a meta analysis of the randomized controlled trials. Eur Neuropsychopharmacol 2007; 17: 79–93
2. Marazziti D, Golia F, Consoli G et al. Effectiveness of long term augmentation with citalopram to clomipramine in treatment resistant OCD patients. CNS Spectr 2008; 13: 971–6
3. Byerly MJ, Goodman WK, Christensen R, High doses of sertraline for treatment resistant obsessive compulsive disorder. Am J Psychiatr 1996; 153: 1232–33
4. Marazziti D, Venlafaxine treatment of obsessive compulsive disorder: case reports. CNS Spectr 2003: 8: 421–2
5. Figueroa Y, Rosenberg DR, Birmaher B et al. Combination treatment with clomipramine and selective serotonin reuptake inhibitors for obsessive compulsive disorder in children and adolescents. J Child Adolesc Psychopharmacol 1998; 8: 61–7
6. Greenberg BD, Malone DA, Friehs G et al. Three year outcomes in deep brain stimulation for highly resistant obsessive compulsive disorder. Neuropsychopharmacol 2006; 31: 2384–93
7. Takano A et al. Psychopharmacol 2006; 185: 395–399

8. Goodman WK, Foote KD, Greenberg BD et al. Deep brain stimulation for intractable obsessive compulsive disorder: pilot study using a blinded staggered-onset design. Biol Psychiat 2010; 67: 535–42

9. Greenberg BD, Rausch SL, Haber SN, Invasive circuitry-based neurotherapeutics: stereotactic ablation and deep brain stimulation for OCD. Neuropsychopharm Rev 2010; 35: 317–336

10. Beer RE, Fitzgerald P, Rosenfeld JV et al. Neurosurgery for obsessive compulsive disorder: contemporary approaches. J. Clin Neurosci 2010; 17: 1–5

11. Dell'Osso B, Altamura AC, Allen A et al. Brain stimulation techniques in the treatment of obsessive-compulsive disorder: current and future directions. CNS Spect 2005; 10: 966–979

12. Bandelow B, The medical treatment of obsessive compulsive disorder and anxiety. CNS Spectr 2008; 13: 9 (suppl 14): 37–46

The Case: The sleepy woman with anxiety

The Question: How can you be anxious and narcoleptic at the same time?

The Dilemma: Finding an effective regimen for recurrent, treatment resistant anxious depression while juggling complex treatments for sleep disorders

Pretest Self Assessment Question (answer at the end of the case)

Which of the following are approved treatments for treatment resistant depression?

A. Deep brain stimulation
B. Transcranial magnetic stimulation
C. Vagal nerve stimulation
D. Aripiprazole (Abilify)
E. Quetiapine (Seroquel)
F. MAO inhibitors

Patient Intake

- 44-year-old woman with a chief complaint of anxiety

Psychiatric History

- The patient had onset of anxiety and depression at about age 15, which she began self-medicating with alcohol
- After graduating from high school, she began college and was about to leave for study abroad when she experienced a panic attack for which she was treated in the emergency room
- She was then hospitalized and treated for alcohol abuse at age 18, and has remained sober ever since, although she does admit to some possible alprazolam (Xanax) abuse in 1999 as well as one overdose with alprazolam
- Her history also includes multiple hospitalizations for major depression
  - Age 19 (approximately one year after her release from the hospital for alcohol abuse) because she became suicidal
  - Age 24 due to recurrence of depression
  - Age 26 with an overdose following a divorce and recurrence of depression
  - Age 27 due to recurrence of depression
  - Age 29 after two miscarriages, with a possible postpartum element and some discontinuation of her medications at that time to try to get pregnant
  - Age 30 when she received electroconvulsive therapy (ECT): 7 sessions as an inpatient and 23 as an outpatient

- Details of medication history unclear from available information and from patient's memory, but has received numerous psychotropic drugs including antidepressants, antipsychotics, and mood stabilizers, all with poor results
- She was much better for several years following her ECT treatment, but had severe memory impairment
- She had a recurrence of her depression one year ago severe enough to become totally disabled, necessitating resignation from a job as an office worker that she had enjoyed
- She continues to be disabled from depression and has a great deal of anxiety, subjectively more disturbed by her anxiety than by her depression

Social and Personal History

- Married since 1996 (second marriage); no children from either marriage
- Non smoker
- Husband an architect, supportive
- Little contact with her family of origin
- Few friends or outside interests

Medical History

- Narcolepsy
- Restless legs syndrome
- Nighttime urinary incontinence possibly related to highly sedating medications
- BMI 26
- BP 120/78
- Normal fasting glucose and triglycerides

Family History

- Grandmother: depression and who has received ECT with good results

Current Medications

- Bupropion (Wellbutrin XL) 450 mg/day (thinks it is helpful as she worsens if she tries to taper)
- Ziprasidone (Geodon, Zeldox) 60 mg in the morning and 180 mg at night (unsure if this is helpful)
- Lamotrigine (Lamictal) 200 mg in the morning and 150 mg at night (thinks it is helpful for her mood)

- Gabapentin (Neurontin) 300 mg in the morning, 600 mg at noon, and 900 mg at night; occasional 100 mg as needed for breakthrough anxiety (experiences intolerable return of anxiety at much lower doses)
- Pramipexole (Mirapex) 1 mg/night for restless legs syndrome (unclear whether helpful)
- Methylphenidate extended-release (Concerta) 54 mg/day for daytime sleepiness (thinks it is helpful)
- Sodium oxybate (Xyrem) 9 mg in one dose at night for narcolepsy and daytime sleepiness (not taken in recommended split dose)
- DDAVP (the peptide Desmopressin) 0.4 mg/night for bedwetting

Based on just what you have been told so far about this patient's history and current symptoms, would you consider her to fall within the bipolar spectrum?
- Yes
- No

Would you continue her "mood stabilizing" medications?
- Yes, continue both ziprasidone (Geodon) and lamotrigine (Lamictal)
- Continue ziprasidone but discontinue lamotrigine
- Continue lamotrigine (Lamictal) but discontinue ziprasidone (Geodon)
- No, discontinue both ziprasidone (Geodon) and lamotrigine (Lamictal)

Attending Physician's Mental Notes: Initial Psychiatric Evaluation

- Nothing unexpected on mental status examination which showed depression and anxiety
- Because she has had numerous recurrences, this makes her illness appear to be somewhat unstable; however, she has not shown any overt signs of bipolarity
- The best diagnosis for this patient may be severe generalized anxiety with major depressive recurrent unipolar disorder
- Nevertheless, tactics that are useful for bipolar mood disorders may be useful in this patient
- Continuing ziprasidone (Geodon) and lamotrigine (Lamictal) may help mitigate the risk of a future relapse
- Thus, these medications were continued at the time of the initial evaluation

Further Investigation:

Is there anything else you would especially like to know about this patient?

- What about details concerning the diagnosis of narcolepsy and of restless legs syndrome, the treatments given and the responses to those treatments?
  - During the past year as her depression has recurred and worsened, she has developed excessive daytime sleepiness
  - She had an overnight sleep polysomnogram done in another city that supposedly showed sleep onset REM (rapid eye movement) periods, but you do not have a copy of the report and do not know if it was done while taking any medications, or after the withdrawal of any medications
  - During the past year she has also complained of restless legs worse in the evening when trying to fall asleep
  - Because of her diagnosis of narcolepsy, she was prescribed methyphenidate extended release (Concerta) which helps a bit for her daytime sleepiness, but because she was still sleepy, sodium oxybate (Xyrem) was added without further improvement of daytime alertness although she gets to sleep right away and also sleeps well through the night now
  - In fact, she sleeps too well through the night now, and has bed wetting, for which she has been prescribed DDAVP (Desmopressin), but it is not very helpful
  - Because of her diagnosis of restless legs syndrome, she is prescribed pramipexole (Mirapex), with equivocal results

Based on what you know so far about this patient's history, current. symptoms, and treatment responses, are you convinced her daytime sleepiness and nighttime restlessness are adequately diagnosed and treated?

- Yes
- No

Would you continue her 4 sleep disorder medications?

- Yes, continue all 4 (methylphenidate (Concerta), sodium oxybate (Xyrem), DDAVP (Desmopressin) and pramipexole (Mirapex))
- No, stop one or more of these

Attending Physician's Mental Notes: Initial Psychiatric Evaluation, Continued

- The patient's complaint of excessive daytime sleepiness can be difficult to assess given all the medications she is taking, especially sodium oxybate (Xyrem) and gabapentin (Neurontin), which can cause excessive daytime sleepiness
- It can also be difficult to determine whether her sleepiness represents narcolepsy or really represents "hypersomnia" as an associated symptom of depression
- It can be similarly difficult to determine whether her restless legs represent restless legs syndrome or really represent psychomotor agitation as an associated symptom of anxiety or whether restless legs represent a side effect of bupropion (Wellbutrin) rather than restless legs syndrome
- It is even possible that her sleep disorder treatments are interfering with her treatments for depression and anxiety
- Thus, her sodium oxybate (Xyrem) was tapered, and then her DDAVP (Desmopressin) discontinued, and her pramipexole (Mirapex) was also tapered over the next month following her initial assessment

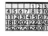

Case Outcome: First and Second Interim Followup Visits, Weeks 2 and 4

- The patient experienced some initial insomnia and restless sleep as sodium oxybate (Xyrem) was withdrawn, but this resolved in several days, as did her incontinence; her daytime sleepiness actually improved somewhat but she continued to have problems falling asleep some nights
- Next, her pramipexole (Mirapex) was tapered without worsening of restless legs, or of insomnia, or mood
- Finally, her daytime gabapentin (Neurontin) was tapered to half dose with improvement in daytime sleepiness, but this was only intermittently tolerated, because of re-emergence of anxiety; however, higher gabapentin (Neurontin) doses caused daytime sleepiness
- She continued to have depression; also, her anxiety continued to wax and wane day and night, with some relief by additional doses of gabapentin (Neurontin), but, unsatisfactory overall results; if anxiety and agitation occur at night, she also has insomnia

Considering her former response and side effects with ECT treatment, would you consider using an alternative non-drug treatment method for her refractory symptoms?

- Yes, consider ECT
- Yes, consider VNS
- Yes, consider TMS
- Yes, consider DBS

Attending Physician's Mental Notes: Second Interim Followup, Week 4

- The patient's prior response to ECT suggests that it, or a similar treatment, may be beneficial
- She is hesitant to try ECT again because of the memory loss she sustained, but may benefit from another alternative treatment strategy
- Vagal nerve stimulation (VNS) (approved for treatment-resistant depression and available at the time of this evaluation)
  - VNS involves surgical implant of a stimulation device in the upper left side of the chest (intended as a permanent implant, though it can be removed)
  - The pulse generator can be programmed to deliver electrical impulses to the vagus nerve at various durations, frequencies, and currents
  - Stimulation typically lasts 30 seconds and occurs every five minutes
  - After an initial wave of enthusiasm for this treatment, use of VNS for depression has waned due to disappointing results, high costs and some complications, include the hassle of having the stimulator and electrode removed
- Transcranial magnetic stimulation (TMS) (approved for treatment-resistant depression)
  - Generally done on an outpatient basis
  - Electromagnetic coil is placed against the scalp near the forehead and turned off and on repeatedly for 30 to 50 minutes per treatment
  - Typical treatment duration is five daily treatments a week for four to six weeks
  - Insurance coverage is variable for a course of this treatment which costs several thousand dollars
  - TMS has been best studied in patients who have failed a single antidepressant, and not for more complicated cases, or in cases with prior good or bad responses to ECT, so it is difficult to predict the chances of success for this patient
- Deep brain stimulation (DBS) (in trials for treatment-resistant depression)

- Involves two surgical procedures, one to implant electrodes in the brain and a second to implant a neurostimulator in the chest
- Stimulation is generally constant but can be temporarily turned off by holding a magnetic device over the area of the chest where the neurostimulator is located
- DBS is an experimental procedure available at only a few medical centers with research protocols that may cover some or all of the costs
- Risks and benefits of DBS remain unknown in treatment resistant depression, so DBS is reserved for patients who have failed many treatments, such as this patient
- After discussion of these options, the patient asked to defer action on them so she could research VNS, TMS and DBS, and in the meantime, she asked to try some other medications

Would you continue her methylphenidate extended release (Concerta) for daytime sleepiness?
- Yes
- No

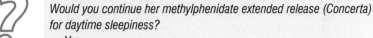

Attending Physician's Mental Notes: Second Interim Followup, Week 4, Continued

- On one hand, methylphenidate extended release (Concerta) seems to be helpful for her daytime sleepiness and one could even consider raising the dose to try to alleviate her depression
- On the other hand, this could risk making her anxiety worse and, to the extent that daytime sleepiness is related to sedating medications' side effects, it may be better to adjust those
- For now, the patient is not willing to stop the stimulant, and after a discussion of risks and benefits, methylphenidate was continued
- Spoke with husband who is supportive and denies any marital conflict

Would you consider adding any of the following medications to her regimen?
- Lithium (to boost mood and mitigate risk of cycling)
- Monoamine oxidase inhibitor (MAOI) (to boost mood)
- Mirtazapine (Remeron) (to boost mood and possibly treat anxiety)
- Quetiapine (Seroquel) (to boost mood and possibly treat anxiety)
- Aripiprazole (Abilify) (to boost mood)
- None of these

Attending Physician's Mental Notes: Second Interim Followup, Week 4, Continued

- Lithium
  - Could help to boost her mood and mitigate risk of future relapse
  - If added it may not be necessary to give her a full dose as she is already on other mood stabilizing medications
- MAOI
  - May help boost mood, as this has been effective for patients with anxious depression
  - However, this could also be activating for some patients and cause problems with sleep and anxiety
  - If added, an MAOI would require discontinuation of bupropion
  - Transdermal selegiline (Emsam) does not require dietary restriction and may be a preferable formulation
- Mirtazapine (Remeron)
  - May boost mood and also potentially treat anxiety
- Quetiapine (Seroquel)
  - May boost mood (approved for depressed phase of bipolar disorder and as adjunct for unipolar depression)
  - May also be helpful for anxiety (anecdotal reports as adjunct)
  - If added, it may require careful dosing to avoid daytime sedation
- Aripiprazole (Abilify)
  - May boost mood (approved as adjunct for unipolar depression)
  - Can be activating and cause problems with anxiety
- The patient was encouraged to switch from bupropion (Wellbutrin) to mirtazapine (Remeron), but instead opted for aripiprazole (Abilify) augmentation of her current medications (bupropion, lamotrigine, gabapentin, methylphenidate), while discontinuing ziprasidone.

Case Outcome: Multiple Interim Followups to Week 24

- Aripiprazole (Abilify) titration from 2 mg to 5 mg while ziprasidone (Geodon) was discontinued showed no real changes good or bad for the first month (week 12)
- Aripiprazole was then increased to 10 mg, with slight improvement (week 16)
- After a second month at 10 mg of aripiprazole, no further improvement in depression and anxiety and overall results not satisfactory (week 20)
- The patient was switched from aripiprazole to quetiapine (Seroquel), which was not associated with improvement of mood or anxiety, and made her sleepiness worse (by week 24)
- The patient was offered a trial of mirtazapine (Remeron) again, and

due to the results with quetiapine, was not willing to take it (at week 24)
- She was offered an MAOI, but said she would rather consider VNS, TMS or another round of ECT (at week 24)
- Insurance approved VNS, and the patient became essentially asymptomatic for more than 4 years

Case Debrief

- The patient has a 25-year history of recurrent anxiety and depression that appears unipolar in nature and has been somewhat responsive to antidepressants and very responsive to ECT in the past
- Her current relapse is causing her disability and is not fully responsive to the 8 medications she was taking on initial referral (bupropion, lamotrigine, ziprasidone, gabapentin, sodium oxybate, DDAVP, methylphenidate and pramipexole)
- It seems possible that her sleep symptoms are more related to her anxious depression rather than to additional diagnoses of narcolepsy and restless legs syndrome and, in any event, her treatments for these sleep disorders did not improve her symptoms; discontinuation of several sleep medications (sodium oxybate, pramipaxole and DDAVP) if anything improved her symptoms; other clinicians may have opted to continue these medications
- Following simplification of her medication regimen from 8 medications to 5, she failed to respond to augmentation with aripiprazole or with quetiapine
- Possibly because of her prior response to ECT (and a first degree relative also responded to ECT), she was an excellent candidate for VNS

Take-Home Points

- It can be difficult to determine whether insomnia with anxiety and psychomotor agitation at night, with simultaneous excessive sleepiness during the day while having poor sleep at night in a patient taking sedating medications, are due to a sleep disorder, to an anxiety disorder, to a depressive disorder or to side effects of medications
- Simplifying medication regimen from 8 medications to 5 may help determine whether some of the symptoms are due to medications and whether all medications are necessary
- The ultimate proof that her symptoms of daytime sleepiness and night time agitation are linked to her anxiety/mood disorder rather than to sleep disorders was that these symptoms abated when her depression and anxiety abated with effective treatment by VNS

Performance in Practice: Confessions of a Psychopharmacologist

- What could have been done better here?
  - Did it take too long to get to the VNS recommendation?
  - Should she have been pushed harder to try mirtazapine or an MAOI rather than augmentation with two additional, three total, atypical antipsychotics?
  - Did it take too long to clarify the sleep issues?
  - Should we have tried harder to get a copy of the written results of the polysomnogram?
- Possible actions for improvement in practice
  - Make sure that augmentation with atypical antipsychotics is not the only option offered, or the only option offered early, since these drugs are expensive and can have notable side effects
  - Despite less robust comparative data, agents such as mirtazapine and MAOIs, and also VNS and ECT, can be considered earlier in the treatment algorithm
  - Get husband more involved as patient is at high risk for long term depression, and he is her major support system
  - Consider psychotherapy earlier rather than after VNS and assess whether the patient is a good candidate for interpersonal or cognitive behavioral approaches

Tips and Pearls

- Treatment with pregabalin (Lyrica), approved for anxiety in Europe but not in the US, rather than gabapentin (Neurontin), not approved anywhere for anxiety, may be less sedating if more expensive
- If the patient requires an MAO inhibitor, best to stop the bupropion and the methylphenidate, but lamotrigrine and gabapentin can be continued. For heroic cases unresponsive to an MAO inhibitor, stimulants such as methylphenidate can sometimes be cautiously added to an MAO inhibitor by experts monitoring cardiovascular status who are sophisticated about weighing risks and benefits

Two-Minute Tute: A brief lesson and psychopharmacology tutorial (tute) with relevant background material for this case
– Classification and testing for narcolepsy, hypersomnia and restless legs syndrome
– Overlap of symptoms in sleep disorders with psychiatric disorders

---

International Classification Of Sleep Disorders Diagnostic Criteria Of Narcolepsy

- Patient complains of excessive sleepiness or sudden muscle weakness

- Recurrent daytime naps or lapses into sleep almost daily for at least 3 months

- Possible sleep-onset REM (rapid eye movement) periods, hypnagogic hallucinations, and sleep paralysis

- With cataplexy
    - Sudden bilateral loss of postural muscle tone in association with intense emotion

- Hypersomnia not better explained by another disorder

- Should be confirmed by PSG (polysomnogram) followed by MSLT (multiple sleep latency test, see below) which should show a mean sleep latency of 8 minutes and two more sleep-onset REM periods (SOREMPs) following normal sleep

- May be confirmed by orexin levels in the cerebrospinal fluid (CSF) <110 pg/ml or, 1/3 of mean normal control levels

---

Narcolepsy is estimated to occur in 0.03–0.16% of the general population, with its development mostly beginning in the teens. Narcoleptic sleep attacks usually occur for 10–20 minutes and, on awakening, the patient can be refreshed for 2–3 hours before feeling the need to sleep again. Although sleep attacks occur most often in a monotonous situation, they can also occur when a person is actively conversing or eating. Symptoms of narcolepsy may include frightening hypnogogic hallucinations and sleep paralysis, which are usually coincident with SOREMPs. Not everyone with narcolepsy will have cataplexy but it is a unique feature of this disorder. An attack normally lasts a few seconds to minutes, during which the person is conscious. Some people have only minimal muscle involvement, while others can have "full-body" attacks; however, the respiratory and ocular muscles are never involved. Excessive sleepiness is the main symptom to continue with age, and it may worsen alongside the development of periodic limb movements and obstructive sleep apnea. In addition, sleep may be disrupted and include frequent awakenings (International Classification of Sleep Disorders, revised, 2001).

Multiple Sleep Latency Test (MSLT)

- Dark comfortable room at an ambient temperature
- Smoking, stimulants and vigorous physical activity avoided during the day, only light breakfast and lunch given
- Instructions are to
    - "Lie quietly in comfy position, keep eyes closed, try to fall asleep"
- Five nap opportunities as 2 hour intervals – initial nap opportunity 1.5–3 hours after termination of usual sleep
- Between naps patient out of bed and awake
- Sleep onset determined by time from "lights out" to first epoch of any sleep stage
- To assess occurrence of REM sleep the test continues for 15 minutes from first sleep epoch
- Session terminated if sleep does not occur after 20 minutes

The Multiple Sleep Latency Test is carried out in sleep laboratories often after a night of PSG and a week filling in a sleep diary.

The Epworth Sleepiness Scale (ESS)

Likelihood of falling asleep or dozing off when:	Chance of Dozing:			
Sitting and reading	0	1	2	3
Watching television	0	1	2	3
Sitting inactive in a public place – theater, meeting	0	1	2	3
As a car passenger for an hour without a break	0	1	2	3
Lying down to rest in the afternoon	0	1	2	3
Sitting and talking to someone	0	1	2	3
Sitting quietly after lunch without alcohol	0	1	2	3
Stopped for a few minutes while driving a car	0	1	2	3
Total Score				

Likelihood scale – rate each from 0–3 and total score

0 – would never doze   2 – moderate chance of dozing
1 – slight chance of dozing   3 – high chance of dozing

Score over 11 indicates abnormal sleepiness

The Epworth Sleepiness Scale (ESS) is a self-rating tool to enable patients and physicians to easily investigate problems with excessive sleepiness. For the most part it can be used both for looking at a day as a whole or for various times throughout a person's wake time to chart their circadian changes. As a self-rating tool, it is of course subjective and may not correlate well with objective test measures.

For the general population the average score on the ESS may be approximately 9 where as scores over 11 indicate excessive sleepiness. Interestingly those with insomnia may have scores lower than the general population, lending further weight to the theory that insomnia is a disorder of the arousal mechanisms that, as well as keeping someone awake at night, can leave someone in a state of hyperarousal during the day.

Cardinal diagnostic features of RLS (restless legs syndrome)

1 Urge to move limbs usually associated with paresthesias or dysesthesias
2 Symptoms start or become worse with rest
3 At least partial relief with physical activity
4 Worsening of symptoms in the evening or at night

Patients with RLS experience an urge to move their legs to rid themselves of unpleasant sensations (prickling, tingling, burning or tickling; numbness; "pins and needles" or cramp-like sensations). This movement typically relieves the sensations, which can occur at any time but are most disruptive when one is trying to fall asleep.

Primary hypersomnia
Differential Diagnosis

- Substance-induced hypersomnia
  Drug of abuse
  Medication use
  Exposure to a toxin
- Psychiatric disorder
  Major depressive disorder
  Depressed phase of bipolar disorder
- Sleep deprivation
  Symptoms reversed with increased sleep
- Post-traumatic hypersomnia
  Head trauma
  CNS injury
- Delay- or advance-phase sleep syndrome
  Circadian rhythm is shifted

Diagnostic measures in narcolepsy and hypersomnia

	ESS	MSLT Lat. (min)	MSLT # SOREMP	CSF Hypocretin pg/ml
Narcolepsy with Cataplexy	18	3.38	3.5	96.5
Narcolepsy without Cataplexy	19	2.75	2.5	277.3
Primary Hypersomnia	17	6	0	226.8
Hypersomnia in Psychiatric Disorders	18	7.83	0	278

(data from Bassetti et al 2003)

ESS = Epworth Sleepiness Scale
MSLT = Multiple Sleep Latency Test
Lat = latency
SOREMP = Sleep onset REM Periods
CSF = Cerebrospinal Fluid

Differential diagnosis in patients with hypersomnia disorders can be difficult, but is important in choosing the best treatment. The diagnosis of primary hypersomnia is reserved for those patients in whom no other factor can be considered causal to the symptom of sleepiness.

Overlap of symptoms in sleep and psychiatric disorders

Disorder \ Symptom	Major Depressive Disorder	Attention Deficit Hyperactivity Disorder	Narcolepsy	Obstructive Sleep Apnea	Shift-Work Sleep Disorder
Mood	+++	−	−	+	−
Sleepiness	+	+	+++	+++	+++
Fatigue	++	+	++	++	++
Concentration	++	+++	++	++	++

+++ Most Common ++ Common + Average − None

Many of the symptoms seen in sleep disorders are common in psychiatric disorders and vice versa. This chart compares the frequency of different symptoms among common sleep and psychiatric disorders, which is useful in making a differential diagnosis. The degree of symptom overlap among many disorders emphasizes the need to be able to recognize and treat a patient's individual symptoms, rather than use a single treatment strategy for all symptoms of a disorder.

Posttest Self Assessment Question: Answer

Which of the following are approved treatments for treatment resistant depression?

A. Deep brain stimulation (in trials for treatment-resistant depression but not approved)
   - Involves two surgical procedures, one to implant electrodes in the brain and a second to implant a neurostimulator in the chest
   - Stimulation is generally constant but can be temporarily turned off by holding a magnetic device over the area of the chest where the neurostimulator is located
   - This is an experimental procedure available at only a few medical centers with research protocols that may cover some or all of the costs
   - Risks and benefits remain unknown so this is reserved for patients who have failed many treatments

B. Transcranial magnetic stimulation (approved for treatment-resistant depression)
   - Generally done on an outpatient basis
   - Electromagnetic coil is placed against the scalp near the forehead and turned off and on repeatedly for 30 to 50 minutes per treatment
   - Typical treatment duration is five daily treatments a week for four to six weeks
   - Insurance coverage is variable for a course of this treatment which costs several thousand dollars
   - TMS has been best studied in patients who have failed a single antidepressant, and not necessarily indicated for more complicated cases, or for cases with multiple antidepressant failures or failure of ECT

C. Vagal nerve stimulation (approved for treatment-resistant depression)
   - Involves surgical implant of a stimulation device in the upper left side of the chest (intended as a permanent implant, though it can be removed)
   - The pulse generator can be programmed to deliver electrical impulses to the vagus nerve at various durations, frequencies, and currents
   - Stimulation typically lasts 30 seconds and occurs every five minutes
   - Studied in patients with more treatment failures than those patients studied with TMS, aripiprazole, or quetiapine
   - After an initial wave of enthusiasm for this treatment, use of VNS for depression has waned due to disappointing results, high

costs and some complications, include the hassle of having the stimulator and electrode removed

D. Aripiprazole (Abilify)(approved for treatment resistant depression)
   – Studied in patients with major depression who did not have an adequate response to one SSRI (Serotonin Selective Reuptake inhibitor) or one SNRI (Serotonin Norepinephrine Reuptake Inhibitor) antidepressant
   – Not known how well it works in patients with failures to more antidepressant treatments

E. Quetiapine (Seroquel)(approved for treatment resistant depression)
   – Also studied in patients with major depression who did not have an adequate response to one antidepressant
   – Also not known how well it works in patients with failures to more antidepressants

F. MAO inhibitors (not approved for treatment resistant depression)
   – Although almost always used for treatment resistant depression and almost never used first line, is currently only approved for first line use and not for treatment resistant depression
   • Clinical practice and numerous anecdotes suggest that some patients who do not respond to one or more antidepressants, including ECT, may respond to MAO inhibitors, but no controlled studies. Activating for some patients and may cause problems with sleep and anxiety

Answer: B, C, D and E

References

1. Stahl SM, Antidepressants, in Stahl's Essential Psychopharmacology, 3rd edition, Cambridge University Press, New York, 2008, pp 511–666
2. Stahl SM, Disorders of Sleep and Wakefulness and their Treatment, in Stahl's Essential Psychopharmacology, Cambridge University Press, New York, 2008, pp 815–862
3. Stahl SM, Aripiprazole, in Stahl's Essential Psychopharmacology The Prescriber's Guide, 3rd edition, Cambridge University Press, New York, 2009, pp 45–50
4. Stahl SM, Quetiapine, in Stahl's Essential Psychopharmacology The Prescriber's Guide, 3rd edition, Cambridge University Press, New York, 2009, pp 459–64
5. Stahl SM, Gabapentin, in Stahl's Essential Psychopharmacology The Prescriber's Guide, 3rd edition, Cambridge University Press, New York, 2009, pp 221–225
6. Silberstein S, Marmura M, Stahl SM (Ed), Pramipexole, in

Neuropharmacology: The Prescriber's Guide, Cambridge University Press 2010, pp 262–265

7. Stahl SM, Diagnosis and Treatment of Sleep Wake Disorders, NEI Press, Carlsbad, California, 2007

8. Stahl SM, Sleep: Excessive Sleepiness, NEI Press, Carlsbad, California, 2005

9. Marangell LB, Martinez M, Jurdi RA et al. Neurostimulation Therapies. Acta Psychiatrica Scandinavica 2007; 116: 174–181

10. Bassetti C, Gugger M, Bischof M et al. The narcoleptic borderland: a multimodal diagnostic approach including cerebrospinal fluid levels of hypocretin-1 (orexinA). Sleep Medicine 2003; 4: 7–12

PATIENT FILE

Lightning Round

The Case: The woman who felt numb

The Question: Are the complaints of a 63-year-old woman with a complex set of psychiatric conditions due to incomplete recovery, or to SSRI induced apathy?

The Dilemma: How to have your cake and eat it, too: namely, remission from psychiatric disorders yet no drug-induced cognitive side effects

Pretest Self Assessment Question (answer at the end of the case)

Which of the following is theoretically false regarding apathy?

A. It can be a residual symptom of depression

B. It can be a side effect of serotonergic antidepressants

C. It is hypothetically due to elevated dopamine

D. It is hypothetically due to elevated serotonin decreasing dopamine

Patient Intake

- 63-year-old woman
- Chief complaint "feeling numb"

Psychiatric History

- Long history since teens of affective, substance abuse and eating disorders
- Depressive episodes since teens
- Alcoholic starting in teens, but sober now for 27 years
- Three suicide attempts, two in her 30s, one in her 40s, overdoses, related to relationship issues when she married and divorced the same man twice
- Restricting anorexia with laxative abuse since teens, with weight as low as 89 pounds as recently as 16 years ago, responsive to inpatient treatment and fluoxetine (Prozac) 60 mg
- Stormy relationship with her mother
- Father with history of depression
- Has developed progressive sense of becoming "numb" over the past 10 years, meaning apathy, loss of memory and problems concentrating
- Numb feelings attributed to fluoxetine, but every time she has stopped it over the past years, began to have "rages" and "panic"
- Currently taking fluoxetine 60 mg because taking it is not as bad as stopping it

Of the following choices, what would you do?
- Switch to another SSRI
- Switch to an SNRI
- Switch to mirtazapine (Remeron)
- Switch to bupropion (Wellbutrin)
- Initiate or refer to psychotherapy

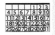

Case Outcome

- Patient switched to bupropion, but developed "rage" and also anxiety while driving
- Switched to lamotrigine (Lamictal), and has done well for many months without recurrent depression, rage, or apathy

Case Debrief

- It appears as though this patient's complaints of numbness were indeed due to her fluoxetine treatment
- Despite her unstable past, she has done well from a psychiatric point of view in recent years except for her apathy and problems concentrating since taking fluoxetine
- She destabilizes when stopping fluoxetine, so some alternative treatment is necessary
- Switching to another SSRI seems very unlikely to be helpful, as would switching to an SNRI, since the apathy is theoretically due to raising of serotonin levels, which can reduce dopamine release in some brain circuits, especially in patients who are very sensitive to this for unknown reasons
- Mirtazapine also raises serotonin
- Bupropion is the most logical choice because it does not raise serotonin, and in fact raises dopamine (and norepinephrine) and even reverses SSRI apathy in patients who are switched to bupropion or who are augmented with bupropion
- This patient may have a contraindication to bupropion in the opinion of some psychopharmacologists because of the remote history of eating disorder; however, this problem is not active, and the patient is at normal body weight, so bupropion can be given safely and prudently
- Surprisingly, bupropion did not work
- Another agent that lacks serotonergic properties is lamotrigine, which may act via blockade of glutamate release
- This patient surprisingly responded well to this switch, possibly because the patient has a bipolar spectrum disorder as part of her complex psychiatric problems, and thus is responsive to an

agent better known for preventing recurrences of depression in bipolar patients

Posttest Self Assessment Question: Answer

Which of the following is theoretically false regarding apathy?

A. It can be a residual symptom of depression
B. It can be a side effect of serotonergic antidepressants
C. It is hypothetically due to elevated dopamine
D. It is hypothetically due to elevated serotonin decreasing dopamine

Answer: C

References

1. Stahl SM, Antidepressants, in Stahl's Essential Psychopharmacology, 3rd edition, Cambridge University Press, New York, 2008, pp 511–666
2. Stahl SM, Bupropion, in Stahl's Essential Psychopharmacology The Prescriber's Guide, 3rd edition, Cambridge University Press, New York, 2009, pp 57–62
3. Stahl SM, Lamotrigine, in Stahl's Essential Psychopharmacology The Prescriber's Guide, 3rd edition, Cambridge University Press, New York, 2009, pp 259–65

The Case: The case of physician do not heal thyself

The Question: Does the patient have a complex mood disorder, a personality disorder or both?

The Dilemma: How do you treat a complex and long-term unstable disorder of mood in a difficult patient?

Pretest Self Assessment Question (answer at the end of the case)

Frequent mood swings are more a sign or symptom of a mood disorder than they are of a personality disorder

A. True
B. False

Patient Intake

- 60-year-old man
- Chief complaint is "being unstable"
- Patient estimates that he has spent about two thirds of the time over the past year being in a mixed dysphoric state and about one third as depressed, but waxing and waning every few days, or even every few hours

Psychiatric History: Childhood and Adolescence

- As a young child, had symptoms of generalized anxiety and separation anxiety
- Also, as a child, remembers "emotional trauma" from mother, herself with recurrent episodes of either unipolar or bipolar depression who was often physically unavailable because of hospitalizations, or emotionally distant when depressed at home
- Has had a lifetime of multiple turbulent interpersonal relationships since childhood, with family members, with friends and especially with women
- As an older child and adolescent, continued to have not only subsyndromal generalized anxiety but developed at least subsyndromal levels of OCD with ruminations, checking and rigidity
- He was told these were good traits and would make him a good student, which he was, with good grades through high school and college, gaining admission to medical school

Psychiatric History: Adulthood

- Diagnosed as major depression for the first time at age 23, early in medical school
  - Was his worst depression so far, as other depressions previously

characterized as unhappiness and transient depressed moods of a few days duration and with more anxiety than depression, improving without treatment
- Actively suicidal and overdosed on his medications at this time but recovered
- In retrospect, patient believes that he has long experienced rejection sensititivity with up to 2 depressive episodes per year since age 16 up to the present
• No clear history of any full syndromal manic or hypomanic episodes
• Since age 23, however, has had many episodes lasting a week or more of irritability, inflated self esteem, increased goal-directed work activity, decreased need for sleep, overtalkativeness, racing thoughts, psychomotor agitation and risky behavior; could also experience euphoria or expansiveness to a significant degree but only for 2 or 3 days at most and usually shorter
• He interpreted these as good traits, indicative of creative persons, and were the reason he was productive as well as creative
• In getting his history, it is not clear whether he has had an irritable dysphoric temperament since childhood, a superimposed episodic subsyndromal dysphoric mixed hypomania, or both
• First marriage ages 32–33
- Depressive episode and overdosed again when first marriage broke up
• Second marriage between 35 and 36
- Another depressive episode after breakup of this marriage
• Third marriage ages 46 to 58
- Another depressive episode after breakup of this marriage

Medication History

• Starting with his first diagnosed episode of depression in medical school, treated off and on with TCAs and benzodiazepines, starting and stopping them over many years in relationship to his symptoms
• First received lithium at age 43, 17 years ago
• Unclear whether this was an augmentation strategy for resistant depression or for bipolar spectrum symptoms
• Was not that helpful according to the patient
• States he has had many, many medication trials since then
• Valproate (Depakote) not tolerated
• Clonazapam (Klonopin) helped sleep
• Oxcarbazapine (Trileptal) caused dysphoria and agitation
• Verapamil caused/worsened depression
• Risperidone (Risperdal) caused depression
• Fluoxetine (Prozac) caused rapid fleeting relief of depression, but also insomnia and headache

- Other SSRIs caused activation and were not tolerated and discontinued after a few doses
- Presents now only taking methylphenidate (Ritalin), which he prescribes for himself as he does not think his physicians know as much about his case, or what he needs, as he does and they will not prescribe it for him

Social and Personal History

- Married and divorced 3 times, currently single
- No children
- Non smoker
- No drug abuse, rarely drinks
- Physician and successful businessman

Medical History

- Crohn's disease

Family History

- Father: sleep disorder
- Mother: either bipolar or unipolar depression, unsure, but successfully treated with ECT
- Maternal uncle: depression
- Maternal aunt: depression
- Maternal grandmother: hospitalized for "manic depressive disorder"

Current Medications

- Azothiaprine and Remicaid for Crohn's
- Methylphenidate

Based on just what you have been told so far about this patient's history what do you think is his diagnosis?

- Recurrent major depression with an anxious/dysphoric temperament
- Bipolar II depression
- Bipolar II mixed episode
- Bipolar NOS
- Bipolar NOS superimposed upon a personality disorder (narcissistic, borderline, other)
- Primarily a cluster B personality disorder (antisocial/histrionic/narcissistic/borderline)

Attending Physician's Mental Notes: Initial Psychiatric Evaluation

- Here is a case that could be a complex combination of a mood disorder plus a personality disorder in someone who has never experienced mania and probably has never reached the threshold of experiencing unequivocal hypomania as defined by DSM IV or ICD10
- It is very difficult to separate the mood disorder from the personality disorder in a one hour initial evaluation session, plus looking at the medical records
- A complete diagnosis will have to await spending more time with the patient, and if possible, having access to the input of other observers as well
- However, seems likely that there is more to this case than a mood disorder, and probably cluster B personality traits if not personality disorder is comorbid

How would you treat him?
- Continue his methylphenidate
- Discontinue his methylphenidate
- Start an antidepressant
- Restart lithium
- Start an anticonvulsant mood stabilizer
- Start an atypical antipsychotic
- Make sure he agrees to weekly insight oriented psychotherapy
- Consider psychoanalysis

Attending Physician's Mental Notes: Initial Psychiatric Evaluation, Continued

- Since the patient lives in another city, psychotherapy will have to be an option via another mental health professional, although some supervision of that plus advice on medications can be possible as a consultant
- The patient is open to pursuing psychotherapy as long as he respects the therapist
- Before recommending psychopharmacologic treatment, it would be good to review what we know from the available history about his response to medications already taken
- As shown from the history of this case, it can be impossible to determine with great accuracy the effects of the medications by taking a history. One should be skeptical of the information as it can be unreliably reported in records and by a patient because it is complex and the medication effects can be subtle

- How many medications were taken long enough to have had a chance to work?
- Did some medications provoke mood instability while others stabilized mood?
- If the person has a mood disorder with an underlying personality disorder, will medications treat only the mood disorder and expose the symptoms of the personality disorder, or
- Will treating the mood disorder with medications allow the patient to recompensate and thus have improvement not only in mood but in personality disorder symptoms?
- These questions are better answered if you live the ups and down along with the patient and experience the signs and symptoms of such a patient in real time
- However, the real question is what can you do to help such a patient and what are the realistic goals of treatment
- Finally, is treatment defined as medications, insight oriented psychotherapy, or both?

• About the only thing solid here is that antidepressants seem to be provocative at times in terms of causing activation and thus should be given cautiously and only concomitantly with mood stabilizing medication

• Has taken numerous mood stabilizing medications that he reported cause depression, especially those that are used to treat mania

• He has a demanding job and is not willing to put up with much sedation and will not accept weight gain

• It is possible that he is a bipolar spectrum patient with more depression than mania and with more pure depressive states alternating with mixed states of dysphoria/irritability superimposed upon depression, but not full syndrome mixed bipolar disorder

• Thus he has four needs"
  - Treat from "below" (i.e., antidepressant)
  - Stabilize from "below: (i.e. prevent cycling into depression)
  - Treat from "above" (in his case, not to treat euphoric mania, but to treat irritability)
  - Stabilize from "above" (i.e. prevent cycling into mixed states of dysphoric/irritable depression)

• Highly unlikely that this will be possible with a single agent

• For now, decided to avoid an antidepressant and to stop the methylphenidate which may help depression but at the expense of destabilizing him and causing cycling into irritable mixed states

• For now, a low side effect mood stabilizing agent with antidepressant and maintenance potential (i.e., treating from below and stabilizing from below) such as lamotrigine seems to be a good bet

- After this is given, might consider adding lithium which he has tolerated in the past although unclear what therapeutic actions it had for him; however, might treat and stabilize him from above in synergy with lamotrigine for a total therapeutic picture

Case Outcome: First Interim Followup, Week 12

- Patient flies back for a followup appointment 3 months later
- Has stopped methylphenidate and his psychiatrist in his home city started lamotrigine by slow upward titration, but a bit faster and to a higher dose than recommended and now taking 400 mg/day
- Mood stabilized but at a level of low grade consistent depression with decreased libido and sexual dysfunction
- Told to reduce lamotrigine to 200 mg and wait another month or two because it can take a while yet for lamotrigine's antidepressant effect to kick in and its mood stabilizing effects may have already started

Case Outcome: Second Interim Followup, Week 16

- Phone consultation
- Learned that the patient decided that lamotrigine was making him depressed and ruining his sex life, so discontinued it and completely relapsed in terms of depression
- Patient agrees to restart lithium after blood and urine tests from his physician

Case Outcome: Third, Fourth, and Fifth Interim Followup Visits, Weeks 20, 24 and 28

- Phone consultations
- Patient has normal labs and starts lithium at week 20 only has a blood level of 0.4, so told to increase dose
- At week 24 calls and states that higher doses give him unacceptable diarrhea and exacerbates his Crohn's disease symptoms, so he is back down to the low dose of lithium
- Also, restarted methylphenidate as needed for dysphoric mood and low energy
- Told to increase his lithium again, more slowly and not to 1800 mg/day which caused diarrhea but only to 1500 mg a day or 1500 mg alternating with 1800 mg/day on alternate days and to stop his methylphenidate
- Also told to restart lamotrigine titrating up to only half his previous dose, namely 200 mg/day with the strategy that both drugs together would allow him to take each in lower tolerable doses for him, yet working together to add their therapeutic effects

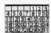

Case Outcome: Sixth and Seventh Interim Followup Visits, Weeks 32 and 36

- Brief phone consults with the patient and his psychiatrist on the phone together
- Getting regular psychotherapy "whatever"
- Monitored by his local psychiatrist monthly face to face appointments
- Lithium level 0.7, occasional tremor and diarrhea but mostly tolerable
- Mood is stable and overall "feels much better"

Case Outcome: Eighth Interim Followup, Week 40

- Emergency phone call
- Can't get a hold of his psychiatrist where he lives
- Patient calls from a football stadium where his alma mater is playing in a big football game
- "I'm in trouble"
- Patient states he has been much troubled recently about always feeling somewhat dysphoric, not really worse recently, but just tired of never being "well"
- Denies psychosocial stressors but feels desperate and suicidal
- Now at the football game, his thoughts are entirely about suicide, making his will, shooting others at the game, and killing himself
- Fortunately, he states he neither has a gun with him nor does he own one
- Has weird reaction to the football game, because when his team scores, he is not euphoric but bursts into tears
- "help me"

What would you do now?

- Tell him to call his local psychiatrist
- Tell him to go to the emergency room
- Tell him to call the suicide hot line
- Tell him to settle down and that you will either call in a prescription for an antipsychotic or coordinate it with his local psychiatrist
- Tell the patient to find another consultant

Case Outcome: Eighth Interim Followup, Week 40, Continued

- Told the patient to settle down and you would call his psychiatrist to meet him at his local emergency room which he agrees to do after the game ends
- Also patient states he feels much better now that he has spoken on the phone, and also now that his team is now winning
- Local psychiatrist sees him in the emergency room and starts him on aripiprazole 2.5 mg increasing if tolerated and not effective to 5.0 mg 1 to 3 days later, increasing to 7.5 mg if tolerated and not effective 1 to 3 days later

Case Outcome: Ninth Interim Followup, Week 41

- One week later, phone consult with his psychiatrist on the line
- Patient states he contacted his local psychiatrist the same day as his phone call from the football stadium, and saw him a week later (which was yesterday)
- Got the prescription for aripiprazole and the next day following the phone call from the football stadium, left on a business trip from California to New York
- In New York, the aripiprazole was not effective at 2.5 mg, so the next day he became desperate and took 20 mg (not an overdose attempt, just to hurry up the therapeutic response)
- Also increased his lamotrigine on his own to 400 mg/day
- Lowered his lithium dose
- Flew back to California
- Had gait disturbance, tremor, word-finding problems, memory loss, yet still verbally provocative, desperate with recurring suicidal and homicidal ideation
- "I want to hang myself"

What would you do now?

- Start another antipsychotic
- Reinstate the original doses of lamotrigine and lithium
- Tell the patient and his local psychiatrist to find another consultant

Case Outcome: Ninth Interim Followup, Week 41, Continued

- Actually, this time, felt as though the patient was manipulating and scolded him with his psychiatrist on the line
- Told him that his psychiatrist is the treating physician, not the consultant, and the consultant's advice is to see his psychiatrist and to have future contacts with the consultant either by phone with his psychiatrist on the line, or face to face with his psychiatrist on the line

- Told to decrease lamotrigine, increase lithium back to previous levels and to discontinuie aripiprazole
- Also advised starting ziprasidone 40 mg at night with food

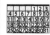

Case Outcome: Tenth Interim Followup, Week 42

- Phone call with local treating psychiatrist and the patient one week later
- Patient was compliant with instructions
- Now states the ziprasidone "turned a switch"
- By this he means that suicidal ideation abated immediately, depression no longer dysphoric but only low grade at worst
- Some fatigue/inertia
- Some tongue chewing suggesting a mild ziprasidone induced EPS
- Dramatically better and very pleased
- Suggest to them that the consultant will now resign from the case
- Did he live happily every after?

Case Outcome: Eleventh Interim Followup, Week 54

- About 3 months later, that is, 1 year after the initial psychiatric evaluation, got phone call from a new psychiatrist in the patient's home city where the patient had transferred his care
- States that the patient decided to add fluoxetine 10 mg, stopped lamotrigine, tried 160 mg of ziprasidone, now back to 40 mg
- The story goes on. . . .

Case Debrief

- This intelligent and manipulative patient with a genuine mood disorder and a personality disorder is decidedly unstable, but able to function as a physician even though not able to maintain long-term interpersonal relationships
- Is not very compliant, often making therapeutic decisions on his own about how to treat his own case, especially when things are not going well
- It is difficult to determine whether his periods of mood stability are related to drug treatment or to the lack of psychosocial stressors, but there is the sense that medications are somewhat helpful for the worst of his mood swings even though the medications are not helpful for his responses to psychosocial stressors

Take-Home Points

- Difficult patients are difficult
- To paraphrase Tolstoy in Anna Karenina
  - "Happy families are all alike; every unhappy family is unhappy in its own way"
  - One could say in cases like this one, "Stable patients are all alike; every unstable patient is unstable in his own way"
- Temperament and personality are factors in bipolar disorder and might even be part of bipolar disorder and are certainly part of the barriers to treatment effectiveness and to treatment compliance/adherence
- A realistic goal in a case like this may be less of a roller coaster, but not full stabilization or true remission, yet well enough to stay employed, have relationships and not be desperate, suicidal or homicidal
- Patients tend to hate depressed states more than mixed states whereas those around patients tend to hate the patient's mixed irritable states more than their depressed states

Performance in Practice: Confessions of a Psychopharmacologist

- What could have been done better here?
  - Should the consultant have stayed engaged after the intial consultation?
  - The involvement of two psychiatrists allowed the patient the opportunity for splitting and chaos
  - Should psychotherapy have played a more prominent role here?
- Possible action item for improvement in practice
  - Make a more concerted effort to define the role of a consultant versus a primary psychiatrist, who is the quarterback of the team, allowing the consultant to play a secondary role, and perhaps in cases like this, try and ensure no direct contact with the consultant without the primary psychiatrist also being present
  - Set realistic goals for a patient like this and realize long term stability may not be attainable

Tips and Pearls

- Lamotrigine, lithium and an atypical antipsychotic can be a useful triple combination for unstable cases of mood and personality disorder and combinations and doses can be found that are relatively tolerable
- Stimulants have no role in a case like this
- Antidepressants can be destabilizing in a case like this
- Physicians can be especially difficult to treat when they are patients as they tend to interfere with their own treatments

Two-Minute Tute: A brief lesson and psychopharmacology tutorial (tute) with relevant background material for this case – Distinguishing personality disorders from mood disorders

Table 1: General symptoms of a personality disorder overlap with general symptoms of a mood disorder, particularly a bipolar spectrum mood disorder

- Frequent mood swings
- Anger outbusts
- Stormy professional and personal relationships
- Social isolation
- Suspicion and mistrust of others
- Difficulty making friends
- Need for instant gratification
- Poor impulse control
- Frequent drug or alcohol abuse

Table 2: Personality disorders vs mood disorders

- Cluster A disorders (paranoid, schizoid personality disorders or schizotypal personality disorder)
  - Tend to overlap with psychotic mood disorders
- Cluster B disorders (antisocial, borderline, histrionic and narcissistic personality disorders)
  - Can be easily confused for a bipolar spectrum disorder
  - Especially if no overt manic episode or any unequivocal hypomanic episode
  - Nevertheless, symptoms can empirically improve when treated with agents for bipolar disorder
  - A very confusing and chaotic condition can be the combination of a bipolar disorder with a cluster B personality disorder
- Cluster C disorders (avoidant, dependent and obsessive compulsive personality disorders)
  - Can be confused with anxiety disorders
  - Often predate the emergence of a mood disorder and can reappear when mood disorder symptoms under control

Posttest Self Assessment Question: Answer

Frequent mood swings are more a sign or symptom of a mood disorder than they are of a personality disorder

A. True
B. False

Answer: False

Mood swings are prominent signs of both mood disorders and personality disorders; not all mood swings are mood disorders

References

1. Stahl SM, Mood Disorders, in Stahl's Essential Psychopharmacology, 3rd edition, Cambridge University Press, New York, 2008, pp 453–510
2. Stahl SM, Antidepressants, in Stahl's Essential Psychopharmacology, 3rd edition, Cambridge University Press, New York, 2008, pp 511–666
3. Stahl SM, Mood Stabilizers, in Stahl's Essential Psychopharmacology, 3rd edition, Cambridge University Press, New York, 2008, pp 667–720
4. Stahl SM, Lamotrigine in Stahl's Essential Psychopharmacology The Prescriber's Guide, 3rd edition, Cambridge University Press, New York, 2009, pp 259–66
5. Stahl SM, Lithium, in Stahl's Essential Psychopharmacology The Prescriber's Guide, 3rd edition, Cambridge University Press, New York, 2009, pp 277–82
6. Stahl SM, Ziprasidone, in Stahl's Essential Psychopharmacology The Prescriber's Guide, 3rd edition, Cambridge University Press, New York, 2009, pp 589–94
7. Stahl SM, Aripiprazole, in Stahl's Essential Psychopharmacology The Prescriber's Guide, 3rd edition, Cambridge University Press, New York, 2009, pp 45–50
8. Schwartz TL and Stahl,SM, Ziprasidone in the treatment of bipolar disorder, in Akiskal H and Tohen M, Bipolar Psychopharmacotherapy: Caring for the Patient, 2nd edition, Wiley Press

The Case: The son whose parents were desperate to have him avoid Kraepelin

The Question: Can you forecast whether an adolescent will become bipolar, schizophrenic or recover?

The Dilemma: Should you treat symptoms empirically when the diagnosis changes every time the patient comes for a visit?

Pretest Self Assessment Question (answer at the end of the case)

Which symptom would better fit a mood disorder spectrum rather than a psychotic disorder spectrum?

A. Affective symptom
B. Cognitive symptom
C. Social symptom

Patient Intake

- 18-year-old male adolescent
- Chief complaint: Depressive mood, with deterioration of social and cognitive performance at school

Psychiatric History: Childhood

- By age 7, patient developed symptoms consistent with attention deficit disorder, and was treated with stimulants from age 7 to 13
- He did very well on stimulants, had good performance in school and adequate peer relationships, although he was somewhat more isolative and less social than his peers

Psychiatric History: Adolescence

- By age 13, he had a decided step off in his function, and became progressively unable to interact with peers at school; his school performance also deteriorated
- This coincided with a series of several surgeries on his sinuses for a chronic fungal infection
- He was evaluated to determine if there was a central nervous system involvement, but that was mostly, although not entirely, ruled out
- From age 13 to age 18, the patient has been evaluated at three different major medical centers and was given numerous diagnoses in that period of time
  - attention deficit hyperactivity disorder
  - schizoaffective disorder
  - major depressive disorder
  - Asperger's syndrome
  - bipolar disorder

- possible neurologic celiac sprue
- possible complications of sinus infections and surgery
- most recently, he has been diagnosed as either prodrome of schizophrenia or an autism spectrum disorder, and has begun clozapine (Clozaril) titration, with some day time sedation
- He has had symptoms of depression, suicidal ideation, alternating with rage and problems of control
- He has not had any overt hallucinations, but has had inappropriate ideas such as being able to move a lock by telekinesis
- He has tried many different antipsychotics, anticonvulsants, lithium, and antidepressants
  - Antidepressants have activated him, similarly to when he used to take stimulants, causing him to be more provokable

Medical History

- Patient's past medical history is significant for sinus infections, which are now resolved
- Possible sprue, although laboratory testing appears to have ruled this out

Family History

- Father: panic attacks
- Sister: attention deficit hyperactivity disorder
- Maternal grandfather: mood swings
- Paternal grandmother: depression
- Uncle: alcoholism
- Cousin: bipolar disorder

Patient Intake

- Patient arrived on time for his appointment, and was accompanied by his mother for the interview
- He was casually dressed in a black T-shirt and appeared to be his stated age
- When engaging in conversations, he had appropriate eye contact, however when the examiner was speaking with his mother, he sat with downcast eyes and appeared to be in some distress
- He seemed to be forlorn, and even depressed
- He seemed to be feeling hopeless in the sense that it was not worth trying and that life no longer had any joy, that he was unable to be happy with the worry that he would never be able to become happy
- He was not suicidal although he had had these thoughts in the past and said he just wished someone would kill him

- His memory and judgment appeared to be intact
- His insight appeared to be limited and the patient appeared to have given up hope
- Current medications
  - Clozapine (Clozaril): 100 mg in the morning and 100 mg at night
  - Escitalopram (Lexapro, Ciprilex): 5 mg per day

Of the following choices, what would be your differential diagnosis?
- Anxiety Disorder
- Asperger like syndrome/autistic spectrum disorder
- Bipolar disorder
- Major depressive disorder
- Prodrome of schizophrenia

Attending Physician's Mental Notes: Initial Psychiatric Evaluation

- No clear diagnosis, and all the diagnoses in the list above could be considered although an anxiety disorder seems the least likely diagnosis
- The patient is clearly a complicated case; but the differential diagnosis should probably be between a prodrome of schizophrenia carrying over from Asperger-like syndrome earlier in development versus a bipolar spectrum disorder with current depressive features
- Diagnosis is perhaps not the issue here, and symptoms may be more important to document, track and treat empirically
- Despite the history and some of the diagnoses given by previous examiners, this case has more of an affective feel than a psychotic one, based on the history gathered here and according to his current clinical state
- This brings up the question of why clozapine is being given
- On the other hand, cases like this can morph between appointments and over time, and although he presents with a more affective spectrum appearance today, perhaps diagnostic judgment should be withheld while monitoring for more psychosis spectrum symptoms over the next few appointments and over the next few months

What factors might help you to make a diagnosis or prognosis that the patients are anxious to have and pressing you to deliver?
- No clear family history of schizophrenia or psychotic illness
- Positive family history of bipolar disorder

Attending Physician's Mental Notes: Initial Psychiatric Evaluation, Continued

- Unfortunately, there are no genetic tests or biological markers to distinguish between a schizophrenic versus a bipolar illness; in fact, many research tests overlap between these two diagnoses, rather than distinguish one from another
- The previous activation by an antidepressant is of interest, and could suggest a bipolar disorder, but antidepressants can often worsen active psychosis
- However, this patient is not actively psychotic and antidepressants can treat prodromal symptoms of schizophrenia
- Seems like the best option here is to keep an open mind about diagnosis and reassure the parents that the best action plan may be to reduce symptom burden empirically while not causing unacceptable side effects
- The immediate therapeutic goal is to improve social and academic performance, and to reduce the patient's and family's current chief complaint, namely depression

How would you treat him now?
- Continue treatment as is
- Decrease or discontinue clozapine
- Increase the dose of clozapine
- Discontinue escitalopram
- Increase the dose of escitalopram
- Add lithium or an anticonvulsant mood stabilizer
- Switch to another atypical antipsychotic

Further Investigation:

Is there anything else you would especially like to know about this patient?

- What about his school placement, vocational placement, how he spends his day, and whether he is participating in psychotherapy or interacting with peers?
  - The patient is living at home, not going to school or working, and spends most of his time in bed or watching TV
  - Denies substance abuse, including alcohol and marijuana
  - Has not had significant psychotherapy
  - Parents are intelligent, well read, and well connected to the elite medical community, proactive, supportive and yet anxious about his outcome and feeling a bit guilty
  - Parents are worried he will develop schizophrenia and want him to avoid this "Kraepelinian" outcome

Attending Physician's Mental Notes: Initial Psychiatric Evaluation, Continued

- The dose of clozapine was reduced to 75 mg in the morning and increased to 125 mg in the evening to determine if the patient tolerated the daytime sedation better
- as the patient had never had his lipids monitored or his body mass index recorded, this procedure was initiated
- The dose of escitalopram was cautiously increased to 10 mg per day to try treating his depressive symptoms
- Suggested referral to a psychotherapist, but this suggestion was not enthusiastically received by either the patient or parents
- The risks, benefits, and alternatives were explained to the patient and his mother and they consented to the treatment plan

Attending Physician's Mental Notes: First Interim Followup, Week 4

- Unfortunately, the patient became activated on the increased dose of escitalopram

What would you do now to address his depressive symptoms?
- Decrease the dose of escitalopram and initiate valproate
- Keep the increased dose of escitalopram and initiate valproate
- Stop escitalopram and initiate valproate

Attending Physician's Mental Notes: First Interim Followup, Week 4, Continued

- The dose of escitalopram was decreased to 5 mg per day
- Valproate (Depakote) was added, and once its titration was complete, the dose of escitalopram was again increased to 10 mg per day

Attending Physician's Mental Notes: Second Interim Followup, Week 8

- The patient's depressive symptoms seemed to resolve over time
- Blood counts normal, no weight gain, some sedation

What would you do now about his clozapine treatment?
- Continue clozapine
- Reduce clozapine dose or discontinue clozapine

Attending Physician's Mental Notes: Second Interim Followup, Week 8, Continued

- Seems like this case is responding as if it is a bipolar disorder, with worsening now for the second time on an antidepressant, this time even in the presence of clozapine, and also responding to valproate even though this medication is better documented to treat mania than depression in bipolar disorder
- On the one hand, "if it ain't broke, don't fix it" and leave well enough alone
- On the other hand, he may be "overtreated" with clozapine and a switch to another antipsychotic could be considered but not a discontinuation of all antipsychotics at the present time
- The parents are quite reluctant to discontinue clozapine, and since the patient is tolerating it reasonably well, that seems prudent for now
- However, if sedation does not improve over time, he may require a dose reduction of clozapine or valproate
- In the long run, depending upon clinical response and whether the patient develops any metabolic problems, clozapine may be switched to another antipsychotic
- Patient is sent for fasting triglycerides to monitor his insulin resistance, as well as a full lipid panel, and glucose
- Now that the patient is in a better space, with more motivation, mother and patient were pressed to pursue weekly psychotherapy at least for support, information, explanation of the treatments, and exploration of how he feels about having this illness and how it is impacting his life and his future

Case Debrief

- When treating complicated child and adolescent cases, with multiple possible diagnoses, it can be challenging to find the appropriate treatment plan.
- In this case, it appeared most useful to treat this patient as an evolving bipolar disorder patient with an antipsychotic, with an anticonvulsant mood stabilizer, and with an antidepressant, although any medication treatment is controversial
- This patient's case is clearly unstable and evolving, with a strong affective nature to the illness and poor social interactions rather than profound current cognitive symptoms
- Over the past few months since his initial evaluation, his condition fits the mood disorder spectrum better than the schizophrenia/autism/psychotic disorder spectrum
- The cognitive and social symptoms are consistent either with a schizophrenia prodrome or with reversible symptoms of an affective

disorder, but it is too soon to tell or to pass long term diagnostic judgment or to make accurate prognostic statements
- For now, it seems logical to first stabilize this patient's mood and see what happens, at least offering short term relief of that symptom
- Although it makes examiners, parents and patients uneasy, the fact remains that only time will tell.

Take-Home Points
- Childhood onset psychiatric disorders are wild cards, and the current state of the art unfortunately is that it is not yet possible to predict with great accuracy the natural history of psychiatric illness in a given individual
- In general, however, the earlier the onset of symptoms, and the more severe, the worse the outcome, especially if poor school performance and peer interactions damage the development of a healthy self esteem
- Genetic and neuroimaging tests of high risk individuals seek to predict who will get schizophrenia, but these remain research tools and not yet very helpful in clinical practice
- No drug is approved for the social withdrawal and cognitive decline of the schizophrenia prodrome, but these same symptoms can be due to an affective disorder for which there are a number of treatments available even in children and adolescents
- It is often best to make an optimistic diagnosis and an optimistic prognosis in cases like this to keep hope alive and to justify attempts at symptomatic therapeutic interventions if risks are outweighed by the potential benefits
- However, there is no documented disease modification by any medication to alter the natural history of whatever illness underlies the symptoms in such cases .

Performance in Practice: Confessions of a Psychopharmacologist
- What could have been done better here?
  - Parents may be interested in research evaluation with neuroimaging, neuropsychological testing, and genetic testing, given that they pursue medical evaluations and second opinions at a number of top medical centers
  - The pursuit of a diagnosis may be a distraction from empiric focus on reducing current symptoms and dealing with the anxiety that is caused by so many unknowns
  - On the other hand, inheriting a patient already on clozapine can seem very aggressive treatment given the state of the evidence supporting that approach

- Possible action item for improvement in practice
  - Supporting the family in getting the best available diagnostic and therapeutic information while helping them work through the crisis of having an uncertain diagnosis with uncertain treatments and uncertain long term outcomes, due to the nature of the state of the art and not due to going to the wrong doctors or medical centers
  - Reassure with distribution of the latest information and cutting edge findings without avoiding the need for here and now treatments of symptoms, for which not only medications but also potentially psychotherapy may be useful. Going to school and working outside the home can also be therapeutic while the ambiguities of the ultimate diagnosis and outcome are still in limbo

Tips and Pearls

- For cases like this, be skeptical of the apparent diagnosis on any given visit
- Track symptoms and their severity, and empirically treat while being careful to monitor side effects
- Affective symptoms may be a better prognostic sign than psychotic or negative or cognitive symptoms, and in this case were apparently responsive to treatment in a family with first degree relatives who have bipolar disorder but no schizophrenia
- Children and adolescents with ever changing psychiatric symptoms and diagnoses without robust treatment responses should be monitored carefully for progression of symptoms
- To treat or not to treat, that is the question
  - Clinicians must decide whether to err on the side of undertreatment (error of omission)
  - or on the side of overtreatment (error of commission) since prodromal cases have unpredictable outcomes
- Genetic testing and biological markers are poised to enter clinical practice but are not understood well enough for routine clinical use
- Ad hoc, ergo propter hoc: just because the patient improves after a given medication does not mean that he improves because of a given medication. That is, symptoms wax and wane spontaneously, and even though the patient was on powerful medications, he may have improved because of a fluctuating illness and not because of treatment response, so keep an open mind as to how to treat him in the future if his symptoms recur or new ones develop, especially on stable medication treatment

Two-Minute Tute: A brief lesson and psychopharmacology tutorial (tute) with relevant background material for this case
– Ultra high risk of psychosis
– Schizophrenia prodromes

Criteria for ultra high risk of psychosis: one or more of the following

1. Attenuated psychotic symptoms, having experienced sub-threshhold attenuated psychotic symptoms during the past year
2. Brief limited intermittent psychotic symptoms, having experienced episodes of frank psychotic symptoms that have not lasted longer than a week and have been spontaneously abated
3. State and trait risk factors, having schizotypal personality disorder or a first-degree relative with a psychotic disorder and have experienced a significant decrease in functioning during the previous year

Neuropsychological functioning in ultra high risk of psychosis

- Global neuropsychological functioning is significantly lower in ultra high risk individuals who progress to psychosis than in those who do not, and is worst in those with a family history of psychosis
- Processing speed is reduced in ultra high risk individuals compared to normal controls
- Verbal learning and memory are reduced in ultra high risk individuals compared to normal controls
- Visuospatial functioning may be relatively spared
- Verbal memory deficits may indicate a prefrontal-hippocampal neurodevelopmental abnormality
- Generalized neurocognitive impairment may be a nonspecific vulnerability marker
- Neurocognitive deficits in schizophrenia are largely uncorrelated with positive symptoms
- Neurocognitive deficits in schizophrenia only modestly improved if at all by antipsychotic treatment

Prodromes: are making a diagnosis and prescribing treatment merciful or ahead of the data?

- Dopamine overactivity may predate the onset of schizophrenia in those with prodromal psychotic symptoms
- Dopamine overactivity may correlate with severity of prodromal symptoms and neurocognitive dysfunction
- Reduced cortical connectivity in schizophrenia is likely to be present from birth
- Hypothetically, if this progresses beyond a critical threshold, psychotic symptoms erupt as a function of normal neuromaturational events such as synaptic pruning during adolescence, and/or environmental insults
- Frequent diagnoses in patients who saw psychiatrists before the diagnosis of schizophrenia
  - Impulse disorder not otherwise specified
  - ADHD
  - Bipolar disorder not otherwise specified

Posttest Self Assessment Question: Answer

Which symptom would better fit a mood disorder spectrum rather than a psychotic disorder spectrum?

A. Affective symptom
B. Cognitive symptom
C. Social symptom

Answer: A

References

1. Stahl SM, Psychosis and Schizophrenia, in Stahl's Essential Psychopharmacology, 3rd edition, Cambridge University Press, New York, 2008, pp 247–326
2. Stahl SM, Antipsychotic Agents, in Stahl's Essential Psychopharmacology, Cambridge University Press, New York, 2008, pp 327–452
3. deKoning MB, Bloemen OJN, va Amelsvoort TAMH et al. Early intervention in patients at ultra high risk of psychosis: benefits and risks. Acta Psychiatrica Scand 2009; 119: 426–42
4. Stahl SM, Prophylactic antipsychotics: do they keep you from catching schizophrenia? J Clin Psychiat 2004; 65: 1445–6
5. McGorry PD, Nelson B, Amminger GP et al. Intervention in individuals at ultra high risk for psychosis: a review and future directions. J Clin Psychiatry 2009; 70: 1206–12

6. Cornblatt BA, Lencz T, Smith CW et al. Can antidepressants be used to treat the schizophrenia prodrome? Results of a prospective-naturalistic treatment study of adolescents. J Clin Psychiatry 2007; 68: 546–57

7. McGlashan TH, Zipursky RB, Perkins D et al. Randomized, double-blind trial of olanzapine versus placebo in patients prodromally symptomatic for psychosis. Am J Psychiatry 2006; 163: 790–9

8. Seidman LJ, Guiliano AJ, Meyer EC et al. Neuropsychology of the prodrome to psychosis in the NAPLS consortium. Arch Gen Psychiatr 2010; 67: 578–88

9. Lencz T, Smith CW, McLaughlin D et al. Generalized and specific neurocognitive deficits in prodromal schizophrenia. Biol Psychiatr 2006; 59: 863–71

10. Howes OK, Montgomery AJ, Asselin MC et al. Elevated striatal dopamine function linked to prodromal signs of schizophrenia. Arch Gen Psychiat 2009; 66: 13–20

11. Stahl SM, Mood Disorders, in Stahl's Essential Psychopharmacology, 3rd edition, Cambridge University Press, New York, 2008, chapter 11, pp 453–510

12. Stahl SM, Clozapine, in Stahl's Essential Psychopharmacology The Prescriber's Guide, 3rd edition, Cambridge University Press, New York, 2009, pp 113–8

13. Stahl SM, Escitalopram, in Stahl's Essential Psychopharmacology The Prescriber's Guide, 3rd edition, Cambridge University Press, New York, 2009, pp 171–5

14. Stahl SM, Valproate, in Stahl's Essential Psychopharmacology The Prescriber's Guide, 3rd edition, Cambridge University Press, New York, 2009, pp 569–74

The Case: The soldier who thinks he is a "slacker" broken beyond all repair after 3 deployments to Iraq

The Question: Are his back injury and PTSD going to end his military career?

The Dilemma: Is polypharmacy with 14 medications including multiple opiates, tranquilizers and psychotropics the right way to head him towards symptomatic remission?

Pretest Self Assessment Question (answer at the end of the case)

What proportion of deployed soldiers and marines return from Iraq/Afghanistan with a psychiatric disorder (depression, PTSD and/or substance abuse)?

A. 5%
B. 10%
C. 15%
D. 20%

Patient Intake

- 39-year-old army sergeant
- Complains of:
  - Dizziness
  - Frequent severe headaches
  - Memory loss
  - Nervousness
  - Habitual stammering
  - Flashbacks and recurrences of images from the war
  - Being emotionally distant from others
  - Nighttime awakenings from nightmares
  - Bilateral knee pain
  - Low back pain

Social and Personal History

- Married 7 years, 2 children
- Smokes cigarettes: one pack a day
- Was a party drinker 5 years ago prior to deployments, no drinks available in Iraq
- Now is binge drinking when angry or when out with buddies one to three times a week
- No other drugs except prescription drugs given to him by medical professionals

Medical History

- None except for current injuries
- Mild allergies

Family History

- No known psychiatric illnesses in first degree relatives

Psychiatric History: Initial Primary Care, Orthopedic and Psychiatric Evaluations

- Soldier served 3 tours of duty in Iraq, 42 out of 60 consecutive months, prior to returning home for the third time 12 months ago
- No medical or mental health contacts between previous tours
- No mental health contacts in combat theater overseas
- Saw a primary care provider for bilateral knee injuries and lower back pain once he returned 12 months ago
- Noted by primary care provider then to have orthopedic injuries but also appeared with a flat facial affect and numerous emotional symptoms as noted above
- Additional history is that he is married and has 2 children ages 6 years and 8 months, the first one born just before his first deployment and the second one born during his third deployment
- Doesn't feel he knows his children or has any real connection with them yet
- Initially referred to orthopedics and started physical therapy
- After several weeks, began drinking heavily
- Arguing with spouse, verbally threatening
- After a few months back in the US, referred to psychiatrist who assigns him a few months later to the Warrior Transition Unit (WTU) for wounded soldiers on his base; thus he avoids his fourth deployment back to Iraq
- This new assignment makes him feel like a loser who is broken beyond all repair and that his combat buddies will just think he is a "slacker" too weak to "man up" and get on with his life
- Will stay in the WTU with the only assignment being "to heal" for several months while the army decides what to do with him
- Now has a primary care provider, a nurse case manager and a fellow soldier (member of the "cadre") all assigned to his case in the WTU
- Sees an orthopedic specialist occasionally
- Has numerous counselors/therapists
- Has been in this unit now for 8 weeks
- Goal is to return to duty in 6 months or to be medically discharged if not fit for duty by then

Medication History

- Gets his pain medications from his primary care provider
- Gets his headache medications from a private doctor off base
- He also sees an army psychiatrist on base for psychotropic medications:
  - Piroxicam (Feldene) 20 mg per day
  - Fexofenidine (Allegra) 180 mg per day
  - Midrin (Isometheptene Mucate 65 mg, a sympathomimetic amine; Dichloralphenazone 100 mg, a mild sedative and Acetaminophen 325 mg, an analgesic) for his headaches
  - Valproate 500 mg at night
  - Seroquel 125–150 mg at night and 25 mg every 6 hours as needed for irritability
  - Clonazepam 0.5 mg three times a day as needed
  - Bupropion SR 150 mg per day

Attending Physician's Mental Notes: Initial Psychiatric Evaluation, 7 Months Post Intake to the Warrior Transition Unit

- Current Treatment Plan:
  - Physical therapy twice weekly
  - PTSD group counseling weekly
  - Anger management class weekly
  - Psychologist counseling weekly
  - Social worker counseling weekly
  - Occupational therapy visits twice, and then as needed
  - Weekly nurse case manager meetings
  - Daily contact with cadre
  - Primary care physician visits as needed
  - Psychiatry med checks monthly
  - TENS (Transcutaneous Electrical Nerve Stimulation) unit for low back pain
  - Medical board process to determine discharge status initiated

Current Medications

- Fexofenidine (Allegra) 180 mg per day for allergies from off base private physician
- Citirizine (Zyrtec) 10 mg at night to help with sleep from army primary care physician
- Piroxicam (Feldene) 20 mg per day for knee and back pain from army orthopedist
- Cyclobenzaprine (Flexeril) for low back pain and spasm from army orthopedist
- Ergotamine (Cafergot) for headaches from off base private physician

- Oxycodone for pain from headaches, knee pain and back pain from army primary care physician
- Vicodin for pain from headaches, knee pain and back pain from off base private physician
- Topiramate (Topamax) for headaches from army psychiatrist
- Venlafaxine (EffexorXR) 75 mg for PTSD from army psychiatrist
- Bupropion (Wellbutrin SR) 150 mg per day for depression from army psychiatrist
- Prazocin (Minipress) 2 mg twice a day for PTSD from army psychiatrist
- Valproate 500 mg at night for headaches from off base private physician
- Clonazepam 0.5–1.0 mg three times a day for PTSD from army psychiatrist
- Seroquel 125–150 mg at night and 25 mg every 6 hours as needed for irritability and PTSD from army psychiatrist

Attending Physician's Mental Notes: Initial Psychiatric Evaluation, Continued

- Had received neuropsychological testing, with results consistent with PTSD
- Continues intermittent abuse of alcohol
- Sometimes takes more opiates than prescribed and sometimes takes opiates when he binges on alcohol
- Calls cadre liaison two-to-three times a week complaining of fighting with spouse
- Withdrawn and feels no emotional attachment to family
- Attends his therapy sessions
- Appears to be compliant with his medications
- Rates his back and knee pain as 6/10 (10 worst)
- Continues having frequent nightmares but can now sleep through them
- Working in a gun department of a sporting goods shop off post
- Risk status upgraded 2 weeks ago by psychiatrist

Based on just what you have been told so far about this patient's history and symptoms, what do you think will be his likely outcome?

- Rejoin his unit for a fourth deployment
- Continue his military career in another capacity
- Be "boarded" out of the army
- Be given access to veterans medical benefits
- Be given a military medical disability pension
- High risk of suicide

- High risk of divorce
- High risk of alcohol dependence/substance abuse
- Find satisfactory civilian employment back in his home town
- Have a smooth transition back to civilian life if boarded out of the army
- Other

Case Debrief

- Combat and repeated deployments have taken a heavy toll on this soldier
- It is not known what his outcome was, but probably was discharged from the army and not certain if he will receive military benefits
- Has PTSD and chronic pain, and remains a high risk patient
- Needs coordination of his therapy and medications once he leaves the army with fewer medications and alcoholism treatment with cautious or no use of opiates
- Prognosis for full recovery would seem to be guarded

Two-Minute Tute: A brief lesson and psychopharmacology tutorial (tute) with relevant background material for this case
– Military and PTSD
– Psychotherapy and medications for PTSD

Table 1: Military Personnel: A population at psychological risk

- Separation from family
- Combat and threat to life
- Witnessing destruction and death
- Access to weapons
- Adjustment to deployment and then to re entry
- One in five with a mental illness post deployment (PTSD, depression and/or substance abuse)
- Record rates of suicides
- Barriers to mental health care
- Insufficient numbers of mental health professionals in the army
- Stigma for getting care
- Most of the cadre in Warrior Transition Units think that most of the soldiers with PTSD are faking or exaggerating
- PTSD likely to present with a number of physical symptoms, especially pain
  - Abdominal, muscle, joint, head pain
  - TMJ (temporomandibular joint) pain
  - CWP (chronic widespread pain)

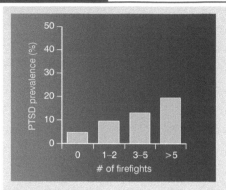

Figure 1: More combat exposure increases the risk of PTSD.
Risk for PTSD may increase with greater exposure to combat (i.e., being shot at, knowing someone who was killed, killing another individual). In fact, a linear "dose response" relationship exists between number of firefights a soldier or marine has been in, and the prevalence of PTSD

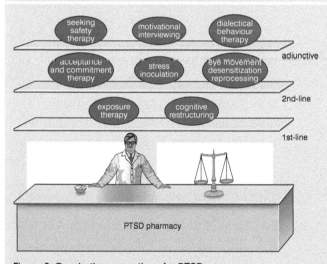

Figure 2: Psychotherapy options for PTSD.
Numerous psychotherapies are being studied in PTSD, with exposure therapy the best documented to have the most robust results, in some cases with effect sizes bigger than medications

Table 2: Exposure therapy for PTSD

- Involves exposing the patient to feared stimuli associated with the traumatic event for repeated and prolonged periods of time.
- Several forms of exposure therapy:
  - Imaginal, which involves repeatedly recounting traumatic memories
  - In vivo, which is exposure to feared stimuli in real life
  - Interoceptive, which involves experiencing feared physical sensations.
- Combining multiple types of exposure therapy is generally most effective.
- Exposure therapy can target
  - Reexperiencing symptoms (by reducing fear associated with thinking about the trauma)
  - Avoidance behaviors (by reducing fear associated with confronting trauma-related stimuli that are not actually dangerous)
  - Reduction of general hyperarousal.
- In addition, by increasing the patient's perceived control over fear, this can facilitate processing of the traumatic memory (help patients "make sense" of it)

Table 3: Cognitive behavioral therapy for PTSD

- A structured form of psychotherapy that includes
  - Behavioral modification strategies
  - Cognitive therapies.
  - Involves exposing the patient to feared stimuli associated with the traumatic event for repeated and prolonged periods of time.
  - Intended to help patients learn new responses to life situations
- Most if not all patients with PTSD should have CBT as part of their treatment regimen

Table 4: Cognitive restructuring therapy for PTSD

- Patients learn to evaluate and modify inaccurate and unhelpful thoughts (e.g., "It was my fault")
- Adjusting how one thinks about a traumatic event can presumably alter one's emotional response to it
- Particularly seems to help address emotions such as shame and guilt
- Can be used alone but is often used as an adjunct to exposure therapy
- Six main steps of cognitive restructuring:
  - Identify a distressing event/thought
  - Identify and rate (0–100) emotions related to the event/thought
  - Identify automatic thoughts associated with the emotions, rate the degree to which one believes them, and select one to challenge
  - Identify evidence in support of and against the thought
  - Generate a response to the thought using the evidence for/against (even though evidence for, in fact is less than evidence against) and rate the degree of belief in the response
  - Re-rate emotion related to the event/thought

Table 5: Stress innoculation training for PTSD

- An anxiety management approach in which patients learn:
  - Relaxation
  - Assertive communication skills
  - Thought stopping (distracting oneself from distressing thoughts)
  - Guided self-dialogue (replacing irrational negative internal dialogue with rational thoughts)

Table 6: Eye movement desensitization and reprocessing (EMDR) for PTSD

- Patients recount traumatic experiences while focusing on a moving object (e.g., the therapist's finger)
- With the intention that this facilitates the processing of the traumatic memory
- Empirical support for this approach, though not as much as for exposure therapy and cognitive restructuring

Table 7: Acceptance and commitment therapy (ACT) for PTSD

- Involves acceptance of thoughts and anxiety as experiences that a person can have while still living a life in accordance with one's values

Table 8: Seeking safety therapy for PTSD

- A technique specifically developed for individuals with substance abuse and trauma histories
- An integrated treatment approach in which both PTSD and substance abuse are addressed simultaneously
- Main goal being to help patients attain safety in their lives (in terms of relationships, thought processes, behaviors, and emotions)
- Offers 25 treatment topics based on four content areas: cognitive, behavioral, interpersonal,and case management
- Can be customized for each individual patient, using whatever combination of treatment topics that best suits the patient's needs
- A clinician guide and client handouts are available for each treatment topic

Table 9: Motivational interviewing for PTSD

- Patient-focused counseling with the direct goal of enhancing one's motivation to change by helping explore and resolve ambivalence (e.g., "I want to stop smoking, but I'm afraid I'll gain weight")
- Originally developed to help individuals with problem drinking but can be used in the treatment of patients with other forms of substance abuse and dependence
- The clinician is a facilitator, helping the patient identify, articulate, and resolve his or her own ambivalence without direct persuasion, confrontation, or coercion.

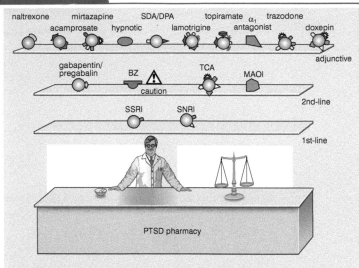

Figure 3: Psychopharmacologic options for PTSD

- First line medications include SSRIs and SNRIs with only paroxetine and sertraline specifically approved by the FDA for PTSD
- Limited evidence for any other medications as monotherapy for PTSD and most medications leave patients with residual symptoms
- Second line treatments include the anticonvulsants gabapentin, pregabalin, benzodiazepines (to be used with caution because of possible substance abuse), TCAs (tricyclic antidepressants) and MAOI (monoamine oxidase inhibitors). Adjunctive treatments include naltrexone and acamprosate for concomitant alcohol abuse and dependency; mirtazapine, hypnotics, atypical antipsychotics (SDAs are serotonin dopamine antagonists and DPAs are dopamine partial agonists), lamotrigine, topiramate, the alpha1 antagonist prazosin for nightmares, trazodone and doxepin.

Posttest Self Assessment Question: Answer

What proportion of deployed soldiers and marines return from Iraq/ Afghanistan with a psychiatric disorder (depression, PTSD and/or substance abuse)?

A. 5%
B. 10%
C. 15%
D. 20%
Answer: D

References

1. Lisi AJ. Management of Operation Iraqi Freedom and Operation Enduring Freedom veterans in a Veterans Health Administration chiropractic clinic: a case series. J Rehab Res Dev 2010; 47(1): 1–6
2. Amin MM, Parisi JA, Gold MS et al. War-related illness symptoms among Operation Iraqi Freedom/Operation Enduring Freedom Returnees. Mil Med 2010; 175(3): 155–7
3. Shaw WS, Means-Christensen AJ, Slater MA et al. Psychiatric disorders and risk of transition to chronicity in men with first onset low back pain. Pain Med 2010; Epub ahead of print
4. Cyders MA, Burris JL, and Carlson CR. Disaggregating the relationship between posttraumatic stress disorder symptom clusters and chronic orofacial pain: implications for the prediction of health outcomes with PTSD symptom clusters. Ann Behav Med 2010; Epub ahead of print
5. Asmundson G, Wright K, McCreary D et al. Post-traumatic stress disorder symptoms in united nations peacekeepers: an examination of factor structure in peacekeepers with and without chronic pain. Cogn Behav Ther 2003; 32(1): 26–37
6. Geisser ME, Roth RS, Bachman JE et al. The relationship between symptoms of post-traumatic stress disorder and pain, affective disturbance and disability among patients with accident and non-accident related pain. Pain 1996; 66(2–3): 207–14
7. Roth RS, Geisser ME, and Bates R. The relation of post-traumatic stress symptoms to depression and pain in patients with accident-related chronic pain. J Pain 2008; 9(7): 588–96
8. Sharp TJ and Harvey AG. Chronic pain and posttraumatic stress disorder: mutual maintenance. Clin Psychol Rev 2001; 21(6): 857-77
9. Beckham JC, Crawford AL, Feldman ME et al. Chronic posttraumatic stress disorder and chronic pain in Vietnam combat veterans. J Psychosom Res 1997; 43(4): 379–89
10. de Leeuw R, Schmidt J, and Carlson C. Traumatic stressors and post-traumatic stress disorder symptoms in headache patients. Headache 2005; 45(10): 1365–74
11. Afari N, Harder LH, Madra NJ et al. PTSD, combat injury, and headache in veterans returning from Iraq/Afghanistan. Headache 2009; 49(9): 1267–76
12. Stahl SM, Mood Disorders, in Stahl's Essential Psychopharmacology, 3rd edition, Cambridge University Press, New York, 2008, pp 453–510
13. Stahl SM, Antidepressants, in Stahl's Essential Psychopharmacology, 3rd edition, Cambridge University Press, New York, 2008, pp 511–666

14. Stahl SM, Anxiety Disorders and Anxiolytics, in Stahl's Essential Psychopharmacology, 3rd edition, Cambridge University Press, New York, 2008, pp 721–72
15. Stahl SM, Stahl's Illustrated Anxiety, Stress and PTSD, Cambridge University Press, New York, 2010
16. Stahl SM, Quetiapine, in Stahl's Essential Psychopharmacology The Prescriber's Guide, 3rd edition, Cambridge University Press, New York, 2009, pp 459–64
17. Stahl SM, Valproate, in Stahl's Essential Psychopharmacology The Prescriber's Guide, 3rd edition, Cambridge University Press, New York, 2009, pp 569–74
18. Stahl SM, Topiramate, in Stahl's Essential Psychopharmacology The Prescriber's Guide, 3rd edition, Cambridge University Press, New York, 2009, pp 535–9
19. Stahl SM, Venlafaxine, in Stahl's Essential Psychopharmacology The Prescriber's Guide, 3rd edition, Cambridge University Press, New York, 2009, pp 579–584
20. Stahl SM, Bupropion, in Stahl's Essential Psychopharmacology The Prescriber's Guide, 3rd edition, Cambridge University Press, New York, 2009, pp 57–62
21. Stahl SM, Clonazepam, in Stahl's Essential Psychopharmacology The Prescriber's Guide, 3rd edition, Cambridge University Press, New York, 2009, pp 97–101
22. Silberstein SD, Marmura MJ, Stahl SM (Ed), Cyclobenzapine, in Essential Neuropharmacology: The Prescriber's Guide, Cambridge University Press, New York, 2010, pp 78–80

The Case: The young man everybody was afraid to treat

The Question: How can you be confident about the safety of combining antihypertensive medications for serious hypertension with psychotropic drugs for serious depression in a patient with a positive urine screen for amphetamine?

The Dilemma: Which antidepressants can you use?

Pretest Self Assessment Question (answer at the end of the case)

Hypertension is a contraindication for treatment with either lithium or with MAO inhibitors.

A. True
B. False

Patient Intake

- 24-year-old male
- Chief complaint: crippling depression

Psychiatric History

- Onset of depression age 13 in 8th grade
- Given fluoxetine with good short-term results
- Discontinued it after it stopped working perhaps two years later
- Began cutting himself, thoughts of self-loathing and self-hatred
- Deteriorated into major depressive episode at age 17; hospitalized
- Diagnosed as bipolar II for unclear reasons and given lithium
- Did well in college for two years, but then progressive worsening of depression past four years
- Recently failed college and relocated to home, unable to study or work
- Treatment over past four years: drugs, doses and duration of medications unclear but best responses reportedly to lithium and mixed amphetamine salts
- Not clear he ever had a diagnosis of ADHD so reasons for giving mixed amphetamine salts similarly unclear
- Poorly documented, marginal responses to aripiprazole (Abilify), venlafaxineXR (Effexor XR), lamotrigine (Lamictal), bupropionSR (Wellbutrin SR) and sertraline (Zoloft), perhaps in part because of compliance issues
- "Some drugs don't work; others that work only do so for a period of time" – however, experiences very few side effects
- Most recently tried ziprasidone (Geodon, Zeldox) 40 mg with no therapeutic effects and no side effects, so discontinued it
- No manic episodes

- "Mood swings" characterized by being "enthusiastic," happy, seeing things clearly and being somewhat better than well
- Five such episodes lasting about a day but never as long as four days
- Has also had many more frequent mood fluctuations, particularly recently, from normal to suicidal over a period of hours

Attending Physician's Mental Notes: Initial Psychiatric Evaluation

- Currently, sleeping 12–14 hours several times a week
- Unbelievable tiredness, all the time, lacking motivation with severely depressed mood and thoughts of death
- Denies active suicidal ideation in the past few weeks yet rates himself 10/10 in severity on a 10-point scale (10 worst)
- Parents are concerned as they have never seen him this depressed before and think he might kill himself even though he denies this

Medical History

- Developed hypertension, noted 4 years ago
- Workup from different renal specialists, diagnosed with "primary hypertension"
- Variable and slightly elevated creatinine and proteinuria
- BP controlled adequately and stable, but requires four meds from four different antihypertensive classes to keep BP < 150/90

Social and Personal History

- Non smoker, denies substance or alcohol abuse
- Few friends or outside interests
- Completed two years of college in another state, then dropped out because of depression
- Trying to go part time to a local community college nearly his parents' home where he is now living

Family History

- Grandmother: depression
- No first degree relatives with early onset hypertension

Current Medications

- Lamotrigine 200 mg/day
- Trazodone 200 mg qhs prn, usually 4x weekly

For hypertension:
- Metoprolol (beta blocker)
- Isradipine (calcium channel blocker)
- Olmesartin (angiotensin II)
- Medoxomil (diuretic)

From the information given, what do you think his diagnosis is?

- Recurrent major depression
- Bipolar II disorder
- Bipolar NOS
- Other

Further Investigation:

Is there anything else you would especially like to know about this patient?

- What about details concerning the diagnosis of bipolar II disorder in the past and about his cutting behaviors?
  - No behaviors elicited from patient or his parents of unequivocal hypomania
  - Patient has experienced mood swings, not reaching the criteria of bipolar disorder I or II
  - Patient is very vague and seems ashamed of prior cutting behaviors, none in the past five years
  - He explains it as wanting to destroy himself then, but without the courage to kill himself, and not that it makes him feel alive or takes away the psychic pain of his depression

Attending Physician's Mental Notes: Initial Psychiatric Evaluation, Continued

- Certainly his depression is recurrent, and no episodes of mania ever, but it is unknown why he was diagnosed as bipolar II in the past
- He might be bipolar II but there is no unequivocal hypomanic episode that the patient relates or that is documented in any available medical records
- Might be best to defer the diagnosis of bipolar spectrum for now and have a provisional diagnosis of recurrent unipolar depression while being vigilant to the possibility of bipolar II disorder, mixed episodes, or bipolar disorder NOS, as well as possible induction of hypomanic, mixed or rapid cycling states by antidepressants
- His rare but definite cutting behaviors are of concern but he denies them currently
- Nothing in the current evaluation that suggests definite borderline personality disorder, but perhaps this is the reason that prior examiners thought he might be bipolar
- Also, no first degree relatives with bipolar disorder
- Nevertheless, cases like this can respond to medications used in bipolar disorder, such as lithium and lamotrigine and atypical antipsychotics

Given his hypertension and slightly elevated creatinine, would you avoid re-treating him now with lithium despite his good response in the past?

- Yes
- No

Of the following choices, which would you utilize at this point?

- Add antipsychotic
- Add antidepressant
- Add anticonvulsant mood stabilizer
- Add lithium
- Add antipsychotic plus antidepressant
- Add mood stabilizer plus antidepressant
- None of the above

If you would give a mood stabilizer/anticonvulsant, which would you add?

- Lithium
- Divalproex
- Lamotrigine
- Carbamazepine
- Oxcarbazepine
- Topiramate
- Levetiracetam
- Zonisamide
- Gabapentin/pregabalin
- I would not add a mood stabilizer/anticonvulsant

If you would give an antipsychotic, which would you add?

- Clozapine
- Risperidone
- Paliperidone
- Olanzapine
- Quetiapine
- Ziprasidone
- Aripiprazole
- Asenapine
- Iloperidone
- Lurasidone
- Conventional antipsychotic
- Depot antipsychotic
- I would not add an antipsychotic

Given his hypertension and slightly elevated creatinine, would you avoid treating him with high doses (225–375 mg/day) of venlafaxine?

- Yes
- No

Given his hypertension and slightly elevated creatinine would you treat him with a MAOI?

- Yes
- No

If you would give an antidepressant, which would you add?

- SSRI (serotonin selective reuptake inhibitor)
- SNRI (serotonin norepinephrine reuptake inhibitor)
- NDRI (bupropion; norepinephrine dopamine reuptake inhibitor)
- NRI (norepinephrine reuptake inhibitor)
- Mirtazapine
- Trazodone
- Tricyclic antidepressant
- MAO inhibitor
- I would not give an antidepressant

Attending Physician's Mental Notes: Initial Psychiatric Evaluation, Continued

- This is a complicated case, given his hypertension and antihypertensive medications
- His hypertension expert physician managing the case is not pleased with the prospect of starting lithium, but agrees this may be justified under the circumstances of the patient's severe and potentially life threatening depression, with a history of having responded to it before
- Restarted lithium 300 mg bid (nephrologist agrees; lithium level 0.3)
- Patient does not want to take anything that could make him sedated as he is already sleeping too much
- Restarted ziprasidone 60 mg twice a day with food
- Lamotrigine and trazodone continued

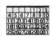

Case Outcome: First Interim Followup, Week 4

- Patient lives in another city, and flies back for an appointment by himself in 4 weeks, without his parents
- On the waiting list of a new psychiatrist in his home city, unable to get in to see him yet
- No antidepressant response in past 4 weeks
- Lithium increased to 900 mg/day (level 0.6)
- No response in 4 weeks to 60 mg twice a day so Ziprasidone increased to 160 mg/day

Case Outcome: Second Interim Followup, Week 8

- Phone appointment
- Still awaiting appointment with psychiatrist
- A "bit of a response" noticeable at 8 weeks

- Rates himself 9/10 on a 10-point scale of severity (10 worst)
- Started transdermal selegiline 6 mg/day

Case Outcome: Third Interim Followup, Week 12

- Phone appointment
- Saw new psychiatrist, who is unwilling to treat him because of his hypertension, concomitant antihypertensive medications, and unease about prescribing especially the MAO inhibitor, but also the lithium
- Still rates himself 9/10 on a 10 point scale (10 worst)
- Increased selegilene to 9 mg/day

Case Outcome: Fourth Interim Followup, Week 16

- Phone appointment
- Now rates himself 4/10
- Several psychiatrists have refused to treat him
- Increased selegilene to 12 mg.day

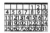

Case Outcome: Fifth Interim Followup, Week 20

- Patient flies in for a face-to-face appointment by himself
- Parents on the phone from their home during the appointment
- Now rates himself 2–3/10; last time this well was 4 years ago
- Still has bad days, "dragged down"
- Still looking for a psychiatrist
- Attending physician now begins to search with him for contacts with another psychiatrist in the patient's city

Case Outcome: Sixth Interim Followup, Week 24

- Phone appointment
- The situation makes him feel both desperate that he will not find psychiatric care and not entirely trusting that the medication choices are the best ones since there is so much turmoil among nephrologists and psychiatrists about how to treat him
- Since the last appointment, he has become concerned both about taking meds and about running out, so on his own cuts doses of lithium and ziprasidone in half, continuing lamotrigine and transdermal selegiline at full doses
- Attending physician thus calls in his prescriptions to a local pharmacy in his town, and recommends increase in lithium and ziprasidone back to full dose since he had responded so well to this combination with his other medications
- The search for a local psychiatrist continues
- The family's primary care physician is also not comfortable managing the patient's medications

Case Outcome: Seventh Interim Followup, Week 28

- On his own, patient decreased transdermal selegiline by half and keeps lithium and ziprasidone at half dose to hoard medications fearing he will run out because he cannot find a doctor
- Severe relapse occurred; parents take him to emergency room; BP normal but urine positive for amphetamine; ER physicians refuse to give him any antidepressants, think he is a drug abuser
- Found a young psychiatrist who trained with the attending physician and who now lives in the patient's city willing to prescribe these meds with some continuing supervision by the attending physician but she is concerned about the safety of this combination and now concerned about the patient's stimulant abuse which he adamantly denies, but neither the parents, the new psychiatrist or the emergency room personnel believe that he did not ingest stimulants

Given his positive urine test for amphetamine and his denial of abuse, is this yet another reason for you to be hesitant to take him on as a psychopharmacology management case?

- Yes
- No

Case Outcome: Seventh Interim Followup, Week 28, Continued

- Phone consult with new psychiatrist: reminded her that selegiline metabolized to methamphetamine and recommended increase of doses of all meds back to levels where he responded
- Positive urine drug screen was from selegiline, not abused stimulants
- Patient continues on transdermal selegiline, ziprasidone, lithium, lamotrigine and trazodone
- The saga continues . . .

Case Debrief

- A complex case of a young man who developed both serious hypertension requiring four antihypertensives from four classes of drugs, plus serious depression unresponsive to standard therapy and requiring heroic psychopharmacological intervention
- Many psychiatrists and internists alike are uncomfortable managing a case like this
- Nevertheless, it is possible to have one's cake and eat it too: namely, control of both hypertension and depression, although with numerous medications

Take-Home Points

- Hypertension is not a contraindication for lithium or for MAO inhibitors
- Use ziprasidone at reasonable doses (120–160 mg/day with food in most cases) or not at all
- MAO inhibitors remain a viable treatment option
- MAO inhibitors by themselves more likely to cause HYPOtension (especially orthostatic) than HYPERtension (unless given with sympathomimetic amines or reuptake inhibitors)
- Difficult cases may justify aggressive treatments

Performance in Practice: Confessions of a Psychopharmacologist

- What could have been done better here?
  - Took too long to find a local psychiatrist willing to manage the case
  - This led to a sense of desperation and lack of confidence, compromising therapeutic alliance and leading to medication nonadherence and relapse
  - The distance of the patient from the original treating physician also interfered with getting psychotherapy established, which could have been helpful in getting patient to adjust to dropping out of college and to his disappointment and anger that depression was interfering with his getting on with his life
- Possible action item for improvement in practice
  - Being more proactive in finding contacts in cities where referred patients live so that local experts can manage the case when referred back
  - Should have told the patient or parents about the urine drug screen for patients taking selegiline and this might have avoided some conflict and tension
  - Should have told the patient or parents about how to extend the use of the transdermal patches (see below) or considered a switch to a less expensive MAOI

Tips and Pearls

- Note that both selegiline and another MAO Inhibitor, tranylcypromine, itself an amphetamine, can show up as positive urine drug screens for stimulants
- Although not approved for use this way, note that each transdermal patch of selegiline actually contains more than 3 days of drug; if patient's skin is not irritated by prolonged administration in a single site, and the adhesive continues to work, costs of this expensive treatment option can be reduced by two or three days use of each patch instead of one

- Also, can switch to another MAOI that is much less expensive
- Modern psychopharmacologists should not be afraid to administer MAOIs for selected cases

Two-Minute Tute: A brief lesson and psychopharmacology tutorial (tute) with relevant background material for this case
– How MAOIs work
– Tips on how to use MAOIs
– see also Case 1 Two-Minute Tute p 8

Table 1: Currently approved MAO inhibitors

Name (trade name)	Inhibition of MAO-A	Inhibition of MAO-B	Amphetamine properties
phenelzine (Nardil)	+	+	
tranylcypromine (Parnate)	+	+	+
isocarboxazid (Marplan)	+	+	
amphetamines (at high doses)	+	+	+
selegiline transdermal system (Emsam)			
brain	+	+	+
gut	+/-	+	+
selegiline low dose oral (Deprenyl, Eldepryl)	-	+	+
rasaligine (Agilect/Azilect)	-	+	-
moclobemide (Aurorix, Manerix)	+	-	-

Table 2: MAO inhibitors with amphetamine actions or amphetamines with MAO inhibitions?

Drug	Comment
amphetamine	MAOI at high doses
tranylcypromine (Parnate)	also called phenylcyclopropylamine, structurally related to amphetamine
selegiline	metabolized to L-methamphetamine
	metabolized to L-amphetamine
	less amphetamine formed transdermally

Table 3: MAO Enzymes

	MAO-A	MAO-B
Substrates	5-HT	Phenylethylamine
	NE	DA
	DA	Tyramine
	Tyramine	
Tissue distribution	Brain, gut, liver, placenta, skin	Brain, platelets, lymphocytes

Table 4: Suggested tyramine dietary modifications for MAO inhibitors*

Food to avoid	Food allowed
Dried, aged, smoked, fermented, spoiled, or improperly stored meat, poultry, and fish	Fresh or processed meat, poultry, and fish
Broad bean pods	All other vegetables
Aged cheeses cheese, yogurt	Processed and cottage cheese, ricotta
Tap and nonpasteurized beers	Canned or bottled beers and alcohol (have little tyramine)
Marmite, sauerkraut	Brewer's and baker's yeast
Soy products/tofu	

*No dietary modifications needed for low doses of transdermal selegiline or for low oral doses of selective MAO-B inhibitors.

Table 5: Potentially dangerous hypertensive combos: agents when combined with MAOIs that can cause hypertension (theoretically via adrenergic stimulation)

Decongestants
phenylephrine (alpha 1 selective agonist)
ephedrine* (ma huang, ephedra) (alpha and beta agonist; central NE and DA releaser)
pseudoephedrine* (active stereoisomer of ephedrine – same mechanism as ephedrine)
phenylpropanolamine* (alpha 1 agonist; less effective central NE/DA releaser than ephedrine)
Stimulants
amphetamines
methylphenidate
Antidepressants with NRI (nonrepinephrine reuptake inhibition)
TCAs
NRIs
SNRIs
NDRIs
Appetite suppressants with NRI
sibutramine*
phentermine

*withdrawn from markets in the United States and some other countries

Table 6: Potentially lethal combos: agents when combined with MAOIs that can cause hyperthermia/serotonin syndrome (theoretically via SERT inhibition)

Antidepressants
SSRIs
SNRIs
TCAs (especially clomipramine)
Other TCA structures
cyclobenzaprine
carbamazepine
Appetite suppressants with SERT inhibition
sibutramine*
Opiods
dextromethorphan
meperidine
tramadol
methadone
propoxyphene

* withdrawn from markets in the United States and some other countries

Table 7: Tyramine content of cheese

Cheese		mg per 15g serving
English STILTON		17.3
Kraft® grated PARMESAN		0.2
Philadelphia® CREAM CHEESE		0

Table 8: Tyramine content of commercial chain pizza

Serving		mg per serving
1/2 medium double cheese, double pepperoni		1.378
1/2 medium double cheese, double pepperoni		0.063
1/2 medium double cheese, double pepperoni		0

Table 9: Tyramine content of wine

Wine		mg per 4-oz serving
Ruffino CHIANTI		0.36
Blue Nun® WHITE		0.32
Cinzano VERMOUTH		0

PATIENT FILE

Posttest Self Assessment Question: Answer

Hypertension is a contraindication for lithium and MAO inhibitors.

A. True
B. False
   – Although many internists and psychiatrists are uncomfortable with this combination, and it has to be used with caution and extensive monitoring by experts, the combination is not contraindicated and can in fact treat both depression and hypertension successfully as in this case

Answer: B

References

1. Stahl SM, Mood Disorders, in Stahl's Essential Psychopharmacology, 3rd edition, Cambridge University Press, New York, 2008, pp 453–510
2. Stahl SM, Antidepressants, in Stahl's Essential Psychopharmacology, 3rd edition, Cambridge University Press, New York, 2008, pp 511–666
3. Stahl SM, Mood stabilizers, in Stahl's Essential Psychopharmacology, 3rd edition, Cambridge University Press, New York, 2008, pp 667–720
4. Stahl SM, Selegilene, in Stahl's Essential Psychopharmacology The Prescriber's Guide, 3rd edition, Cambridge University Press, New York, 2009, pp 489–96
5. Stahl SM and Felker A. Monoamine oxidase inhibitors: a modern guide to an unrequited class of antidepressants. CNS Spectrums 13: 10, 855–70
6. Stahl SM, Lithium, in Stahl's Essential Psychopharmacology The Prescriber's Guide, 3rd edition, Cambridge University Press, New York, 2009, pp 277–82
7. Stahl SM, Ziprasidone, in Stahl's Essential Psychopharmacology The Prescriber's Guide, 3rd edition, Cambridge University Press, New York, 2009, pp 589–94
8. Schwartz TL and Stahl,SM, Ziprasidone in the Treatment of Bipolar Disorder, in Akiskal H and Tohen M, Bipolar Psychopharmacotherapy: Caring for the Patient, 2nd edition, Wiley Press, in press

The Case: The young woman whose doctors could not decide whether she has schizophrenia, bipolar disorder or both

The Question: Is there a such thing as schizoaffective disorder?

The Dilemma: Does treatment depend upon whether the diagnosis is schizophrenia, bipolar disorder or schizoaffective disorder?

Pretest Self Assessment Question (answer at the end of the case)

In recent studies, the classical discontinuity hypothesis for schizophrenia and affective disorders has been consistently:

A. Corroborated
B. Rejected
C. None of the above

Patient Intake

- 26-year-old female arrives with both her parents
- Chief complaint: "I'm here because of my parents; I'm completely normal and I do not need medications"
- The patient has a four-year history of psychotic illness; and according to her parents has had a progressive downhill course following the onset of her illness
- She has delusions and hallucinations, which seem not to be treatable in a robust way with usual doses of antipsychotics

Psychiatric History

- Prior to onset of psychotic symptoms, thought to have an anxiety disorder at age 20, and given diazepam (Valium), but a few months later clearly had a psychotic break

Psychiatric History of First Psychotic Break: Schizophrenia

- Onset of psychotic illness characterized by delusions and hallucinations without prominent affective symptoms at age 21, when she was a junior in college, diagnosed as schizophrenic
- She was hospitalized and given haloperidol initially, followed by risperidone (Risperdal)
- Risperidone seemed not to work, so she was switched to olanzapine (Zyprexa) plus escitalopram (Lexapro) and clonazepam (Klonopin), which she received as an outpatient after leaving the hospital
- She was well enough after this to start as a teacher's aide, but was not well enough to go back to college

Psychiatric History of Second Psychotic Break: Mania

- After a brief time she stopped her medications and relapsed into what was diagnosed as a manic episode, but with clear psychotic symptoms as well
- She had ideas of reference, particularly about God controlling her and that she was a prophet, and had themes of religiosity
- She reinstituted olanzapine and added lamotrigine (Lamictal), and then moved away from home

Psychiatric History of Third Psychotic Break: Mania

- Because of weight gain she switched to ziprasidone (Geodon, Zeldox) while maintaining lamotrigine, but then stopped ziprasidone and developed recurrent manic/psychotic symptoms diagnosed as bipolar disorder

Psychiatric History of Unremitting Psychosis: Schizoaffective Disorder

- She was hospitalized for six months at a residential treatment center and diagnosed as schizoaffective disorder
- She refused medications until forced to take them by legal proceedings
- She was then given ziprasidone, lamotrigine, haloperidol (Haldol), lorazepam (Ativan), and lithium
- Brief trials with aripiprazole (Abilify) and lithium were unimpressive
- She was then switched to olanzapine plus lamotrigine
- She was doing poorly, apparently unresponsive to her medications despite several months of treatment, so her parents took her out of the long term residential treatment facility and brought her home

Psychiatric History: Treatment Resistant Schizoaffective Disorder

- The patient comes in for her initial psychiatric evaluation 6 months after leaving the residential treatment facility. She is still living at her parents' home and continues to take olanzapine 30 mg/day and lamotrigine 400 mg/day
- Her response has been poor
- She is not experiencing weight gain; her only significant side effect is gastrointestinal (GI) discomfort

Social and Personal History

- Non smoker
- Some girlfriends, some dating in high school but little dating in college
- Denies use of drugs, alcohol, marijuana

Medical History

- Normal BMI and BP
- Routine blood tests including fasting glucose and triglycerides are normal

Family history

- Paternal uncle: "mentally unstable"
- Maternal uncle: posttraumatic stress disorder (PTSD) and paranoid state
- Paternal grandmother: hospitalized long ago for some sort of psychotic break

Patient Intake

- During evaluation she seems a bit hebephrenic
- She is somewhat tangential and incoherent and is quite disruptive
- She exhibits inappropriate laughter and constant interruptions as well as occasional affective irritability
- She states, "My fiancé is a beautiful butterfly; there are caterpillars in the world. I don't want you talking to my parents. God is talking to me."
- She is not able to track direct questions; she sits silently for 30 seconds or longer after direct questioning and then goes on talking with psychotic content
- By the end of the interview she is leaning forward, her head on her hands and knees, unresponsive to attempts to explain things to her
- She is not currently suicidal but is also not extremely responsive to direct questioning

Do you find the designation of schizoaffective disorder useful in your practice?

- Yes
- No

Based on the information provided, how would you diagnose this patient?

- Bipolar I disorder
- Schizoaffective disorder
- Schizophrenia

Attending Physician's Mental Notes: Initial Psychiatric Evaluation

- Current evaluation confirms psychotic disorder, with lack of insight, probably more schizophrenic than schizoaffective, with bipolar disorder doubtful
- By history she seems to have had some affective episodes, so at this time her best working diagnosis may be schizoaffective disorder
- Seems to have had psychotic episodes not only when manic, but also when depressed and even when mood apparently normal

Do you treat schizoaffective disorder differently than you do schizophrenia?
- Yes
- No

Of the following options, which antipsychotic would you choose for this patient?
- Increase dose of olanzapine (currently at 30 mg/day)
- Switch to quetiapine (Seroquel)
- Switch to clozapine (Clozaril)
- Switch to an intramuscular formulation of one of the antipsychotics
- Get plasma drug levels of her current olanzapine and lamotrigine to see if she is absorbing them and/or is compliant

Attending Physician's Mental Notes: Initial Psychiatric Evaluation, Continued

- She has affective and psychotic symptoms over the past 5 years, often at the same time, episodically, and clearly disabling and at times requiring hospitalization
- The history is not clear in terms of what symptoms she had at what times, and the parents, patient and medical records are conflicting as to whether this is more consistent with schizophrenia, mania or schizoaffective disorder during various episodes
- Regardless of her actual diagnosis, the most striking thing is that she has an apparent lack of response to antipsychotics, with waxing and waning of psychotic symptoms not clearly changing when medications given, but also not clear how compliant she has been
- The patient is not currently out of control, and her parents believe that hospitalization is not necessary
- Decided to keep medication treatment unchanged and find out what her plasma drug levels are

Case Outcome: First Interim Followup, Week 4

- Her lamotrigine level is high normal and her olanzapine level is within the therapeutic range; thus, she is compliant and absorbing her medications at the present time despite stating she does not need to take medications
- Her lamotrigine dose is decreased from 400 mg/day to 200 mg/day
  - There is not much evidence to suggest that 400 mg is more effective than 200 mg for bipolar disorder and the patient believes her GI upset is due to the higher dose of lamotrigine
- Her olanzapine dose is increased to 40 mg/day

Case Outcome: Second Interim Followup, Week 8

- No improvement in psychosis or affect, but patient believes her GI symptoms are better
- Instructed to increase her olanzapine dose to 50 mg/day

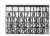

Case Outcome: Third Interim Followup, Week 12

- No improvement, so instructed to increase her olanzapine to 60 mg/day

Case Outcome: Fourth Interim Followup, Week 16

- No improvement, but sedated; no notable weight gain
- Switched to clozapine

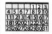

Case Outcome: Fifth Interim Followup, Week 20

- Still no improvement, but continues on clozapine plus lamotrigine

Case Debrief

- There is current debate surrounding the clinical utility of schizoaffective disorder as a diagnosis
- An unequivocal definition of schizoaffective disorder does not exist, with differences between ICD-10 and DSM-IV. Diagnostic reliability is also relatively low, with many patients changing their diagnosis over time to bipolar disorder or schizophrenia
- At the neurobiological level there is evidence both in favor of and against separation of psychotic and affective disorders, depending on the dimension studied
- Whatever the diagnosis, there is apparent treatment resistance to antipsychotics so far

Take-Home Points

- Schizoaffective disorder may be a way for a clinician to avoid making a decision as to whether the patient has either schizophrenia or bipolar disorder
- Few hints from neuroimaging or genetics studies exist to help differentiate schizophrenia from bipolar disorder, let alone from schizoaffective disorder
- Kraepelin proposed a classical dichotomy, of two separate diseases to explain severe mental illness, one with a poorer outcome (schizophrenia or dementia praecox) and one with a better outcome (manic depressive illness or bipolar disorder)
- What about cases in between? Even Kraepelin recognized numerous such cases
- It can be very difficult in practice to determine whether a patient is schizophrenic, bipolar or schizoaffective, particularly at the beginning of the illness, and particularly if the same examiner has not observed the patient over time and in different clinical states
- The diagnostic debate may be more of an academic exercise than a clinically useful designation
- Empirically, it is important to search for mood symptoms in psychotic patients, and to treat these with mood stabilizers as well as antipsychotics

Performance in Practice: Confessions of a Psychopharmacologist

- What could have been done better here?
  - More active efforts to retrieve old medical records or to speak directly with clinicians who managed her case over the past 5 years may have thrown light on the diagnosis
  - Such information may also help clarify if the patient really has failed to respond to medications or if some medications were more effective than others, or indeed whether she was noncompliant at times
  - In fact, times when she knowingly discontinued medications were associated with recurrent psychosis and rehospitalization, so even though medication did not restore her to full asymptomatic function, her medications may have been useful in preventing acute relapses
- Possible action item for improvement in practice
  - Focus on treatment rather than diagnosis
  - Search more carefully for mood symptoms over her past course of illness
  - Emphasize mood stabilizers such as valproate or lithium rather than antipsychotics, since antipsychotics are not robustly restoring her function

– Look into vocational rehabilitation now that the patient is in a stable living situation at home

Tips and Pearls

- Chaos is chaos no matter what you call it
- There is no such thing as schizoaffective disorder. Long live schizoaffective disorder (see references to this debate at the end of this case)
- The question of diagnosis can distract the clinician and family from efforts to restore function and even attain a symptomatic and functional recovery from a psychotic illness of any kind

Two-Minute Tute: A brief lesson and psychopharmacology tutorial (tute) with relevant background material for this case – Schizophrenia vs bipolar vs schizoaffective

The dichotomous disease model and schizoaffective disorder

- The dichotomous disease model in the tradition of Kraepelin proposes that schizophrenia and bipolar disorder are separate and distinct diseases
- In the Kraepelinean model, schizophrenia is a chronic unremitting illness with a poor outcome and a decline in function (non restitutio ad integrum) whereas bipolar disorder is a cyclical illness with a better outcome and good restoration of function between episodes (restitution ad integrum)
- However, there is great debate as to how to define the borders between these two illnesses
- One notion is that cases with overlapping symptoms and intermediate disease courses can be seen as a third illness, schizoaffective disorder
- Today, many define this border with the idea that "even a trace of schizophrenia is schizophrenia"
- From this "schizophrenia centered perspective," many overlapping cases of psychotic mania and psychotic depression might be considered to be either forms of schizophrenia, or to be schizo-affective disorder with schizoaffective disorder seen as a form of schizophrenia with affective symptoms
- A competing point of view within the dichotomous model is that "even a trace of mood disturbance is a mood disorder"
- From this "mood/affective-centered perspective," many overlapping cases of psychotic mania and psychotic depression might be considered to be either forms of a mood/affective/bipolar disorder or to be schizo-affective disorder with schizoaffective disorder seen as a form of mood/affective/bipolar disorder with psychotic symptoms
- Where patients have a mixture of mood symptoms and psychosis, it can be difficult to tell whether they have a psychotic disorder like schizophrenia, a mood disorder like bipolar or a schizoaffective disorder, or even whether these are distinctions without a difference
- Proponents of the dichotomous model point out that treatments for schizophrenia differ from those for bipolar disorder, since lithium is rarely helpful in schizophrenia, and anticonvulsant mood stabilizers have limited efficacy for psychotic symptoms in schizophrenia, and perhaps only as augmenting agents
- Treatments for schizoaffective disorder can include both treatments for schizophrenia and treatments for bipolar disorder
- The current debates within the dichotomotous model are: If you have bipolar disorder do you have a good outcome and if you have schizophrenia do you have a poor outcome? What genetic and biological markers rather than clinical symptoms can distinguish one from another?

The single disease continuum model and schizoaffective disorder

- The single disease model proposes that schizophrenia and bipolar disorder are opposite ends of the spectrum of the same disease, with schizoaffective disorder in the middle of this spectrum
- Today, it is not clear whether psychotic mood disorders, either mania or depression, are phenotypically or genotypically distinguishable from the traditional conceptualization of schizophrenia
- The current debate within the continuum model is whether this is a multifaceted expression of a single disease or whether the spectrum consists of many different diseases, with overlapping genetic, epigenetic and biomarkers as well as overlapping clinical symptoms and functional outcomes
- Basic science may be telling us there is only one highly complex disease
- Proponents of the continuum model point out that treatments for schizophrenia overlap greatly now with those for bipolar disorder, since second generation atypical antipsychotics are effective in the positive symptoms of schizophrenia and in psychotic mania and psychotic depression, and are also effective in nonpsychotic mania and in bipolar depression and unipolar depression
- These same second generation atypical antipsychotics are effective for the spectrum of symptoms in schizoaffective disorder
- From the single disease perspective, failure to give mood stabilizing medications may lead to suboptimal symptom relief in patients with psychosis, even those whose prominent psychotic symptoms mask or distract clinicians from seeing underlying and perhaps more subtle mood symptoms
- In the one disease model, schizophrenia can be seen as the extreme end of a spectrum of severity of mood disorders and not a different disease
- Schizophrenia and schizoaffective disorder can both therefore have severe psychotic symptoms that obscure mood symptoms and a chronic course that eliminates cycling, shows resistance to antipsychotic treatments, and prominent negative symptoms, yet be just a severe form of the same illness
- In this one disease model, schizoaffective disorder would be a milder form of the illness with less severe psychotic features and more severe mood features
- The debate rages on . . .

Posttest Self Assessment Question: Answer

In recent studies, the classical discontinuity hypothesis for schizophrenia and affective disorders has been consistently:

A. Corroborated

B. Rejected

C. None of the above

Answer: C

References

1. Bora E, Yucel M, Fornito A et al. Major psychoses with mixed psychotic and mood symptoms: are mixed psychoses associated with different neurobiological markers? Acta Psychiatr Scand 2008; 118: 172–87
2. Maier W. Do schizoaffective disorders exist at all? Acta Psychiatr Scand 2006; 13: 369–71
3. Maier W. Common risk genes for affective and schizophrenic psychoses. Eur Arch Psychiatry Clin Neurosci 2008; 258 (suppl 2): 37–40
4. Vollmer-Larsen A, Jacobsen TB, Hemmingsen R et al. Schizaffective disorder—the reliability of its clinical diagnostic use. Acta Psychiatr Scand 2006; 113: 402–7
5. Robinson DG, Woerner MG, McMeniman M et al. Symptomatic and functional recovery from a first episode of schizophrenia or schizoaffective disorder. Am J Psychiatry 2004; 161: 473–9
6. Azorin JM, Long term treatment of mood disorders in schizophrenia, Acta Psychiatr Scand 1995; 91 suppl 388: 20–3
7. Hafner H, Maurer K, Trendler G et al. Schizophrenia and depression: challenging the paradigm of two separate diseases – a controlled study of schizophrenia. depression and healthy controls. Schiz Res 2005; 77: 11–24
8. Lake CR, The validity of schizophrenia vs bipolar disorder. Psychiatric Annals 2010; 40: 77–87
9. Laursen TM, Labouriau R, Licht RW et al. Family history of psychiatric illness as a risk factor for schizoaffective disorder: a Danish register based cohort study. Arch Gen Psychiat 2005; 62: 841–8
10. Maier W, Zobel A, Wagner M, Schizophrenia and bipolar disorder: differences and overlaps. Current Opinion in Psychiatry 2006; 19: 165–70
11. Stahl SM, Psychosis and Schizophrenia, in Stahl's Essential Psychopharmacology, 3rd edition, Cambridge University Press, New York, 2008, pp 247–326

12. Stahl SM, Antipsychotic Agents, in Stahl's Essential Psychopharmacology, Cambridge University Press, New York, 2008, pp 327–452
13. Stahl SM, Clozapine, in Stahl's Essential Psychopharmacology The Prescriber's Guide, 3rd edition, Cambridge University Press, New York, 2009, pp 113–8
14. Stahl SM, Lamotrigine, in Stahl's Essential Psychopharmacology The Prescriber's Guide, 3rd edition, Cambridge University Press, New York, 2009, pp 171–5

Lightning Round

The Case: The scary man with only partial symptom control on clozapine

The Question: How to manage breakthough positive symptoms as well as chronic negative symptoms in a 48-year-old psychotic patient with history of homicide and suicide attempts?

The Dilemma: What do you do when even clozapine does not work adequately?

Pretest Self Assessment Question (answer at the end of the case)

What are potential evidence-based treatment strategies for psychotic patients with inadequate responses to clozapine?

A. Maintain plasma clozapine levels between 200–300 ng/ml
B. Raise clozapine dose up to 900 mg/day
C. Maintain plasma clozapine levels between 400–600 ng/ml
D. Augment with lamotrigine
E. Augment with a second antipsychotic

Patient Intake

- 48-year-old man diagnosed with schizophrenia, disorganized type, has a 31-year history of psychotic illness
- Referred by his treating psychiatrist for consideration of augmentation of clozapine with another agent because he continues to have breakthough symptoms of threatening behavior to himself and to others with a history of acting upon these threats
- Hospitalized in a forensic unit with hallucinations, ideas of reference, bizarre behavior, severe psychomotor agitation and self destructive behavior, including numerous suicide attempts in the past such as swallowing razor blades and jumping from a motorcycle; also elopement from psychiatric facilities and assault on others, including murdering his friend by hammering him in the head because he thought he was a vampire
- Found mentally incompetent to stand trial and now resides in a forensic facility

Psychiatric History

- After partial and inadequate responses to many antipsychotics, clozapine (Clozaril) treatment (300 mg twice a day, with plasma concentrations in the presumed optimal range of 400–600 ng/ml) has improved many positive symptoms, but the patient continues to have prominent negative symptoms as well as denial of illness and denial of the murder of his friend
- Upon provocation he rapidly develops threatening behavior to himself and others

- Higher doses of clozapine may have more efficacy but also more side effects including seizures
- There is little guidance for what to do when clozapine at adequate doses is not sufficiently efficacious
- Patient is also taking fluvoxamine (Luvox, Favrin) 25 mg twice a day for depressive symptoms, a medication that can itself raise clozapine levels by blocking CYP450 1A2 which partially metabolizes clozapine

Of the following choices, what would you do?
- Switch to another antipsychotic
- Increase clozapine dose to attain plasma concentrations > 600 ng/ml
- Augment with lamotrigine (Lamictal)
- Augment with risperidone (Risperdal)
- Augment with a benzodiazepine
- Increase fluvoxamine dose
- Leave well enough alone

Case Outcome

- Patient was too dangerous to himself and others to do nothing, yet high clozapine doses were deemed too dangerous for him
- Lamotrigine was given, titrating up to 200 mg twice a day over a few months, but no improvement was seen after 3 months and several acting out episodes in the interim required restraint
- Lithium was considered as a potential adjunct for self injurious and suicidal behavior, but clozapine is also useful for suicidal behavior, and a more rapid and robust plan was needed to prevent assaults on other patients and staff
- Augmentation with a second antipsychotic was considered, including intramuscular acute dosing of haloperidol (Haldol), olanzapine (Zyprexa) or ziprasidone (Geodon, Zeldox), but this was not practical for long term treatment
- He was instead given oral risperidone, the one antipsychotic best studied in combination with clozapine, but with mixed results in the literature
- With a step-wise increase to 3 mg/day of risperidone augmenting clozapine 300 mg twice a day, the patient experienced only rare break through symptoms, and was not as provocable

Case Debrief

- It appears as though this patient has a very malignant psychotic illness associated with violent and dangerous behaviors

- The patient's symptoms were only partially controlled by clozapine, but prior antipsychotics were even less effective
- Not clear what therapeutic role fluvoxamine is playing here nor whether it needs to be continued long term
- Lamotrigine augmentation failed but risperidone augmentation was successful
- This suggests that, for this patient, despite supposedly fully therapeutic doses of clozapine, D2 dopamine receptors are not fully saturated and that additional D2 antagonism by risperidone was therapeutic
- If the patient relapses on current treatment regimen, his response to risperidone augmentation suggests that he might be a candidate either for an even higher dose of risperidone or even a dose increase of clozapine
- Also, amisulpride (not available in the US) augmentation of clozapine has been studied with some good results reported

Posttest Self Assessment Question: Answer

What are potential evidence-based treatment strategies for psychotic patients with inadequate responses to clozapine?

A. Maintain plasma clozapine levels between 200–300 ng/ml
  – This is clearly not the way to go because this is considered subtherapeutic
B. Raise clozapine dose up to 900 mg/day
  – Not a first choice, since will likely result only in more side effects and not necessarily more therapeutic effects
C. Maintain plasma clozapine levels between 400–600 ng/ml
  – This is already being done, so seems like a necessary but not sufficient answer
D. Augment with lamotrigine
  – This is reasonable and has some evidence to support it
E. Augment with a second antipsychotic
  – This might also be reasonable, if expensive and with potentially additive side effects. Risperidone might be the best choice but other agents in this class could be rationally considered

Answer: C, D and E

References

1. Stahl SM, Lamotrigine, in Stahl's Essential Psychopharmacology The Prescriber's Guide, 3rd edition, Cambridge University Press, New York, 2009, pp 259–65
2. Stahl SM, Clozapine, in Stahl's Essential Psychopharmacology The Prescriber's Guide, 3rd edition, Cambridge University Press, New York, 2009, pp 113–8
3. Stahl SM, Risperidone, in Stahl's Essential Psychopharmacology The Prescriber's Guide, 3rd edition, Cambridge University Press, New York, 2009, pp 475–81
4. Goff DC, Keefe R, Citrome L et al. Lamotrigine as add-on therapy in schizophrenia, J Clin Psychopharmacol 2007; 27: 582–9
5. Stahl SM, Antipsychotics, in Stahl's Essential Psychopharmacology, 3rd edition, Cambridge University Press, New York, 2008, pp 327–452
6. Stahl SM, Grady MM. A critical review of atypical antipsychotic utilization: comparing monotherapy with polypharmacy and augmentation. Cur Med Chem, 11, 313–26
7. Stahl SM. Focus: antipsychotic polypharmacy – evidence based prescribing or prescribing based evidence? Int J Neuropsychopharmacol 2004; 7(2): 113–6.

The Case: 8-year-old girl who was naughty

The Question: Do girls get ADHD?

The Psychopharm Dilemma: How do you treat ADHD with oppositional symptoms?

Pretest Self Assessment Question (answer at the end of the case)

What is true about oppositional symptoms in patients with ADHD

A. They can be part of the diagnostic criteria for ADHD in children
B. They can be confused with impulsive symptoms of ADHD
C. They can be part of oppositional defiant disorder (ODD) which can be comorbid with ADHD
D. They can be part of conduct disorder (CD) which can be comorbid with ADHD

Patient Intake

- 8-year-old girl brought to her pediatrician by her 26-year-old mother
- Chief complaint: fever and sore throat

Psychiatric History

- While evaluating the patient for an upper respiratory infection, the pediatrician asks if school is going well
- The patient responds "yes" but in the background the mother shakes her head "no"
- The mother states that her daughter is negative and defiant at home and she has similar reports, mostly of disobedience, from her teacher at school
- The patient has had temper tantrums since age 5 but these have decreased over the past 3 years, especially the past year
- Still angry and resentful since her little sister was born 6 years ago
- Academic problems
- Fights with other children, mostly arguments and harsh words with other girls at school

Social and Personal History

- Goes to public school
- Has a younger sister age 6
- Does not see her father much, lives in a nearby city
- Not many friends
- Spends most of her time with her sister and either her mother or her maternal grandmother who helps with after school supervision and baby sitting

Medical History

- None

Family History

- None known for medical or psychiatric disorders other than the father who drinks a bit too much and his father (paternal grandfather) who some think might be an alcoholic
- Mother was adopted and no family history known

Pediatrician's Notes: Initial Evaluation

- Not enough time to do any more evaluation
- Instead, the mother is given the parent and teacher version of the Conners ADHD rating scale and is instructed to bring the completed forms to the followup visit
- A variety of rating scales are available, some without charge (see http://www.neurotransmitter.net/adhdscales.html).
- The Connors scale charges a fee but other rating scales available at this link, or listed in the Two-Minute Tute below are free.

Pediatrician's Notes: Followup Visit Week 3

- At the followup visit, the mother admits to having been too busy to fill out the parent form
- Also admits to having forgotten to send the rating form to the teacher
- Mother acknowledges being more disorganized since her second child started school this year
- Since then it has also been extremely difficult to keep the patient organized and focused on school
- The mother is on the verge of tears
- "Two children are too much for a single mother"
- The pediatrician offers to send the teacher form to the school and gives the mother tips on how to remember to fill out her own form
- When the teacher form is sent back to the pediatrician's office the mother will be contacted for a followup visit

Pediatrician's Notes: Followup Visit Week 6

- At the followup visit, the mother comes alone
- Teacher's ADHD rating scale responses state that the patient has significant problems with
  - Talking excessively
  - Sustaining attention
  - Being organized
  - Being distracted
  - Being forgetful

- Following instructions
- Making careless errors (except when it comes to her homework)
- The teacher also complains of the patient being more argumentative and disobedient than the other children in her class
- The mother's responses on the ADHD rating scales are similar to the teacher's but she endorses only five symptoms as significantly impairing
- Checked "severe" for ability to listen (rated only mild by the teacher)
- Upon further questioning by the pediatrician, it becomes clear that the mother is compensating for her daughter by
  - Double checking her homework
  - Making sure homework is in her backpack
  - Helping the patient be organized
- Eventually, symptoms that were originally determined to be "mild" by the mother are changed to "significantly impairing"
- Mother confirms that the patient argues a lot with her, especially when the mother is trying to oversee her work, and that the patient still occasionally has temper tantrums similar to when she was five years old, but milder

Based on just what you have been told so far about this patient's history what do you think is her diagnosis?

- ADHD
- ODD (oppositional defiant disorder)
- CD (conduct disorder)
- ADHD comorbid with ODD
- ADHD comorbid with CD
- A child acting out again her mother's divorce and against having to share her mother with her sister
- Other

Pediatrician's Mental Notes: Followup Visit, Week 6, Continued

- The patient is diagnosed with ADHD, mostly inattentive type, comorbid with symptoms of oppositional defiant disorder
  - ADHD symptoms include inattention but not hyperactivity
  - Some of her impulsive symptoms such as being argumentative and disobedient overlap with her ODD symptoms but the ODD symptoms seem to be willful and on purpose rather than truly thoughtlessly impulsive
- To be diagnosed with conduct disorder, the patient would need to exhibit symptoms similar to ODD plus have aggression towards animals, destruction of property, deceitfulness or theft, and serious violations of rules, symptoms of a type and severity that neither the teacher nor the mother brought up

How would you treat her?

- Cognitive behavioral therapy
- Parent training
- d-methylphenidate XR (Focalin) 5 mg once daily in the morning titrated in 5 mg increments each week to optimization
- OROS methylphenidate (Concerta) 18 mg once daily in the morning titrated in 18 mg increments each week to optimization
- Mixed salts of amphetamine XR (Adderall XR) 10 mg once daily in the morning titrated in 10 mg increments each week to optimization
- Lisdexamfetamine (Vyvanse) 30 mg once daily in the morning titrated in 10–20 mg increments a week to optimization
- Other

Pediatrician's Mental Notes: Followup Visit Week 6, Continued

- Mother is initially uncomfortable with the diagnosis of ADHD with ODD and is far from ready to accept medication treatment for her daughter
- Wants different options
- Pediatrician suggests cognitive behavioral therapy and parent training
- Pediatrician also offers to write a letter to the school to implement strategies to help her daughter such as
  - Allowing extra time on tests and assignments
  - Placing child nearest to the teacher
  - Devising signals between teacher and child to redirect child's attention without embarrassing the child

Pediatrician's Mental Notes: Followup Visit Week 10

- Mother learns that closest CBT specialist is one-hour drive away from their home so this option falls through
- Also, while the teacher is happy to implement the strategies suggested by the pediatrician, she admits to already using them with the patient, given her experience with other ADHD students
- The lack of non-pharmacological treatment options helps the mother reconsider the risks versus the benefits of ADHD medications
- All the options listed as stimulants in the list above, plus some nonstimulants, are approved for the treatment of ADHD and have shown some efficacy for ODD symptoms
- D-methylphenidate XR is chosen

Pediatrician's Mental Notes: Followup Visits Weeks 12 and 14

- The dose of d-methylphenidate is titrated to 20 mg/day with some improvement in classroom behavior according to the teacher

- However, the patient develops problems with initial insomnia
  - Sometimes the effects of stimulants later in the day can actually improve sleep, especially in hyperactive individuals who have problems slowing down for bedtime routines
  - Some studies suggest that OROS methylphenidate lasts even longer (up to 12 hours) compared to d-methylphenidate XR, which seems to be more effective in the first 8 hours; thus OROS methylphenidate would be a potential option in such cases
  - However, this is not this patient's presentation
  - Since this patient did not have problems with sleep prior to starting d-methylphenidate XR, the initial insomnia is likely due to the stimulant
- Also, even though classroom behavior seems to be improving according to the teacher, the patient remains defiant with the mother, tears up some toys of her younger sister to upset her and screams more than ever at her mother while doing homework, seeming delighted when her mother gets upset and yells back
- The mother is instructed to give the medication another month to see if the improvements in the classroom begin to be seen in the home and is instructed about sleep hygiene including
  - Keeping regular schedules for going to bed and waking up
  - Avoiding the patient's favorite caffeinated sodas, especially in the late afternoon
  - Providing quiet activities as part of a bedtime routine
  - Having the patient leave her room to do another quiet activity if she does not fall asleep within 30 minutes

Pediatrician's Mental Notes: Followup Visit Week 18

- The mother herself is often overwhelmed and disorganized and so has a difficult time keeping regular schedules for going to bed and waking up, even during the week but especially on weekends
- Despite trying the behavioral approach, the initial insomnia remains a problem
- So does the defiant behavior at home
- Also, reports last week that the patient shoved somebody who she said was crowding in line, causing her classmate to cut her knee, requiring stitches/sutures
- Was not sorry or remorseful

How would you treat her now?
- Refer to a psychiatrist for further evaluation and psychopharmacological management
- Refer to a psychologist for therapy

- Switch to dl-methylphenidate immediate release (classical Ritalin) 10 mg twice daily, then titrate to optimized dose
- Switch to the methylphenidate transdermal patch (Daytrana) starting at 10 mg, then titrate to optimized dose
- Switch to the prodrug lisdexamfetamine (Vyvanse) starting at 30 mg once in the morning, then titrate to optimized dose
- Switch to atomoxetine (Strattera) 10–18 mg per day, then titrated to optimized dose
- Switch to guanfacineXR (Intuniv) 1 mg/day, then titrated to optimized dose
- Other

Pediatrician's Mental Notes: Followup Visit Week 18, Continued

- Each treatment option has specific considerations to take into account:
  - In general, the active d enantiomer of methylphenidate (which the patient was originally prescribed) may be slightly more than twice as potent as racemic d,l-methylphenidate; so, if side effects persist on d-methylphenidate it may be useful to switch to immediate release d, l methylphenidate which might require a "sculpted dose" with a higher morning than afternoon dose
  - The methylphenidate patch needs to have the patient and mother follow instructions and in this patient's case, may need to remove the patch before the suggested nine-hour wear time is over, if insomnia or other adverse events emerge; the patch should not be cut as a way to lower the dose
  - Lisdexamfetamine should be titrated by increasing the dose in 10–20 mg increments each week; 10–12 hours of clinical action can be expected, so might be less favorable in patients who already have problems with insomnia
  - Atomoxetine can have a longer onset of action but does not cause insomnia
  - Guanfacine/guanfacineXR should start at 1 mg and titrate by 1 mg increments to a maximum of 4 mg/day but an 8 year old will not likely need or tolerate the highest dose, which may cause sedation
- The mother prefers the methylphenidate patch approach, as it seems to be the most convenient way to address the sleep problems
- Additionally, sometimes the patient refuses to swallow pills and will take the medication only if convinced to do so, or possibly if sprinkled on food. This confrontation over medications adds too much extra time to the mother's already hectic morning schedule
- The patient likes the novelty of the patch, which reminds her of a sticker

Pediatrician's Mental Notes: Followup Visit Week 20

- The 10 mg patch with an eight hour or shorter wear time addresses the classroom ADHD symptoms without causing insomnia
- However, on the days when the mother forgets to remove the patch before 3 pm, insomnia returns
- That is resolved by setting her cell-phone alarm to remind her to remove the patch every day at 3 pm after applying it at 7 am
- At first the patient and her mother are impressed with the novelty of the patch and its flexibility and the resolution of the patient's insomnia
- However, she is still argumentative, including some evenings at bedtime, and this can interfere with getting to bed on time even though the patient no longer has insomnia
- The patient scratched her sister's face last week with her fingernails because her sister was playing with the patient's dolls
- Thinks it is funny that her sister's face is scratched
- "She looks like she has warpaint on her cheek"
- The pediatrician feels like only a bit of progress has been made with several months of medication treatment, including two different stimulants
- Even though inattentive symptoms in the classroom are reportedly improved, oppositional symptoms both at school and at home are not improved and if anything, are the main problem now
- Furthermore, the patches are expensive, not covered well by the mother's insurance and frequently are pulled off by the patient or her classmates tormenting her in response to her fighting/arguing with them
- Refers the patient and her mother to a psychiatrist

Attending Psychiatrist's Mental Notes: Initial Psychiatric Evaluation

- Seems like the patient needs more stimulant during the day and less at night
- Also, seems like the oppositional symptoms may require special therapeutic focus
- Considerations include:
  - Developing a platform of stimulant to optimize treatment with another oral medication
  - Increasing the dose during the day to see if oppositional symptoms will respond to this
  - If not, consider augmentation strategies for the oppositional symptoms
    - Psychotherapy (too expensive and too time consuming, mother cannot miss work, and too far away)

- Atypical antipsychotic (controversial, for use of atypical antipsychotics is not approved for ADHD or for oppositional symptoms of ADHD/ODD
- guanfacine XR – approved for ADHD with some evidence for use in oppositional as well as inattentive/hyperactive symptoms of ADHD but not approved for ODD
- Suggested switching back to an oral medication from the patch
- Trial of lisdexamfetamine 30 mg once in the morning

Attending Physician's Mental Notes: First and Second Interim Followups, Weeks 4 and 8

- Only partial efficacy but no insomnia
- Rather than increase dose of lisdexamfetamine, added 5 mg of dextroamphetamine at 7 am, then 10 mg, then 15 mg, became nauseous, reduced to 10 mg on top of lisdexamphetamine 30 mg in the morning
- Sometimes a second 5 mg dose of the dextroamphetamine after school is necessary
- This regimen does not cause insomnia
- ADHD better but oppositional symptoms persist
- Augmentation with guanfacine XR 1 mg/day

Case Outcome: Followup Weeks 12 to 20

- No side effects
- Titration to 2 mg/day
- Continues lisdexamfetamine 30 mg in the morning
- Plus dextroamphetamine 5 mg in the morning
- Plus occasional dextroamphetamine 5 mg additional daytime dose
- Oppositional symptoms improved slowly but surely over 2 months
- Psychiatrist asks whether the patient's sister has any problems in school, and the mother states that she is "spacey" but not oppositional
- Psychiatrist suggests to bring in the sister the next time the patient comes and gives mother screening forms for ADHD and asks her to consult with her other daughter's teacher to see if there are symptoms of ADHD in that daughter as well
- Psychiatrist asks mother to make an appointment for herself because it is obvious that she has undiagnosed and untreated ADHD
  - Given adult ADHD rating form for mother to fill out
  - Symptoms of ADHD in the mother are obvious during various interviews
    - Mother misses appointments or is late for appointments
    - Often appears disorganized

- Did not fill out her child's forms on time
- Did not deliver forms to her child's teacher, forgot, lost them
- Admits being very disorganized since her second child started school
- Feels overwhelmed by two children and her life circumstances
- Could also have some signs of depression
- Can't get organized to take her child to CBT
- Has a hard time keeping a regular schedule and also keeping her daughter on a regular schedule of going to bed and waking up
- Was unable to remember to remove the daughter's skin patch unless she set a cell phone alarm
- All these suggest further evaluation of the mother is indicated since ADHD commonly runs in families and has a very high genetic contribution
- See the following Case 14, p 151 for presentation of the mother's case

Case Debrief

- The patient is an 8-year-old with ADHD, inattentive type with comorbid ODD
- High doses of stimulants reduce inattention but cause insomnia and do not adequately treat oppositional symptoms
- "Top up" with the alpha 2A selective noradrenergic agonist (guanfacine XR) improves oppositional symptoms and the patient has stabilized

Take-Home Points

- ADHD with ODD comorbidity can be a difficult combination of behaviors to treat in children
- Combining stimulants with alpha 2A selective agonist actions may be useful in some patients with this combination of symptoms not adequately responsive to stimulants alone

Performance in Practice: Confessions of a Psychopharmacologist

- What could have been done better here?
  - Should the father have been included in the medical decisions?
  - Whether or not he has legal medical rights, he has visitation rights and could feel upset or vindictive if left out
  - It is possible that the patient is still dealing with her parents' divorce and still adjusting to her sister taking some of her mother's time and attention; some of the oppositional symptoms may not be due to ODD but to family conflict and possibly family

or individual psychotherapy involving the patient, her mother and/
or her sister could be productive here
- Possible action item for improvement in practice
  - Make a concerted effort to involve the father
  - Perhaps this patient should have been sent to a specialist
    psychopharmacologist earlier and symptom improvement may
    have occurred earlier
  - Perhaps a trial of atomoxetine would have been beneficial

Tips and Pearls

- Although guanfacine XR is approved as a monotherapy for ADHD,
  some studies and clinical anecdotes suggest that it can be combined
  with stimulatnts for patients with difficult oppositional comorbid
  symptoms
- "Sculpted therapy" combining long acting with immediate acting
  formulations of stimulants may optimize treatment for some cases
  with inadequate responses to long acting formulations alone

Two-Minute Tute: A brief lesson and psychopharmacology tutorial (tute) with relevant background material for this case
– Rating scales
– Oppositional Defiant Disorder vs Conduct Disorder
– NE and DA in prefrontal cortex in ADHD

Table 1: ADHD Rating Scale-IV – home version

Child's Name _____

Child's Age _____   Sex: M F   Grade_____   Child's Race_____

Completed by: Mother   Father   Guardian   Grandparent

Circle the number that *best describes* your child's home behavior over the
last 6 months

	never or rarely	sometimes	often	very often
1. Fails to give close attention to details or makes careless mistakes in schoolwork.	0	1	2	3
2. Fidgets with hands or feet or squirms in seat.	0	1	2	3
3. Has difficulty sustaining attention in tasks or play activities.	0	1	2	3
4. Leaves seat in classroom or in other situations in which remaining seated is expected.	0	1	2	3

5. Does not seem to listen when spoken to directly.	0	1	2	3
6. Runs about or climbs excessively in situations in which it is inappropriate.	0	1	2	3
7. Does not follow through on instructions and fails to finish work.	0	1	2	3
8. Has difficulty playing or engaging in leisure activities quietly.	0	1	2	3
9. Has difficulty organizing tasks and activities.	0	1	2	3
10. Is "on the go" or acts as if "driven by a motor."	0	1	2	3
11. Avoids tasks (e.g., schoolwork, homework) that require sustained mental effort.	0	1	2	3
12. Talks excessively	0	1	2	3
13. Loses things necessary for tasks or activities.	0	1	2	3
14. Blurts out answers before questions have been completed.	0	1	2	3
15. Is easily distracted.	0	1	2	3
16. Has difficulty awaiting turn.	0	1	2	3
17. Is forgetful in daily activities.	0	1	2	3
18. Interrupts or intrudes on others.	0	1	2	3

Table 2: ADHD rating scale-IV – school version

Child's Name _____

Child's Age _____   Sex: M F   Grade_____   Child's Race_____

Completed by: Mother   Father   Guardian   Grandparent

Circle the number that *best describes* your child's home behavior over the last 6 months

	never or rarely	sometimes	often	very often
1. Fails to give close attention to details or makes careless mistakes in schoolwork.	0	1	2	3
2. Fidgets with hands or feet or squirms in seat.	0	1	2	3
3. Has difficulty sustaining attention in tasks or play activities.	0	1	2	3
4. Leaves seat in classroom or in other situations in which remaining seated is expected.	0	1	2	3
5. Does not seem to listen when spoken to directly.	0	1	2	3
6. Runs about or climbs excessively in situations in which it is inappropriate.	0	1	2	3
7. Does not follow through on instructions and fails to finish work.	0	1	2	3
8. Has difficulty playing or engaging in leisure activities quietly.	0	1	2	3
9. Has difficulty organizing tasks and activities.	0	1	2	3
10. Is "on the go" or acts as if "driven by a motor."	0	1	2	3
11. Avoids tasks (e.g., schoolwork, homework) that require sustained mental effort.	0	1	2	3
12. Talks excessively	0	1	2	3
13. Loses things necessary for tasks or activities.	0	1	2	3
14. Blurts out answers before questions have been completed.	0	1	2	3
15. Is easily distracted.	0	1	2	3
16. Has difficulty awaiting turn.	0	1	2	3
17. Is forgetful in daily activities.	0	1	2	3
18. Interrupts or intrudes on others.	0	1	2	3

Table 3: Oppositional defiant disorder

- Aggressiveness
- Tendency to purposefully bother and irritate others
- Negativistic, hostile and defiant behavior lasting at least 6 months which according to DSM IV must have 4 or more of the following:
  - Often loses temper
  - Often argues with adults
  - Often actively defies or refuses to comply with adults' requests or rules
  - Often deliberately annoys people
  - Often blames others for his or her mistakes or misbehavior
  - Is often touchy or easily annoyed by others
  - Is often angry and resentful
  - Is often spiteful and vindictive

Table 4: Conduct disorder

- Some think that conduct disorder is a worse version of ODD
- Approximately 6–10% of boys and 2–9% of girls
- Can be comorbid with ADHD
- Can go away by adulthood
- Can progress into antisocial personality disorder
- Can be comorbid with many other disorders including substance abuse
- Violation of basic rights of others and rules of society, which according to DSM IV at least three of the following must be present in the last 12months and at least one in the last 6 months
  - Aggression to people and animals
  - Destruction of property
  - Deceitfulness or theft
  - Serious violations of rules

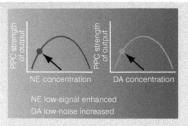

Figure 1. ADHD: Hypothetically Low Signals and/or High Noise in the Prefrontal Cortex (PFC) in ADHD.
Theoretically, ADHD with inattention, hyperactivity and/or impulsiveness is due to the prefrontal cortex being "out of tune" with both DA (dopamine) and NE (norepinephrine) being too low, and causing signals to be low and/or "noise" to be too high and drown out signals, thus creating the symptoms of ADHD

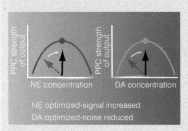

Figure 2. ADHD: Treatment to Increase NE, Increase DA.
Stimulants increase both NE (norepinephrine) and DA (dopamine) actions in prefrontal cortex, increasing signals and reducing noise and thus hypothetically reducing the symptoms of ADHD

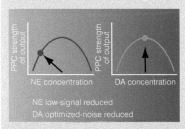

Figure 3. ADHD: Hypothetically Low Signals Due to Low NE.
Although many cases of ADHD may be due to low DA and NE as shown in Figure 1, some may hypothetically be due to only low NE

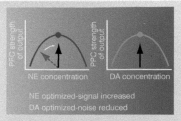

Figure 4. ADHD: Treatment with Alpha 2A Agonist.
In cases where ADHD is due predominantly to low NE activity, as shown in Figure 3, selective NE enhancing agents such as the alpha 2A selective noradrenergic agonist guanfacine XR may be helpful in treating ADHD symptoms without necessarily needing to interact with DA

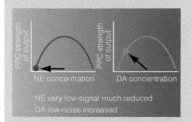

Figure 5. ADHD and Oppositional Symptoms: Hypothetically Very Low Signals in VMPFC (Ventromedial Prefrontal Cortex).
Cases of ADHD with comorbid ODD (oppositional defiant disorder) may differ from classical ADHD shown in Figure 1. With ADHD and ODD, there may hypothetically be very low NE signals and low DA levels with increased noise.

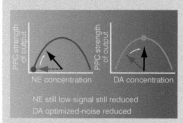

Figure 6. ADHD and Oppositional Symptoms: Treatment with a Stimulant.
When ADHD with ODD (Figure 5) is treated with a stimulant, this improves both NE and DA levels, but is theoretically suboptimal tuning of NE. Thus, NE is still low, signals still reduced while DA optimized because noise is reduced. This may explain why stimulants can improve some ADHD symptoms in patients with comorbid ADHD but not their ODD symptoms. Raising the dose of the stimulant would put NE into balance, but would put DA too high and thus out of balance

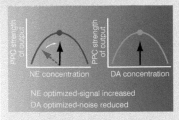

NE concentration   DA concentration

NE optimized-signal increased
DA optimized-noise reduced

Figure 7. ADHD and Oppositional Symptoms: Augment a Stimulant with an Alpha 2A Agonist.
After treatment of ADHD comorbid with ODD (Figure 5) with stimulants (Figure 6), the prefrontal cortex is still not adequately tuned (Figure 6), so that ADHD symptoms may be improved but oppositional symptoms persist. Adding an alpha 2A selective noradrenergic agonist such as guanfacine XR to the stimulant will improve NE tone selectively, and hypothetically enhance the therapeutic actions of the stimulant so that both ADHD and ODD symptomst are improved

Posttest Self Assessment Question: Answer

What is true about oppositional symptoms in patients with ADHD

A. They can be part of the diagnostic criteria for ADHD in children
   - False. The diagnostic criteria are inattentive, hyperactive and impulsive, not oppositional; some patients have oppositional symptoms insufficient to meet the criteria for ODD but they are not part of the diagnostic criteria for ADHD
B. They can be confused with impulsive symptoms of ADHD
   - True. Oppositional symptoms, however, are purposeful and without remorse whereas impulsive symptoms are thoughtless and cause remorse after the fact
C. They can be part of oppositional defiant disorder (ODD) which can be comorbid with ADHD
   - True
D. They can be part of conduct disorder (CD) which can be comorbid with ADHD
   - Although true, oppositional symptoms are not sufficient for the diagnosis of conduct disorder which requires additional symptoms as well for the diagnosis to be made

Answer: B, C and D

References

1. Franke B, Neale BM, and Faraone SV. Genome-wide association studies in ADHD. Hum Genet 2009; 126(1): 13–50
2. Haberstick BC, Timberlake D, Hopfer CJ et al. Genetic and environmental contributions to retrospectively reported DSM-IV

childhood attention deficit hyperactivity disorder. Psychol Med 2008; 38(7): 1057–66

3. McLoughlin G, Ronald A, Kuntsi J et al. Genetic support for the dual nature of attention deficit hyperactivity disorder: substantial genetic overlap between the inattentive and hyperactive-impulsive components. J Abnorm Child Psychol 2007; 35(6): 999–1008

4. Todd RD, Rasmussen ER, Neuman RJ et al. Familiality and heritability of subtypes of attention deficit hyperactivity disorder in a population sample of adolescent female twins. Am J Psychiatry 2001; 158(11): 1891–8

5. Faraone SV, Advances in the genetics and neurobiology of attention deficit hyperactivity disorder, Biol Psychiatry 2006; 60: 1025–7

6. Stahl SM, Stahl's Illustrated Attention Deficit Hyperactivity Disorder, Cambridge University Press, New York, 2009

7. Stahl SM, Attention Deficit Hyperactivity Disorder and its Treatment, in Stahl's Essential Psychopharmacology, 3rd edition, Cambridge University Press, New York, 2008, pp 863–98

8. Stahl SM, Lisdexamfetamine, in Stahl's Essential Psychopharmacology The Prescriber's Guide, 3rd edition, Cambridge University Press, New York, 2009, pp 271–6

9. Stahl SM, Atomoxetine, in Stahl's Essential Psychopharmacology The Prescriber's Guide, 3rd edition, Cambridge University Press, New York, 2009, pp 51–5

10. Stahl SM, Guanfacine XR, in Stahl's Essential Psychopharmacology The Prescriber's Guide, 3rd edition, Cambridge University Press, New York, 2009, pp 233–5

11. Stahl SM, d-Methylphenidate, in Stahl's Essential Psychopharmacology The Prescriber's Guide, 3rd edition, Cambridge University Press, New York, 2009, pp 323–7

12. Stahl SM, d,l Methylphenidate, in Stahl's Essential Psychopharmacology The Prescriber's Guide, 3rd edition, Cambridge University Press, New York, 2009, pp 329–35

13. Stahl SM, Mixed Salts of d,l amphetamine, in Stahl's Essential Psychopharmacology The Prescriber's Guide, 3rd edition, Cambridge University Press, New York, 2009, pp 39–44

14. Stahl SM, d-amphetamine, in Stahl's Essential Psychopharmacology The Prescriber's Guide, 3rd edition, Cambridge University Press, New York, 2009, pp 33–8

The Case: The scatter-brained mother whose daughter has ADHD, like mother, like daughter

The Question: How often does ADHD run in families?

The Dilemma: When you see a child with ADHD should you also evaluate the parents and siblings?

Pretest Self Assessment Question (answer at the end of the case)

Patients with comorbid ADHD and anxiety should in general not be prescribed stimulants

A. True
B. False

Patient Intake

- 26-year-old woman
- Has a daughter with ADHD
- Psychiatrist noted symptoms in the mother and suggested she come in for her own evaluation
- See the previous Case 13, p 133 for presentation of the daughter's case

Psychiatric History

- During interviews with the patient's daughter (also attended by the patient) over the past several months, it was not only noted that the daughter has ADHD with comorbid ODD, but that the mother also exhibited multiple symptoms consistent with lifelong and undiagnosed ADHD including
    - Mother misses appointments or is late for appointments
    - Often appears disorganized
    - Did not fill out her child's forms on time
    - Did not deliver forms to her child's teacher, forgot, lost them
    - Admits being very disorganized since her second child started school
    - Feels overwhelmed by two children and her life circumstances
    - Could also have some signs of depression
    - Can't get organized to take her child to CBT
    - Has a hard time keeping a regular schedule and also keeping her daughter on a regular schedule of going to bed and waking up
    - Was unable to remember to remove the daughter's skin patch unless she set a cell phone alarm
    - All these suggest further evaluation of the mother is indicated since ADHD commonly runs in families and has a very high genetic contribution

- Has always done poorly academically
- Has always felt intimidated by any type of testing
- In addition, reports that she has always been worried about the future and financial stability of her family
- Says she sometimes mentally "freezes when it gets to be too much"
- When her eight year old daughter was diagnosed with ADHD, she suddenly realized that she had similar problems as a child
- The psychiatrist explained to her that ADHD was highly heritable and that there was a 75% chance of having a child with ADHD if both parents have ADHD and thus was asked to fill out an Adult ADHD screening form

Social and Personal History

- High school drop out, age 17 after getting pregnant
- Married age 17, divorced 2 years later
- Two children, ages 8 and 6
- Smoker
- No drug or alcohol abuse
- Single mother works full time in retail
- Father not much involved with his children

Medical History

- None notable
- BP normal
- BMI normal
- Normal lab tests

Family History

- 8-year-old daughter: recently diagnosed with ADHD
- Other family history unknown as the patient was adopted
- See the previous Case 13, p 133 for presentation of the daughter's case

Patient Intake

- The last time the patient brought her child to see the psychiatrist, the mother was asked to fill out her own checklist, the Adult ADHD Self Report Scale Symptom Checklist
  - She endorsed many items, mostly inattentive but not really hyperactive or impulsive such as:
    - Having trouble wrapping up the final details of a project once the challenging parts have been done
    - Difficulty getting things in order
    - Difficulty remembering appointments or obligations

- Making careless mistakes on difficult projects
- Difficulty keeping attention on repetitive work
- Misplacing things at home and work
- Distracted by activity around her
- Difficulty unwinding and relaxing when having time to herself
- Difficulty focusing/listening during conversations

- Earlier, the mother was also requested to obtain copies of her report cards from first and second grade
  - Her own mother had kept these in storage
  - Showed grades that were quite low
  - Her teachers had commented on some of the problems endorsed in the adult ADHD checklist that she continues to experience as an adult
- Asked how these problems affect her life, she states that:
  - They cause great difficulty managing family matters
  - She used to be unable to stay focused in conversations with her ex-husband, which made him feel she did not care about him
- Additional complaints include:
  - Constantly feeling overwhelmed with taking care of the two children while working fulltime
  - Blaming herself for her daughter's academic difficulties
  - Feeling very emotional and overwhelmed
    - "I'm sorry, doctor, but two kids are just too much for this single mom"
- Having difficulty sleeping and being irritable with the children at night, which she regrets later on
- Has many worries, about finances, about the future, about her children's futures, about getting a better job, about getting her own education, about finding a new partner

Based on just what you have been told so far about this patient's history and symptoms, what do you think is her diagnosis?

- Appropriate response to her circumstances with her severe psychosocial stressors
- Mostly just stress and anxiety
- ADHD
- ADHD and stress
- Generalized anxiety disorder (GAD)
- Major depressive episode
- ADHD and GAD
- Other

Attending Physician's Mental Notes: Initial Psychiatric Evaluation

- Here is a case that indeed is ADHD, but her symptoms also suggest that she suffers from GAD
  - Constant worry
  - Feeling on edge
  - Fatigue
  - Difficulty concentrating and her mind going blank
  - Irritability
  - Trouble sleeping
- Most adults with ADHD are comorbid for a second psychiatric disorder, and the most common is GAD
- Also, this patient is a smoker which may be related to her ADHD since a disproportionate number of ADHD patients smoke, perhaps because of the therapeutic effects of nicotine on ADHD symptoms

How would you treat her?
- Stimulant for her ADHD
- SSRI/SNRI for her GAD
- Benzodiazepine as need for GAD and insomnia
- Stimulant plus an SSRI/SNRI or benzo for both ADHD and GAD
- CBT for both ADHD and GAD
- Other

Attending Physician's Mental Notes, Initial Psychiatric Evaluation, Continued

- It seems as though the primary disorder is ADHD and it will be simplest if this is treated first, with a single drug, probably a stimulant
- An SSRI/SNRI and/or benzodiazepine can be added at a later time once the actions of the stimulant are evident
- Even though patients with GAD alone or even normal controls may be "over stimulated" by a stimulant, in many cases of ADHD comorbid with GAD, the stimulant is paradoxically calming and well tolerated and even works for GAD symptoms as well as ADHD symptoms without having to prescribe a second medication for the GAD
- Any stimulant could be chosen but not all are explicitly approved for treatment of ADHD in adults
- She was started on mixed salts d,l amphetamine XR (Adderall XR)
- She was referred to a local mental health training program where she could possibly get CBT for free or for a reduced rate from a trainee receiving supervision

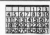

Case Outcome: First, Second, and Third Interim Followup Visits, Weeks 4, 8 and 12

- Due to scheduling issues, by the time the patient had her first CBT session, she had already been titrated to 20 mg of mixed salts of d,l – amphetamine XR
- She thought that the medication had already started to help her and in fact that she would not have been able to cooperate with the CBT assignments had she not been on the medication
- Because of lack of side effects but continuing ADHD and GAD symptoms, the dose of d,l-amphetamine XR increased to 30 mg (off label since the maximum approved dosage for adults is 20 mg)
- Her BP and pulse were stable on the 30 mg dose but she felt jittery particularly in the morning and around noon; she also felt very anxious about her job situation and being able to provide for her family
- Dose lowered to 25 mg, but the jitteriness persisted so the dosage was further lowerd to 20 mg
- The jitteriness abated but her ADHD symptoms were not well controlled on the 20 mg dose anymore
- Instructed to stay on 20 mg for two more weeks as she is going on vacation and not to change the dose until after her vacation and then retry the 25 mg dose again
- Complained of feeling overwhelmed and irritable
- For most patients, a week between dosing adjustments for a stimulant being used to treat ADHD is quite adequate
- Weekly intervals give patients and clinicians a chance to see the way that the dosage is working though the spectrum of challenges that occur in a typical week
- As vacations do not represent typical activities for a week, special consideration must be given to the effectiveness of medication changes that are done while a patient is on vacation
  - Many adults with ADHD may relax on vacation and not challenge themselves with cognitive loads and multitasking so may appear to be better even without a medication change
  - Other adults with ADHD, especially women with young children, may actually find vacation more challenging
  - For example, a parent with ADHD taking a family vacation with several children in tow may find the planning and organization for the trip more taxing than anything encountered at work or during the normal routine at home
  - It can also be difficult to manage timing the medication appropriately when traveling to different time zones

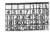

Case Outcome: Fourth Interim Followup, Week 16

- "Glad to be back from vacation"
- "I don't think I could have even got through our vacation without my medication, but I still have a hard time holding things together"
- On at least 20 mg/day dosage of d,l-amphetamine XR combined with CBT for 12 weeks, including a couple of weeks back from vacation, the patient still has problems with
  - Organizing her day
  - Procrastinating
  - Following instructions
  - Losing items such as her keys which make her late for appointments/activities
- On the few days that the patient missed, and thus skipped, her medication inadvertently she realized that the medication was really helping her concentrate and get through the day even though she remains symptomatic
- Knowing that she could achieve better functioning on medication she asked if other medications might accomplish this without the jittery and anxious feelings
- While other medication options were discussed, the CBT was continued which was slightly less helpful

How would you treat her now?

- Start lisdexamfetamine 30 mg once in the morning and titrate the dosage by 20 mg each week until an optimal dosage is achieved
- Start d-methylphenidate XR 10 mg once in the morning and titrate the dosage by 10 mg each week until an optimal dosage is achieved
- Start OROS methylphenidate 18 mg once in the morning and titrate the dosage by 18 mg each week until an optimal dose is achieved
- Start atomoxetine 40 mg a day and increase to 80 mg after one week

Attending Physician's Mental Notes: Fourth Interim Followup, Week 16

- Lisdexamfetamine, d-methylphenidate XR, OROS methylphenidate, and atomoxetine are all FDA-approved for the treatment of adults with ADHD
- On the one hand, the patient found her amphetamine-based stimulant to be very effective, and thus another long-acting stimulant would be reasonable
- On the other hand, she had jitteriness with the stimulant, and thus a non-stimulant would be equally reasonable
- After explaining the options, the patient elected to try another long-acting stimulant

- d-methylphenidate uses a bead-based technology similar to the mixed salts amphetamine XR in that 50 percent of the beads are immediate-release and 50 percent delayed-released
- Methylphenidate LA and d-methylphenidate XR employ the same patented SODAS technology in their delivery systems, but other long-acting forms of stimulants with beaded delivery systems vary due to proprietary differences in their manufacturing processes
- For instance, one formulation of methylphenidate utilizes a capsule that contains a ratio of 30 percent immediate-release beads and 70 percent delayed-released beads
- Although the different technologies used in beaded forms of stimulants can have clinical implications in individual cases, they all follow a similar design scheme:
  - A bolus of stimulant medication becomes bioavailable rather quickly as the immediate-release beads dissolve
  - Over time, the coating on the delayed-release beads deteriorates, allowing the stimulant contained within the bead to be released
  - The medication within the delayed-release bead becomes bioavailable about four hours after the patient swallows the capsule
- Lisdexamfetamine is the only stimulant preparation that is a prodrug:
  - In its prodrug form, a lysine molecule is attached to dextroamphetamine
  - Dextroamphetamine will not be active until the lysine is cleaved from it
  - Cleaved lysine is an amino acid that does not contribute to the clinical efficacy of this medication
- Lisdexamfetamine could be a good choice for multiple reasons:
  - It uses a different delivery system that appears to have a more consistent interval to maximum concentration (Cmax)
- It is conceivable that the jitteriness this patient was experiencing was related more to the l-isomer than to the d-isomer
- A nonstimulant such as atomoxetine may be particularly useful in a patient who has stimulant related side effects, because atomoxetine does not cause these side effects
- Also, atomoxetine may be particularly useful in patients with comorbid anxiety

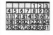

Case Outcome: Fourth Interim Followup, Week 16, Continued

- In the end, the patient and the attending physician agreed upon a trial of OROS methylphenidate (Concerta)
- Main reasons for this choice:
  - To be able to compare the benefits the patient experienced on an amphetamine preparation with those of a methylphenidate

preparation since patients may experience differing tolerabilities as well as efficacies on methylphenidate versus amphetamine
- To be able to test the uniqueness of the OROS delivery system in terms of attained efficacy with better tolerability
• OROS methylphenidate uses a delivery system that is quite different from beaded delivery systems:
- Coating of OROS methylphenidate contains 32 percent of the medication
- Remainder of medication is contained within a permeable membrane that allows water from the gut to enter once the coating of methylphenidate dissolves away
- Different concentrations of methylphenidate in gel form are contained in two compartments
- A push compartment absorbs water and expands like a sponge does, pushing the methylphenidate gel out of the hole at the opposite end

Case Outcome: Fifth Interim Followup, Week 20
• The patient's dose was titrated from 18 mg to 72 mg over the course of four weeks
• Although she did not feel jittery, OROS methylphenidate 72 mg once a day did not seem to work as well as the mixed salts amphetamine at 30 mg a day
• She voiced concerns that the dosage was more than double that of the mixed salts amphetamine dosage that was tried
• The psychiatrist explained that methylphenidate compounds are half as potent as amphetamine ones, and that 72 mg/day is an approved dose in adults
• She was reminded that her blood pressure and pulse had remained in the normal range throughout the titration, and she was told that some of the methylphenidate gel may remain inside the delivery system and not be bioavailable (inherent properties of OROS technology)
• After documenting that information about off-label use was given to the patient, the psychiatrist recommended to further increase the dose of OROS methylphenidate to 90 mg

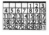

Case Outcome: Sixth Interim Followup, Week 24
• The patient felt that 90 mg of OROS methylphenidate worked at least as well as 30 mg of the mixed salts of d,l amphetamine XR
• Her blood pressure and pulse increased a bit from baseline, but they were still in the middle of the normal range

- She still has some problems with organization and losing items, but she indicates she would continue CBT to address these
- Similar to when she was on the amphetamine compound, once her ADHD symptoms abated, her anxious feelings became more prominent
  - "It's like now that I can concentrate on my daily tasks, I also feel much more anxious about the financial security of my children, and I often feel my throat tighten when I think about the financial impact of the girls going to college"
  - "The thought of losing my job or getting sick frightens me . . . what would happen to the girls?"
  - She has trouble falling asleep at night, as her mind does not shut off

ADHD is often comorbid with other psychiatric disorders and one disorder can mask the symptoms of another. In the present case, this patient exhibits symptoms of anxiety, probably generalized anxiety disorder, especially more prominent every time her ADHD symptoms abate. How would you address the patient's anxiety at this point?

- Augment with a benzodiazepine
- Augment with buspirone
- Augment with a selective serotonin reuptake inhibitor (SSRI) or SNRI
- Incorporate techniques to resolve anxiety into ongoing CBT

Case Outcome: Seventh and Eighth Interim Followup, Weeks 24 and 36

- Incorporating techniques to resolve anxiety into the patient's ongoing CBT would likely be most appropriate, prior to attempting to add a medication
- A letter was sent suggesting this to the CBT therapist, but after 12 weeks, this led to limited benefit, and thus medication augmentation was considered
- Benzodiazepines, buspirone, and SSRIs/SNRIs can all be used to treat generalized anxiety disorder and are not contraindicated with stimulants
- After discussion of the options, paroxetine was prescribed to augment her stimulant and her CTB

Case Outcome: Ninth Interim Followup, Week 48

- After three months on OROS methylphenidate and paroxetine, while continuing her CBT, at first the patient stated that she "had her life back"
- Then, after thinking back over the past year of treatment, and to how she had been since childhood she stated, "No, I don't have my life back – I finally have a life!"

Case Debrief

- It took a long time to get both the ADHD and GAD recognized
- It took over a year of trial and error and combination treatment to attain a remission of symptoms
- Real remission will come when sustained improvement of symptoms leads to better functional outcomes, not only less subjective distress, but now perhaps the chance for an education, a better job, and having enough emotional reserve to develop another relationship
- Stopping smoking might be a goal to tackle in the next year as well

Take-Home Points

- ADHD is highly heritable
- It is not uncommon for adults with previously undiagnosed ADHD to recognize their own symptoms once their child is diagnosed
- A multigenerational approach should be considered for parents who have ADHD and who care for children with ADHD
- In the patient's case, by addressing her own ADHD issues, she also felt she could be a better parent to her daughter with ADHD

Performance in Practice: Confessions of a Psychopharmacologist

- What could have been done better here?
  - Perhaps ADHD could have been recognized earlier
  - Perhaps CBT could have been implemented earlier
  - Perhaps she should have been more actively engaged or have had more serious discussions about smoking cessation already
- Possible action item for improvement in practice
  - Make a concerted effort to keep contact with low cost CBT resources in the community
  - Make a more concerted effort to encourage smoking cessation

Tips and Pearls

- Prescribing stimulants to an ADHD patient is very much like tailoring a "bespoke" treatment, one case at a time
- That is, some patients respond very differently to amphetamine than they do to methylphenidate
- Many patients respond very differently to one controlled dosage pattern versus another
- Look for comorbidities in adult ADHD, including both anxiety disorders and substance dependence/abuse (especially smoking)
- True remission means reduction not just in symptoms of ADHD, but in the comorbid conditions as well

Two-Minute Tute: A brief lesson and psychopharmacology tutorial (tute) with relevant background material for this case
– ADHD rating scales for adults
– Contributions of genetics to ADHD

Table 1: Adult ADHD Self-Report Scale (ASRS-v1.1) Symptom Checklist Instructions

The questions on the back page are designed to stimulate dialogue between you and your patients and to help confirm if they may be suffering from the symptoms of attention-deficit/hyperactivity disorder (ADHD).

Description: The Symptom Checklist is an instrument consisting of the eighteen DSM-IV-TR criteria. Six of the eighteen questions were found to be the most predictive of symptoms consistent with ADHD. These six questions are the basis for the ASRS v1.1 Screener and are also Part A of the Symptom Checklist. Part B of the Symptom Checklist contains the remaining twelve questions.

Instructions:

Symptoms

1. Ask the patient to complete both Part A and Part B of the Symptom Checklist by marking an X in the box that most closely represents the frequency of occurrence of each of the symptoms.

2. Score Part A. If four or more marks appear in the darkly shaded boxes within Part A then the patient has symptoms highly consistent with ADHD in adults and further investigation is warranted.

3. The frequency scores on Part B provide additional cues and can serve as further probes into the patient's symptoms. Pay particular attention to marks appearing in the dark shaded boxes. The frequency-based response is more sensitive with certain questions. No total score or diagnostic likelihood is utilized for the twelve questions. It has been found that the six questions in Part A are the most predictive of the disorder and are best for use as a screening instrument.

Impairments

1. Review the entire Symptom Checklist with your patients and evaluate the level of impairment associated with the symptom.

2. Consider work/school, social and family settings.

3. Symptom frequency is often associated with symptom severity, therefore the Symptom Checklist may also aid in the assessment of impairments. If your patients have frequent symptoms, you may want to ask them to describe how these problems have affected the ability to work, take care of things at home, or get along with other people such as their spouse/significant other.

History

1. Assess the presence of these symptoms or similar symptoms in childhood. Adults who have ADHD need not have been formally diagnosed in childhood. In evaluating a patient's history, look for evidence of early-appearing and long-standing problems with attention or self-control. Some significant symptoms should have been present in childhood, but full symptomology is not necessary.

Adult ADHD Self-Report Scale (ASRS-v1.1) Symptom Checklist

Patient Name		Today's Date						

Please answer the questions below, rating yourself on each of the criteria shown using the scale on the right side of the page. As you answer each question, place an X in the box that best describes how you have felt and conducted yourself over the past 6 months. Please give this completed checklist to your healthcare professional to discuss during today's appointment.

	Never	Rarely	Sometimes	Often	Very Often
1. How often do you have trouble wrapping up the final details of a project, once the challenging parts have been done?					
2. How often do you have difficulty getting things in order when you have to do a task that requires organization?					
3. How often do you have problems remembering appointments or obligations?					
4. When you have a task that requires a lot of thought, how often do you avoid or delay getting started?					
5. How often do you fidget or squirm with your hands or feet when you have to sit down for a long time?					
6. How often do you feel overly active and compelled to do things, like you were driven by a motor?					

Part A

	Never	Rarely	Sometimes	Often	Very Often
7. How often do you make careless mistakes when you have to work on a boring or difficult project?					
8. How often do you have difficulty keeping your attention when you are doing boring or repetitive work?					
9. How often do you have difficulty concentrating on what people say to you, even when they are speaking to you directly?					
10. How often do you misplace or have difficulty finding things at home or at work?					
11. How often are you distracted by activity or noise around you?					
12. How often do you leave your seat in meetings or other situations in which you are expected to remain seated?					
13. How often do you feel restless or fidgety?					
14. How often do you have difficulty unwinding and relaxing when you have time to yourself?					
15. How often do you find yourself talking too much when you are in social situations?					
16. When you're in a conversation, how often do you find yourself finishing the sentences of the people you are talking to, before they can finish them themselves?					
17. How often do you have difficulty waiting your turn in situations when turn taking is required?					
18. How often do you interrupt others when they are busy?					

Part B

The Value of Screening for Adults With ADHD

Research suggests that the symptoms of ADHD can persist into adulthood, having a significant impact on the relationships, careers, and even the personal safety of your patients who may suffer from it.[1-4] Because this disorder is often misunderstood, many people who have it do not receive appropriate treatment and, as a result, may never reach their full potential. Part of the problem is that it can be difficult to diagnose, particularly in adults.

The Adult ADHD Self-Report Scale (ASRS-v1.1) Symptom Checklist was developed in conjunction with the World Health Organization (WHO), and the Workgroup on Adult ADHD that included the following team of psychiatrists and researchers:

- **Lenard Adler, MD**
  Associate Professor of Psychiatry and Neurology
  New York University Medical School

- **Ronald C. Kessler, PhD**
  Professor, Department of Health Care Policy
  Harvard Medical School

- **Thomas Spencer, MD**
  Associate Professor of Psychiatry
  Harvard Medical School

As a healthcare professional, you can use the ASRS v1.1 as a tool to help screen for ADHD in adult patients. Insights gained through this screening may suggest the need for a more in-depth clinician interview. The questions in the ASRS v1.1 are consistent with DSM-IV criteria and address the manifestations of ADHD symptoms in adults. Content of the questionnaire also reflects the importance that DSM-IV places on symptoms, impairments, and history for a correct diagnosis.[4]

The checklist takes about 5 minutes to complete and can provide information that is critical to supplement the diagnostic process.

References:
1. Schweitzer JB, et al. Med Clin North Am. 2001;85(3):10-11, 757-77.
2. Barkley RA. Attention Deficit Hyperactivity Disorder: A Handbook for Diagnosis and Treatment. 2nd ed. 1998.
3. Biederman J, et al. Am J Psychiatry.1993;150:1792-8.
4. American Psychiatric Association: Diagnostic and Statistical Manual of Mental Disorders, Fourth Edition, Text Revision. Washington, DC, American Psychiatric Association. 2000: 85-93.

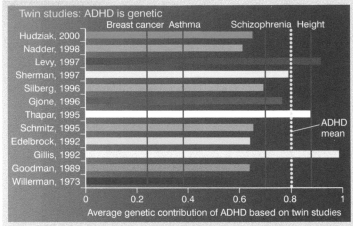

Figure 1: Average Genetic Contribution of ADHD Based on Twin Studies

ADHD is one of the most genetically loaded medical or psychiatric conditions, higher than schizophrenia, asthma or breast cancer.

Posttest Self Assessment Question: Answer

Patients with comorbid ADHD and anxiety should in general not be prescribed stimulants

A True
B False

Answer: B

References

1. Franke B, Neale BM, and Faraone SV. Genome-wide association studies in ADHD. Hum Genet 2009; 126(1): 13–50

2. Haberstick BC, Timberlake D, Hopfer CJ et al. Genetic and environmental contributions to retrospectively reported DSM-IV childhood attention deficit hyperactivity disorder. Psychol Med 2008; 38(7): 1057–66

3. McLoughlin G, Ronald A, Kuntsi J et al. Genetic support for the dual nature of attention deficit hyperactivity disorder: substantial genetic overlap between the inattentive and hyperactive-impulsive components. J Abnorm Child Psychol 2007; 35(6): 999–1008

4. Todd RD, Rasmussen ER, Neuman RJ et al. Familiality and heritability of subtypes of attention deficit hyperactivity disorder in a population sample of adolescent female twins. Am J Psychiatry 2001; 158(11): 1891–8

5. Faraone SV, Advances in the genetics and neurobiology of attention deficit hyperactivity disorder, Biol Psychiatry 2006; 60: 1025–7

6. Stahl SM, Stahl's Illustrated Attention Deficit Hyperactivity Disorder, Cambridge University Press, New York, 2009

7. Stahl SM, Attention Deficit Hyperactivity Disorder and its Treatment, in Stahl's Essential Psychopharmacology, 3rd edition, Cambridge University Press, New York, 2008, pp 863–98

8. Stahl SM, Atomoxetine, in Stahl's Essential Psychopharmacology The Prescriber's Guide, 3rd edition, Cambridge University Press, New York, 2009, pp 51–5

9. Stahl SM, d,l methylphenidate, in Stahl's Essential Psychopharmacology The Prescriber's Guide, 3rd edition, Cambridge University Press, New York, 2009, pp 329–35

10. Stahl SM, Mixed Salts of d,l Amphetamine, in Stahl's Essential Psychopharmacology The Prescriber's Guide, 3rd edition, Cambridge University Press, New York, 2009, pp 39–44

11. Stahl SM, Paroxetine, in Stahl's Essential Psychopharmacology The Prescriber's Guide, 3rd edition, Cambridge University Press, New York, 2009, pp 409–15

The Case: The doctor who couldn't keep up with his patients

The Question: Is cogntitive dysfunction following a head injury due to traumatic brain injury or to depression?

The Psychopharm Dilemma: How can treatment improve his functioning at work?

Pretest Self Assessment Question (answer at the end of the case)

Agents that enhance DA and NE in prefrontal cortex may be useful in treating executive dysfunction of a residual head injury, but not for the cognitive dysfunction of depression and anxiety.

A. True
B. False

Patient Intake

- 52-year-old man
- Chief complaints: anxiety, depression, problems concentrating

Psychiatric History

- Anxiety since college, waxing and waning, bothersome but never disabling, treated with psychotherapy and no meds
- Became a physician in a very stressful high-volume practice eight years ago with an increase of anxiety
- Trial of nefazodone (Serzone) not helpful
- Switch to sertraline (Zoloft) which caused akathisia on two consecutive doses, so discontinued it and reinstituted psychotherapy with good results

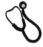

Medical History

- Developed angina five years ago, diagnosed as coronary artery disease and had a stent placement
- Post-operatively had more anxiety, treated with fluoxetine (Prozac) 20 mg with "fabulous" results except moderate sexual dysfunction
- Not obese but diagnosed with obstructive sleep apnea and restless legs syndrome, treated with CPAP (continuous positive airway pressure) and clonazepam (Klonopin) 0.5 mg at night

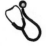

Head Injury

- Bicycle accident two years ago with flaccid right hemiparesis (later with full right sided motor recovery), prolonged loss of consciousness, seizure, ICU (intensive care unit) hospitalization and documented left prefrontal brain contusion on MRI brain scan

- Neuropsychological testing documents
  - Average memory
  - Average psychomotor speed
  - Average reaction time
  - Average complex attention
  - Average cognitive flexibility
  - However, might be low for performance for that expected of a physician
- Able to understand oral and visual information better than written information
- Does not make errors when able to work slowly and methodically
- Becomes frustrated and overwhelmed when presented information too quickly or forced to perform multitasking
- Fully disabled for four months
- Returns to work part-time as an internist in a well known HMO (health maintenance organization) outpatient clinic
- Partially disabled for eight months, i.e., works full-time but fewer patients scheduled per day than for a normal full time physician to allow him additional time for charting and to take short breaks between appointments with every other Friday off
- HMO performance standards for a full-time physician schedule 11 patients an hour, juggling no-shows, phone calls and time-consuming new patients or patient crises as necessary

Social and Personal History

- Married for 28 years
- 2 children
- Non smoker, no substance of alcohol abuse
- Interested in photography as a hobby
- Many friends

Family History

- No history of depression in the family
- First degree relatives with premature deaths from cardiovascular disease

Psychiatric History: Following the Head Injury

- Upon returning to work part-time four months after the head injury, noted to be somewhat disinhibited emotionally, with some low-grade anxiety and depression
- Increased fluoxetine to 30 mg and noted side effects: falling backward, occasional myoclonus, fasciculations in the day, worsening restless legs at night

- Reduced fluoxetine to 10 mg and noted periods of waxing and waning depression (maximum severity 4/10 on a 10-point scale with 10 worst; lasting a few days) followed by a near recovery for a few days
- Notes slowness of problem-solving skills, difficulty reading medical journals
- Over the next year after returning to work, tries to raise work productivity under increased pressure to do so
- Repeat neuropsychological testing six months after brain injury shows no further improvement; still only average memory but slightly below-average complex motor speed, complex attention and cognitive flexibility
- Trial of methylphenidate (Ritalin) in an attempt to improve subjective cognitive performance and work productivity back to baseline: causes activation and paranoia
- Trials of a number of SSRIs, SNRIs, tricyclic antidepressants to improve mood and anxiety either did not work or were not tolerated
- Referred to you for evaluation and management

Current Medications

- Citalopram (Celexa) 10 mg/day
- Clonazepam (Klonopin) 0.5 mg/day
- ACE (angiotensin converting enzyme) inhibitor for hypertension
- Statin for hypercholesterolemia
- Omeprazole for GERD (gastroesophageal reflex disease)
- Aspirin
- CPAP

From the information given, what do you think the diagnosis for this patient's mood disorder is?

- Unipolar major depression with anxiety
- Bipolar spectrum disorder
- Organic affective disorder
- Unipolar major depression with anxiety and organic effective disorder
- Bipolar spectrum disorder and organic effective disorder
- Other

Attending Physician's Mental Notes: Initial Psychiatric Evaluation

- Seems to have had a good recovery so far from a potentially devastating head injury
- However, recovery from head injury does appear to be incomplete
- He is undoubtedly frustrated at incomplete recovery although thankful for avoiding the worst case outcome

- Nevertheless, he is now nearly a year out from his head injury and it is likely that the majority of his recovery has already occurred, or at least that the pace of any further recovery is likely to be very slow and over many months
- He may have some organic cognitive symptoms, but his mood disorder is likely to be linked both to his mild pre-existing mood and anxiety disorder, plus the psychosocial stressor of the head injury, requiring an adjustment in the workplace, rather than to an organic affective disorder
- His disinhibition does suggest, however a mild organic component to his mood

From the information given, what do you think is the cause of his continuing low work productivity?

- Secondary to anxious depression, pre-existing but currently not in remission
- Subtle and now permanent organic brain syndrome
- Laziness in an MD clever enough to try to exploit his head injury to work at an easier pace
- Unreasonable and diabolical, profit-motivated HMO productivity demands!
- All the above

Attending Physician's Mental Notes: Initial Psychiatric Evaluation, Continued

- The cognitive deficiency from his head injury is now subtle and seems only to be unmasked under situations where the limits of anyone would be exposed
- He was able to handle this schedule previously, so his problems do represent a problem linked to incomplete recovery from his head injury and not likely to be due to his mild to moderate depression
- Further recovery is possible, but not a good idea to over-work but to set his pace and see if he gets better over the next year
- Unfortunately, business is business and his colleagues and his employer expect him to "pull his weight" and he is asked to take a pay cut in proportion to his reduced productivity
- The patient is upset and his wife thinks he should consult an employment lawyer
- The patient thinks this will poison the work environment for him, so refuses to do so

Given his head injury and single seizure, would you avoid treating him with bupropion?

- Yes
- No

Of the following choices, what would you do?

- Add another antidepressant
- Switch to another antidepressant
- Add a mood stabilizer
- Add modafinil (Provigil) or armodafinil (Nuvigil)
- None of the above

If you would give an antidepressant, which would you add?

- SSRI (serotonin selective reuptake inhibitor)
- SNRI (serotonin norepinephrine reuptake inhibitor)
- NDRI (bupropion; norepinephrine dopamine reuptake inhibitor)
- NRI (norepinephrine reuptake inhibitor)
- Mirtazapine
- Trazodone
- Tricyclic antidepressant
- MAO inhibitor
- I would not give an antidepressant

Attending Physician's Mental Notes: Initial Psychiatric Evaluation, Continued

- Most likely his cognitive problems are linked to his head injury, but he is moderately depressed, so we might get lucky and improve his cognition if his depression goes into complete remission
- In many ways, cognitive symptoms linked to depression might be the most treatable cognitive symptoms he could have and also the fastest to respond to effective treatment, so it is definitely worth trying
- In selecting an antidepressant, best to avoid one that is either sedating or that causes sexual side effects
- Although any antidepressant that improves his depressive episode sufficient for a complete remission would be able to concomitantly improve the cognitive symptoms of depression, choosing an agent with pro-dopaminergic effects might be preferable
- Although immediate release formulations of bupropion have an increased incidence of seizures, controlled release formulations of bupopion do not
- Thus, he was started on bupropion XL 150 mg once daily

Case Outcome: First Interim Followup, Week 4

- Four weeks later "99% success"
- Depression, rumination, anxiety gone; staying up later; more energy, getting more done at work (increased work load) and at home (photography hobby)
- Sometimes a bit overactivated, especially with caffeine
- Has to stop drinking coffee now
- Has some continuing sexual dysfunction (continued his citalopram)
- Notes forgetting of some phone calls with clonazepam 1.0 mg qhs, so reduces again to 0.5 mg qhs but experiences some insomnia
- Switch to zolpidem (Ambien) from clonazepam for sleep
- Reduced citalopram to 5 mg

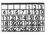

Case Outcome: Second Interim Followup, Week 12

- In another eight weeks, patient reports continuing sexual dysfunction and muscle twitching and headaches even on 5 mg citalopram. When he stops it on his own, immediately these side effects are gone
- Citalopram discontinued
- Increased bupropion XL to 300 mg

Case Outcome: Third Interim Followup, Week 28

- After another four months, doing very well except for slight mood reactivity with depression and anxiety when under more stress
- Sees up to 10 patients per hour, but under pressure from HMO and colleagues/partners to pull full weight and get back to 11
- Gets flustered occasionally at slightly reduced workload, and too exhausted to extend work hours
- Employer considering reduction of pay for full-time work with only 10/11 productivity; patient considering disability litigation
- And so it goes for practicing medicine in the 21st century. . . .

Case Debrief

- This patient with mild pre-existing depression and anxiety not needing psychopharmacological management, developed depression in response to a head injury that left him disabled for a while, and now appears to be headed for a robust but incomplete recovery
- Treatment of residual symptoms of depression definitely improved his cognition, his frustration tolerance, and sense of well being

Take-Home Points

- Bupropion in sustained-release formulations is not demonstrably more pro-convulsant than any other antidepressant (1/1000), but patient should be advised and get his/her consent
- It can be difficult to see the consequences of closed head injury in a high-functioning patient unless (s)he is pushed to the limits of his/her high function
- Affective disorder can compound the effects of a head injury and may be the most treatable component of patients with both
- Nevertheless, agents that enhance DA and NE in prefrontal cortex may be useful in the executive dysfunction of residual head injury as well as in the executive dysfunction of depression and anxiety

Performance in Practice: Confessions of a Psychopharmacologist

- *What could have been done better here?*
  - Perhaps some intervention with his employers to ensure that they understand his limits would take some pressure off him
  - Trying to resolve this situation without litigation with his employer or his disability carrier would be ideal, since losing his job or prolonged litigation is likely to make his depression, and possibly even his cognition, worse
  - Perhaps earlier treatment of his depression with bupropion would have been helpful
- Possible action item for improvement in practice
  - Make sure he has a support mechanism with psychotherapy for his frustrations
  - More active involvement of his wife may have been indicated, so getting spouse involved early in treatment could be an item for improvement

Tips and Pearls

- The dorsolateral prefrontal cortex is the site where problem solving and executive functioning is regulated
- This is the exact area of the brain he damaged on his bicycle and is also the same area of the brain thought to be involved in the cognitive symptoms of depression
- Improving the efficiency of information processing in this part of the brain, buy boosting dopamine and/or norepinephrine neurotransmission, can lead to subjective and objective improvement in executive functioning just as in ADHD

Posttest Self Assessment Question: Answer

Agents that enhance DA and NE in prefrontal cortex may be useful in treating executive dysfunction of a residual head injury, but not for the cognitive dysfunction of depression and anxiety.

A. True

B. False

Answer: B. False

These agents can be useful for executive dysfunction from both of these as well as other causes.

References

1. Stahl SM, Antidepressants, in Stahl's Essential Psychopharmacology, 3rd edition, Cambridge University Press, New York, 2008, pp 511–666
2. Stahl SM, Bupropion, in Stahl's Essential Psychopharmacology The Prescriber's Guide, 3rd edition, Cambridge University Press, New York, 2009, pp 57–62

The Case: The computer analyst who thought the government would choke him to death

The Question: Can you tell the difference between schizophrenia, delusional disorder and obsessive compulsive disorder?

The Dilemma: What do you do when antipsychotics do not help delusions?

Pretest Self Assessment Question (answer at the end of the case)

Which disorder(s) listed below have hallucinations associated with them?

A. OCD
B. Delusional disorder
C. Schizophrenia
D. Simple schizophrenia
E. Schizotypal personality disorder

Patient Intake

- 38-year-old man referred for evaluation of his chief complaint that "the government is out to get me and there is a grand conspiracy against me"

Psychiatric History

- Uneventful childhood but became "suspicious" with some strange thoughts and sexual ideas diagnosed as OCD and for which he retained insight that they were excessive and not true
- He would look at people in the face and develop disturbing sexual thoughts, so began to avoid eye contact
- Given SSRIs with equivocal improvement
- Some affective instability variably diagnosed as bipolar disorder or schizoaffective disorder
- Main treatment was psychotherapy between ages 19 and 27 which the patient believes helped him greatly "hold things together"
- After college, got a job as a computer analyst for the government, but quit precipitously a few months ago after he began to think that the government was against him and they would "do him in" by which he thought he would be choked to death
- Is currently preoccupied by police cars, thinking they are after him
- He now regrets resigning from his job but has no doubt that the government is actually after him, even though he admits no one else, including his wife, believes this
- Affect somewhat flat but not overtly depressed
- No other delusions, no hallucinations and no thought disorder

Social and Personal History

- College graduate
- Successful computer analyst for 15 years
- Married
- No children
- No drug or alcohol abuse

Medical History

- Obese
- Smoker

Family History

- Sister: schizophrenia
- Paternal aunt: schizophrenia

Current Medications

- Topiramate (Topamax) 300 mg/day
- Buproprion SR (Wellbutrin SR) 300 mg/day
- Buspirone (Duspar) 60 mg/day
- Paroxetine (Paxil, Seroxat) 60 mg/day
- Aripiprazole (Abilify) 40 mg/day
- Risperidone (Risperdal) 8 mg/day

What do you think is his diagnosis?

- OCD
- Paranoid schizophrenia
- Schizoaffective disorder
- Delusional disorder
- Simple schizophrenia
- Schizophreniform disorder
- Schizotypal personality disorder
- Obsessive compulsive personality disorder
- Schizoid personality disorder

Attending Physician's Mental Notes: Initial Psychiatric Evaluation

- Seems like early OCD evolving into paranoia, but of a delusional nature, not of a paranoid schizophrenia nature
- Does not seem like simple schizophrenia
  - Even though no hallucinations present
  - Not much functional decline yet

- Also, this is an ICD10 and not a DSM IV concept
- However, the patient is still young and if his symptoms progress, simple schizophrenia might be a future diagnostic consideration
- Since he has delusions, this is not schizotypal personality disorder
  - However, he may have had some premorbid schizotypal features with his early OCD symptoms, such as unusual perceptual experience, odd thinking, suspiciousness, lack of many close friends and excessive social anxiety

How would you treat him?
- Try another SSRI
- Try another atypical antipsychotic
- Raise the dose further of his current SSRI
- Raise the doses further of his current antipsychotics
- Reduce the doses of his antipsychotics
- Discontinue one of his antipsychotics
- Refer for psychotherapy

Attending Physician's Mental Notes: Initial Psychiatric Evaluation, Continued

- He seems excessively medicated, probably in an attempt to get better control of his delusion about the government, but obviously without much benefit
  - Should his medications be decreased?
  - Should he try heroic doses of different medications?
- Decided to recommend discontinuation of both bupropion SR and paroxetine, cross tapering them with fluvoxamine, an agent with sigma 1 properties reported to work both in OCD and in delusional/psychotic depression
- For now, leave other medications alone

Case Outcome: First Interim Followup, Week 12

- His local psychiatrist switched his bupropion and paroxetine to fluvoxamine 200 mg/day without notable changes in symptoms

Attending Physician's Mental Notes: First Interim Followup, Week 12

- Sometimes responses to SSRIs are slow, so plan to keep with fluvoxamine for a few more months
- The question is whether to reduce his antipsychotics, or switch him to another heroic dosing trial with another antipsychotic

- Since aripiprazole has higher affinity for D2 dopamine receptors than risperidone, and is only a partial agonist, it can theoretically interfere with the actions of risperidone
- The first thing to try is to reduce aripiprazole and maintain risperidone and see if, despite lowering the total dose of the two antipsychotics, that he might actually show improvement
- If this does not work, there are anecdotal reports, but very little data, that some patients with schizophrenia seem to respond to very high doses of olanzapine or quetiapine, so maybe that is worth a try even though there is essentially no evidence of the results of this approach in patients with delusional disorder

Case Outcome: Second Interim Followup, Week 24

- His local psychiatrist stopped his aripiprazole (it takes a few weeks to wash out aripiprazole since it has a 2 to 3 day half life with an active metabolite with a similarly long half life), and his doctor tapered it down although aripiprazole tapers itself and can be stopped at once
- Amazingly, the patient seems somewhat better, but not dramatically so
- Opted to continue to observe, possibly increase his fluvoxamine while keeping risperidone dose stable and see if there is further improvement over the next few months

Case Debrief

- This patient was a first degree relative of two family members with schizophrenia
- His disorder is consistent with being related to schizophrenia, as a lower severity and later onset condition such as delusional disorder
- However, some epidemiological studies suggest that delusional disorder may not be increased in family members of patients with schizophrenia
- If the patient has some odd thoughts that he knows are false (i.e., obsessions) and other odd thoughts that only he thinks are true (i.e., delusions), it is possible that he has evolved from a case of OCD, perhaps with some schizotypal personality features, into a case of comorbid delusional disorder plus OCD that may be on the way to becoming a case of simple schizophrenia
- Delusional disorder typically has onset around age 40, whereas schizophrenia generally starts much earlier
- Delusional disorder can be impervious not only to reason, but also to antipsychotics
- Combination of aripiprazole with other psychotics such as risperidone can actually reduce the efficacy of risperidone since aripiprazole successfully competes for D2 receptors with risperidone

Performance in Practice: Confessions of a Psychopharmacologist

- What could have been done better here?
  - Should neuropsychological testing have been done in his teens and then repeated more recently as additional symptoms evolved?
  - Should he get neuropsychological testing now as a baseline in case his condition evolves further with cognitive decline, to document his current functioning and have a potential quantitative assessment of cognitive functioning for comparison in the future?
- Possible action items for improvement in practice
  - Did he evolve into too high dosing and too many drugs in a desperate attempt to help him?
  - Sometimes it is better to accept the limits of the drugs, especially antipsychotics, and not overtreat because this may generate more side effects in the long run than justified by meager therapeutic effects
  - Psychotherapy has helped this patient in the past, and rather than challenge his delusion, use psychotherapy to help him learn not to talk about this delusion at work or in social settings so it does not compromise potential future employment or friends

Two-Minute Tute: A brief lesson and psychopharmacology tutorial (tute) with relevant background material for this case – Differential diagnosis of delusional disorder

Delusional disorder according to DSM IV and ICD 10

- Nonbizarre delusions
- Patients do not have simultaneous hallucinations, disorganized speech, negative symptoms
- Functioning is not markedly impaired
- Behavior not obviously odd or bizarre
- If mood disorder has occurred, episodes are brief compared to duration of delusions
- Not due to a substance

Delusional Disorder

- Mean age of onset 40 years
- Rare (schizophrenia prevalence 1%; delusional disorder 0.03%)
- Kendler (1985) found no increased incidence of schizophrenia or schizoid-schizotypal personality disorder in first degree relatives of delusional disorder patients, unlike this patient and his family
- Persecutory type which this patient has, is the most common type (other types are erotomanic, grandiose, jealous, and somatic)
- Delusions are systematized, coherent and defended with clear logic, in contrast to many persecutory delusions of schizophrenia
- Patients with OCD show varying degree of insight into their obsessions and compulsions; if reality testing is lost and conviction in their beliefs reaches the level of delusions, both disorders may be present
- Psychopharmacological myth is that the antipsychotic pimozide may be more effective than other treatments, but this has not held up to further studies, and pimozide has enhanced cardiovascular risks from drug interactions and overdose compared to other antipsychotics

Simple Schizophrenia

- A concept in ICD10 used in Europe and other parts of the world, but not a concept in DSM IV and not used as a concept as much in the United States
- An uncommon disorder
- Insidious but progressive onset of oddities of conduct, inability to meet the demands of society and decline in total performance
- Delusions and hallucinations not evident
- Negative symptoms of schizophrenia develop without being preceded by any overt psychotic symptoms
- With increasing social impoverishment, vagrancy may ensue and the individual become self absorbed, idle and aimless

Schizotypal Personality Disorder

- May be the DSM equivalent of simple schizophrenia, except simple schizophrenia is generally progressive
- Pervasive social and interpersonal deficits
- Reduced capacity for close relationships
- Cognitive or perceptual distortions, eccentricities of behavior beginning by early adulthood
- Ideas of reference
- Odd beliefs, magical thinking
- Inconsistent with subcultural norms (superstitious, clairvoyant, telepathic)
- Unusual perceptual experiences
- Odd thinking and speech (vague, circumstantial, metaphorical, overelaborate or stereotyped)
- Suspicious or paranoid ideation
- Inappropriate or constricted affect
- Odd, eccentric, peculiar behavior
- Lack of close friends or confidants
- Excessive social anxiety

Posttest Self Assessment Question: Answer

Which disorder(s) listed below have hallucinations associated with them?

A. OCD
   – No hallucinations
B. Delusional disorder
   – No hallucinations
C. Schizophrenia
   – According to either ICD10, DSM-IV or both, this is the only one of these five diagnoses with hallucinations
D. Simple schizophrenia
   – No hallucinations
E. Schizotypal personality disorder
   – No hallucinations

Answer: C

References

1. Stahl SM, The sigma enigma: can sigma receptors provide a novel target for disorders of mood and cognition? J Clin Psychiatry 2008; 69: 1673–4
2. Stahl SM, Antidepressant treatment of psychotic major depression: potential role of the sigma receptor. CNS Spectrums 2005; 10: 319–23
3. Hayashi T and Stahl SM, The sigma1 receptor and its role in the treatment of mood disorders. Drugs of the Future 2009; 34: 137–46
4. Manschreck TC, Khan NL. Recent advances in the treatment of delusional disorder. Can J Psychiatry 2006; 51(2): 114–9
5. Kendler KS. Demography of paranoid psychosis (delusional disorder): a review and comparison with schizophrenia and affective illness. Arch Gen Psychiatry 1982; 39(8): 890–902
6. Kendler KS, Maserson CC, Davis KL. Psychiatric illness in first-degree relatives of patients with paranoid psychosis, schizophrenia and medical illness. Br J Psychiatry 1985;147: 524–31
7. O'Connor K, Stip E, Pelissier MC, et al. Treating delusional disorder: a comparison of cognitive-behavioural therapy and attention placebo control. Can J Psychiatry 2007; 52(3): 182–90
8. Liberman RP. Recovery from Disability: Manual of Psychiatric Rehabilitation. Arlington VA. Amer Psychiatric Publishing Inc; 2008.
9. Stahl SM, Risperidone, in Stahl's Essential Psychopharmacology The Prescriber's Guide, 3rd edition, Cambridge University Press, New York, 2009, pp 475–81
10. Stahl SM, Aripiprazole, in Stahl's Essential Psychopharmacology The Prescriber's Guide, 3rd edition, Cambridge University Press, New York, 2009, pp 45–50
11. Stahl SM, Fluvoxamine, in Stahl's Essential Psychopharmacology The Prescriber's Guide, 3rd edition, Cambridge University Press, New York, 2009, pp 215–20
12. Citrome L, Kantrowitz JT, Olanzapine dosing above the licensed range is more efficacious than lower doses: fact or fiction? Expert Reviews Neurother 2009; 9: 1045–58
13. Stahl SM, Antipsychotics, in Stahl's Essential Psychopharmacology, 3rd edition, Cambridge University Press, New York, 2008, pp 327–452
14. Citrome L, Quetiapine: dose response relationship to schizophrenia CNS Drugs 2008; 22: 69–72
15. Lindenmayer J-P, Citrome L, Khan A, Kaushik S, A randomized double-blind, parallel-grou, fixed dose, clinical trial of quetiapine 600 mg/day vs 1200 mb/day for patients with treatment-resistant

schizophrenia or schizoaffective disorder. Abstracts of the Society for Biological Psychiatry, 2010, New Orleans, Louisiana

16. Stahl SM, Grady MM. A critical review of atypical antipsychotic utilization: Comparing monotherapy with polypharmacy and augmentation. Cur Med Chem 11: 313–26

17. Stahl SM and Buckley PF. Negative Symptoms of Schizophrenia: a problem that will not go away. Acta Scandinavia Psychiatria 2007; 115: 4–11

18. Buckley PF and Stahl SM. Pharmacological Treatment of negative symptoms of schizophrenia: therapeutic opportunity or Cul-de-Sac? Acta Scandinavia Psychiatria 2007: 115: 93–200

The Case: The severely depressed man with a life insurance policy soon to lose its suicide exemption

The Question: Is unstable depression without mania or hypomania a form of unipolar depression or bipolar depression?

The Dilemma: Do mood stabilizers work for patients with very unstable mood even if the patient has no history of mania or hypomania?

Pretest Self Assessment Question (answer at the end of the case)

What percentage of depressed patients are now considered to have either bipolar I depression, bipolar II depression or a mixed/bipolar spectrum/bipolar not otherwise specified (NOS) diagnosis and how many have unipolar major depression?

A. About 2% bipolar I depression, 2% bipolar II depression, 10% bipolar spectrum/NOS and 86% unipolar depression
B. About 2% bipolar I depression, 10% bipolar II depression, 15% bipolar spectrum/NOS and 73% unipolar depression
C. About 2% bipolar I depression, 15% bipolar II depression, 33% bipolar spectrum/NOS and 50% unipolar depression

Patient Intake

- 28-year-old man
- Chief complaint: tiredness and depression

Psychiatric History

- Onset of depressive symptoms: at age 11, in the sixth grade; possibly related to the break-up with a girlfriend
- Symptoms of depression waxed and waned ever since then, but no recall of feeling fully well ever since age 11 except for a short period of time in recent months while on antidepressants
- In college, at age 21, had a more serious and sustained major depressive episode, and recovered without treatment to his usual level of incomplete remission
- Experienced a great deal of waxing and waning mood throughout the rest of his 20s
- Graduated from college as a software programmer, married at age 24, and had a child at age 26
- Did not get any treatment until 2 years ago, after his child was born, as he thought he should get some help due to the increased responsibilities of being a father and as he saw his wife have an excellent response to antidepressant treatment after her own postpartum depressive episode
- Has tried various antidepressants over the past 2 years

- Trial of venlafaxine (Effexor XR)
  - no response until 300 mg
  - at 300 mg, felt "wired" with possibly a mild hypomanic reaction but it was dysphoric and so he discontinued the venlafaxine
- Trial of nortriptyline (Pamelor)
  - no effect
- Trial of citalopram (Celexa)
  - no effect
- Trial of phenelzine (Nardil)
  - excellent initial and fast onset response according to him
  - as the dose went to 60 mg he became "speedy Gonzales" according to his wife
  - had energy and motivation
  - this was out of character as though he has been suddenly "switched on"
  - However, mood itself was not high
  - Not entirely clear whether he was just activated or had hypomania
  - Felt as good as he remembered feeling at age 10 before all his depression
  - Subjectively did not feel euphoric or high
  - Lasted for several months, then the effect wore off
- Switched to another monoamine oxidase inhibitor, tranylcypromine (Parnate), but it did not restore his full recovery or cause activation
- Upon discontinuation of tranylcypromine, he crashed to a much lower state of depression with lack of motivation
- Started divalproex (Depakote); did not tolerate it and discontinued one month later
- Most recently, started on bupropion (Wellbutrin SR) which has helped a bit

Patient Intake

- Continues to complain of longstanding symptoms of low energy and hypersomnia associated with physical tiredness and depressed mood
- Continues to work full time but without enthusiasm
- Patient discloses thoughts of suicide
- He has long planned to leave his family enough money to live without his income by purchasing a large insurance policy on his life when his child was born
- However, has a 2-year exclusion clause for suicide, and in order to pay out to his family, he must not commit suicide before this date
- Admits that he knows the exact date that his family could collect on his policy after which he can commit suicide, which is in about a year
- Is sure he will not act on suicidal ideas before then, but unwilling to make any promises for what would happen after that

Social and Personal History

- Married, one child a year old
- College graduate
- Computer programmer
- Non smoker
- No drug or alcohol abuse

Medical History

- BP normal
- BMI normal
- Normal fasting glucose and lipids

Family History

- Father: high anxiety
- One sister: depression; another sister with anxiety
- Paternal aunt: seasonal depression
- No unequivocal history of first degree relative with bipolar disorder

From the information given, what do you think is his diagnosis?

- Recurrent major depression
- Rapid-cycling bipolar disorder
- Bipolar II disorder
- Bipolar spectrum/NOS
- Other

Attending Physician's Mental Notes: Initial Psychiatric Evaluation

- Not a classic case of either bipolar or unipolar depression
- Began as perhaps a case of dysthymia, or cycling between major depression and dysthymia and poor interepisode recovery until worst ever episode in his 20s, which could be considered a type of unipolar depression sometimes called "double depression"
- On the other hand, he could also have one of the bipolar spectrum disorders in the absence of overt mania or hypomania, such as what Akiskal would call Bipolar II1/2 (See Figure 3), namely cyclothymia with superimposed major depression
- The point is, that major depression would hypothetically respond to an antidepressant whereas a bipolar spectrum disorder would potentially get worse on an antidepressant and require mood stabilizers
- As a young adult, he may have had recurrent major depressive episodes, but his lack of response to antidepressants plus overly robust activation, and even possible antidepressant induced mania/

hypomania suggest that he might have progressed to a bipolar spectrum disorder that Akiskal would call bipolar III (see Figure 4)
- There is even concern that his mood disorder may have become progressive with long term symptoms over many years and inadequate symptomatic improvement (Figure 10)
- In any event, this pattern suggests cautious use of antidepressants and weighs in favor of a mood stabilizer trial even though not either bipolar I or unequivocally bipolar II

Of the following choices, what would you do?
- Add antipsychotic
- Add another antidepressant
- Add anticonvulsant mood stabilizer
- Add lithium
- Start supportive psychotherapy to explore suicidal ideation
- None of the above

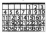

Case Outcome: First 12 Weeks of Followup Visits

- Patient agrees to supportive psychotherapy
- Sessions alone and some with his wife acknowledge his feelings and his plans
- Patient discusses openly his suicidal ideation and plans with his wife in therapy sessions
- Agrees to give treatment time to work
- The best he can do is agree not to commit suicide until at least 3 months after the life insurance policy becomes payable for suicide
- After several sessions, drops out of psychotherapy because of expense and time away from work, but agrees to continue psychopharmacology followup visits monthly
- Started lamotrigine (Lamictal) with slow upward titration over several weeks while receiving weekly psychotherapy
- Continued his bupropion SR 150 mg twice daily and then increased it to 200 mg twice daily

Case Outcome: Second Interim Followup, Week 20

- Seen 2 months later
- More energy, more stable; not very enthusiastic about results, however
- Feels low most of the time, but not low enough for suicidal thoughts which are better
- Continued lamotrigine 200 mg/day plus bupropion SR 200 mg twice a day

Case Outcome: Third Interim Followup, Week 24

- Seen one month later, no improvement, demoralized, got a cold, and if anything feels worse, but not suicidal
- Hard to tell what is happening, but since he has experienced overall improvement from the initiation of lamotrigine despite his recent setback, decide to continue medications and re-evaluate once his upper respiratory infection (URI) is resolved

Case Outcome: Fourth Interim Followup, Week 32

- Seen 2 months later
- 50% responder overall; not impressed with results, however
- Wife is more enthusiastic about his progress
- Still has viral URI (upper respiratory infection) still hanging on and that also makes him feel sluggish and low
- Trial of modafinil (Provigil) 100–200 mg per day

Case Outcome: Fifth Interim Followup, Week 36

- One month later, reports that one or two doses modafinil makes him feel more awake and less tired
- Tapered bupropion on his own to half dose (200 mg SR) "because I don't think it works"
- Agrees to bring wife to next appointment
- Agrees to continue lamotrigine and bupropion at full doses until then

Case Outcome: Sixth Interim Followup, Week 44

- Seen 2 months later, still feels tired
- Pharmacy had made an incredible mistake dispensing topiramate (Topamax) rather than lamotrigine and patient got very tired on it!
- Error discovered after a few doses and reinstituted lamotrigine
- Overall, feels slightly better than at last appointment
- URI is resolved which is helping his subjective well-being
- Wife is very relieved that maybe the danger has passed but recognizes patient has a long way to go for remission
- Wife reveals that one of the reasons he decreased bupropion dose was to save money
- Given some samples of the most expensive medication (modafinil) and patient agrees to continue full doses until next visit

Case Outcome: Seventh Interim Followup, Week 52

- 2 months later, namely, 10 months after starting lamotrigine, patient feels that his progress has stalled at an unacceptable level of depression
- Trial of venlafaxine augmentation to bupropion, lamotrigine, and modafinil

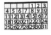

Case Outcome: Eighth Interim Followup, Week 56

- Venlafaxine not tolerated, with insomnia and headaches; discontinued with some withdrawal effects and then back to incomplete recovery

Case Outcome: Ninth and Subsequent Interim Interim Followup, Weeks 56 to 108

- Maintained lamotrigine, bupropion and intermittent modafinil over the next year; patient perception is not improving, but wife's perception is a steady improvement
- Finally reached full remission with no waxing and waning about 18 months after initiating lamotrigine, maintaining bupropion, now with very little modafinil
- Has hinted at wanting to stop treatment, but is seen twice yearly and now in full remission for over eight years; continuing full time in software, now 38-years-old with second child

Case Debrief

- Even patients with bipolar NOS may respond to mood stabilizers
- Many patients have bipolar NOS, but there are no approved medications for it
- Lamotrigine often works as the "stealth" antidepressant, meaning that since it has a long titration period and does not immediately help sleep or provide energy, the recovery seems to "sneak up on you" and only appear dramatic in retrospect
- Patients with long-standing symptoms, such as this patient for over 14 years, may not have a full recovery in 8 weeks
- May require many months to respond, especially if there is the possibility of hippocampal cell loss from the stress of uncontrolled symptoms, and the need for hippocampal neurogenesis to provide input to full recovery, taking many months to occur (at least in theory).

Take-Home Points

- Major depression can be recurrent, and recurrences can possibly indicate disease progression potentially manifested as shorter and shorter periods of wellness between subsequent episodes, with eventually poor interepisode recovery, and ultimately, treatment resistance
- This may be linked to changes in brain structure and neurotrophic factors
- Patients with 3 or more episodes of depression should be treated indefinitely with antidepressant maintenance

Performance in Practice: Confessions of a Psychopharmacologist

- What could have been done better here?
  - Perhaps explaining at the outset that improvement from long term depression might take months or even a year or two rather than weeks
  - Setting expectations may allow the patient to await recovery without getting demoralized, or taking desperate measures
  - Perhaps finding a way for the patient and his wife to continue some form of psychotherapy, even through counseling services or their church would have been helpful here
- Possible action item for improvement in practice
  - Setting better expectations, not only for initial response and remission in a case like this, but for life long treatment
  - The patient remains at high risk of dropping out of treatment and stopping his medications and thus having a relapse

Tips and Pearls

- Lamotrigine can take months and months to work
- Dramatic responses to antidepressants are frequently transient and not sustained
- Remaining on treatment to stay well and prevent relapse is as important as getting well and attaining remission
- Sustained remission is the goal of treatment

PATIENT FILE

Two-Minute Tute: A brief lesson and psychopharmacology tutorial (tute) with relevant background material for this case
– Bipolar subtypes
– Bipolar vs unipolar depression

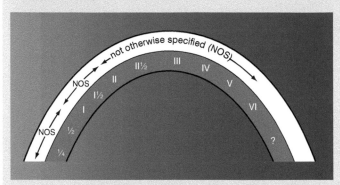

Figure 1: The Bipolar Spectrum. The only formal unique bipolar diagnoses identified in the Diagnostic and Statistical Manual of Mental Disorders, fourth edition (DSM-IV) are bipolar I, bipolar II, and cyclothymic disorder, with all other presentations that include mood symptoms above the normal range lumped together in a single category called "not otherwise specified (NOS)." However, there is a huge variation in the presentation of patients within this bipolar NOS category. It may be more useful instead to think of these patients as belonging to a bipolar spectrum and to identify subcategories of presentations, as has been done by Akiskal and other experts.

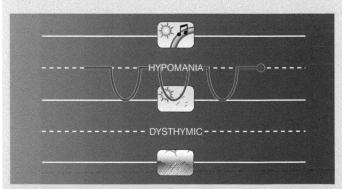

Figure 2: Bipolar I½. A formal diagnosis of bipolar II disorder requires the occurrence not only of hypomanic episodes but also depressive episodes. However, some patients may experience recurrent hypomania without having experienced a depressive episode, a presentation that may be termed bipolar I½. These patients may be at risk of eventually developing a depressive episode and are candidates for mood stabilizing treatment although no treatment is formally approved for this condition.

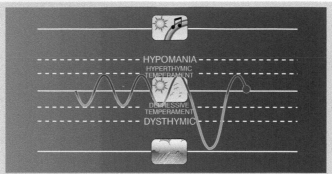

Figure 3: Bipolar II½. Patients may present with a major depressive episode in the context of cyclothymic temperament, which is characterized by oscillations between hyperthymic or hypomanic states (above normal) and depressive or dysthymic states (below normal) upon which a major depressive episode intrudes (bipolar II½). Individuals with cyclothymic temperament who are treated for the major depressive episodes may be at increased risk for antidepressant-induced mood cycling.

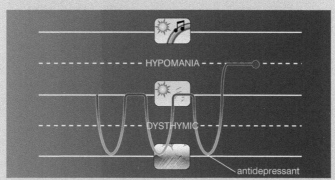

Figure 4: Bipolar III. Although the Diagnostic and Statistical Manual of Mental Disorders, fourth edition (DSM-IV) defines antidepressant-induced hypomania as substance-induced mood disorder, some experts believe that individuals who experience substance-induced hypomania are actually predisposed to these mood states and thus belong to the bipolar spectrum (bipolar III).

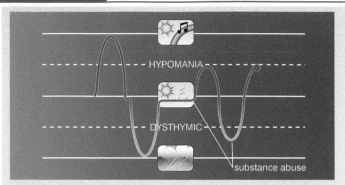

Figure 5: Bipolar III½. Bipolar III½ is bipolar disorder with substance abuse, in which the substance abuse is associated with efforts to achieve hypomania. Such patients should be evaluated closely to determine if hypomania has ever occurred in the absence of substance abuse.

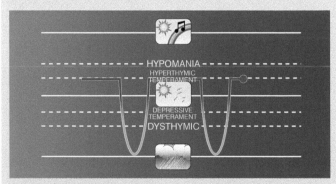

Figure 6: Bipolar IV. Bipolar IV is seen in individuals with long standing and stable hyperthymic temperament in which a major depressive episode intrudes. Individuals with hyperthymic temperament who are treated for depressive episodes may be at increased risk for antidepressant-induced mood cycling and may instead respond better to mood stabilizers.

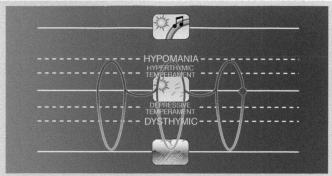

Figure 7: Bipolar V. Bipolar V is defined as major depressive episodes with hypomanic symptoms occurring during the major depressive episode, but without the presence of discrete hypomanic episodes. Because the symptoms do not meet full criteria for mania, these patients would not be considered to have a full mixed episode but nonetheless exhibit a mixed presentation and may require mood stabilizer treatment as opposed to antidepressant monotherapy.

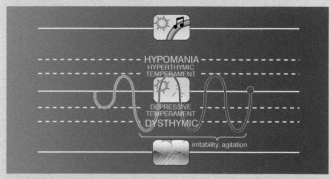

Figure 8: Bipolar VI. Another subcategory within the bipolar spectrum may be "bipolarity in the setting of dementia," termed bipolar VI. Mood instability here begins late in life, followed by impaired attention, irritability, reduced drive, and disrupted sleep. The presentation may initially appear to be attributable to dementia or be considered unipolar depression, but is likely to be exacerbated by antidepressants and may respond to mood stabilizers.

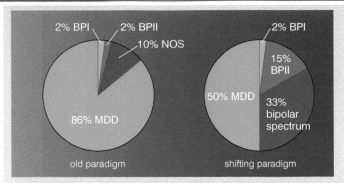

Figure 9: Prevalence of mood disorders. In recent years there has been a paradigm shift in terms of recognition and diagnosis of patients with mood disorders. That is, many patients once considered to have major depressive disorder (MDD) (old paradigm, left) are now recognized as having bipolar II disorder or another form of bipolar illness within the bipolar spectrum (shifting paradigm, right).

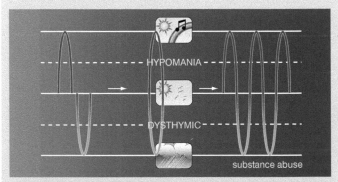

Figure 10: Is bipolar disorder progressive? There is some concern that undertreatment of discrete manic and depressive episodes may progress to mixed and dysphoric episodes and finally to rapid cycling and treatment resistance.

Table 1: Is it unipolar or bipolar depression?

- No foolproof way to tell
- No genetic test yet
- No reliable neuroimaging test yet
- The presenting symptoms of a major depressive episode in bipolar illness may be completely indistinguishable from those of a major depressive episode in unipolar depression. Thus, analysis of the current presentation is not sufficient for making the differential diagnosis between a unipolar and a bipolar disorder. Additional information that is needed includes family history, symptom and treatment-response history, and feedback from a friend or relative.
- Patterns of past symptoms as well as treatment-response history may aid in distinguishing between unipolar and bipolar illness. Although two patients may both present with major depressive episodes, they may have divergent histories that suggest a unipolar illness for one and a bipolar illness for the other
- Although all symptoms of a major depressive episode can occur in either unipolar or bipolar depression, some symptoms may present more often in bipolar vs. unipolar depression, providing hints if not diagnostic certainty that the patient has a bipolar spectrum disorder.
  - increased time sleeping
  - overeating
  - comorbid anxiety
  - psychomotor retardation
  - mood lability during episode
  - psychotic symptoms
  - suicidal thoughts.
- Even in the absence of any previous hypomanic episodes, there are often specific hints in the untreated course of illness that suggest depression is part of the bipolar spectrum. These include
  - early age of onset
  - high frequency of depressive episodes
  - high proportion of time spent ill
  - acute onset or abatement of symptoms
  - behavioral symptoms such as frequent job or relationship changes
- Treatment-response history, particularly prior response to antidepressants, may provide insight into whether depression is unipolar or bipolar. Prior responses that suggest bipolar depression may include
  - multiple antidepressant failures
  - rapid response to an antidepressant
  - activating side effects such as insomnia, agitation, and anxiety

Posttest Self Assessment Question: Answer

What percentage of depressed patients are now considered to have either bipolar I depression, bipolar II depression or a mixed/bipolar spectrum/bipolar not otherwise specified diagnosis and how many have unipolar major depression?

A. About 2% bipolar I depression, 2% bipolar II depression, 10% bipolar spectrum/NOS and 86% unipolar depression

B. About 2% bipolar I depression, 10% bipolar II depression, 15% bipolar spectrum/NOS and 73% unipolar depression

C. About 2% bipolar I depression, 15% bipolar II depression, 33% bipolar spectrum/NOS and 50% unipolar depression

Answer: C

References

1. Stahl SM, Mood Disorders, in Stahl's Essential Psychopharmacology, 3rd edition, Cambridge University Press, New York, 2008, pp 453–510

2. Stahl SM, Antidepressants, in Stahl's Essential Psychopharmacology, 3rd edition, Cambridge University Press, New York, 2008, pp 511–666

3. Stahl SM, Mood Stabilizers, in Stahl's Essential Psychopharmacology, 3rd edition, Cambridge University Press, New York, 2008, pp 667–720

4. Stahl SM, Lamotrigine, in Stahl's Essential Psychopharmacology The Prescriber's Guide, 3rd edition, Cambridge University Press, New York, 2009, pp 259–66

5. Stahl SM, Bupropion, in Stahl's Essential Psychopharmacology The Prescriber's Guide, 3rd edition, Cambridge University Press, New York, 2009, pp 57–62

6. Stahl SM, Modafinil, in Stahl's Essential Psychopharmacology The Prescriber's Guide, 3rd edition, Cambridge University Press, New York, 2009, pp 359–63

7. Judd LL, Akiskal HS, Maser JD et al. Major depressive disorder: a prospective study of residual subthreshold depressive symptoms as predictor of rapid relapse. J Affect Disord 1998; 50(2–3): 97–108

8. Kendler, KS, Thornton, LM, Gardner, CO. Stressful life events and previous episodes in the etiology of major depression in women: an evaluation of the "kindling" hypothesis. Am J Psychiatry 2000; 157: 1243–51

9. Angst J. (2007) The bipolar spectrum. British Journal of Psychiatry 190; 189–91

10. Judd LL, Akiskal HS, Schettler PJ et al. A prospective investigation of the natural history of the long term weekly symptomatic status of bipolar II disorder. Arch Gen Psychiatry 60; 261–9.

11. Merikangas KR, Akiskal HS, Angst J et al. Lifetime and 12-month prevalence of bipolar spectrum disorder in the national Comorbidity Survey replication. Arch Gen Psychiatry 2007; 64(5): 543–52

12. Benazzi F and Akiskal HS. How best to identify bipolar-related subtype among major depressive patients without spontaneous hypomania: superiority of age at onset. J Affect Disord 2008; 107(1–3): 77–88

13. Ng B, Camacho A, Lara DR et al. A case series on the hypothesized connection between dementia and bipolar spectrum disorders: bipolar type VI? J Affect Disord 2008; 107(1–3): 307–15

14. Akiskal HS and Benazzi F. Continuous distribution of atypical depressive symptoms between major depressive and bipolar II disorder: dose-response relationship with bipolar family history. Psychopathology 2008; 41(1): 39–42

15. Vázquez GH, Kahn C, Schiavo CE et al. Bipolar disorders and affective temperaments: a national family study testing the "endophenotype" and "subaffective" theses using the TEMPS-A Buenos Aires. J Affect Disord 2008; 108(1–2): 25–32

16. Oedegaard KJ, Neckelmann D, Benazzi F et al. Dissociative experiences differentiate bipolar-II from unipolar depressed patients: the mediating role of cyclothymia and the Type A behavior speed and impatience subscale. J Affect Disord 2008; 108(3): 207–16

17. Savitz J, van der Merwe L and Ramesar R. Dysthymic and anxiety-related personality trait in bipolar illness. J Affect Disord 2008; 109(3): 305–11

18. Correa R, Akiskal H, Gilmer W et al. Is unrecognized bipolar disorder a frequent contributor to apparent treatment resistant depression? J Affect Disord 2010; 127(1–3): 10–8

The Case: The anxious woman who was more afraid of her anxiety medications than of anything else

The Question: Is medication phobia part of this patient's anxiety disorder?

The Dilemma: How do you treat a patient who has intolerable side effects with every medication?

Pretest Self Assessment Question (answer at the end of the case)

Which of the following is available as a liquid formulation?

A. Citalopram (Celexa)
B. Duloxetine (Cymbalta)
C. Escitalopram (Lexapro)
D. Fluvoxamine (Luvox)

Patient Intake

- 33-year-old woman with a chief complaint of "extreme anxiety"

Psychiatric History

- The patient was well until about age 20 when, as an undergraduate in college, she developed a major depressive episode (perhaps related to seasonal depression)
- She responded to paroxetine (Paxil, Seroxat) and continued treatment with it for two years
- After stopping medication, she had at least two emergency room visits for panic attacks but received no treatment
- Over the next seven years she received no treatment despite experiencing a great deal of generalized anxiety and feeling tense and overwhelmed
- Because of relapse of her depression in the last two years she started again on various SSRIs
- Restarted paroxetine but unlike the first time she took it, could not tolerate it after 2 weeks and discontinued it
  - Had fatigue and blurred vision
- Trial of sertraline (Zoloft)
  - Had worsening anxiety and discontinued it after a week
  - Started CBT
- Trial of fluoxetine (Prozac)
  - First dose caused a panic attack and discontinued it
  - Continued CBT
- Trial of venlafaxine (Effexor XR)
  - Vomited on the first dose and discontinued it
  - Continued CBT

- Trial of fluvoxamine (Luvox)
  - Made her tired and stopped after 3 days
  - Continued CBT
- Trial of duloxetine (Cymbalta)
  - Racing pulse and palpitations after first dose and discontinued it
  - Continued CBT
- Trial of escitalopram (Lexapro)
  - Insomnia and agitation and stopped after 3 days

Social and Personal History

- Single, no children
- Non smoker
- No drug or alcohol abuse
- College graduate
- Unemployed, supported by wealthy parents

Medical History

- Mitral valve prolapse
- BP normal
- BMI normal
- Normal fasting glucose and lipids

Family History

- Father: posttraumatic stress disorder (PTSD) and depression
- Maternal grandparents: alcoholism and anxiety
- Paternal grandparents: bipolar disorder; grandmother received electroconvulsive therapy (ECT)

Current Medication

- Lorazepam 0.5 mg, up to 1.0 mg/day

Attending Physician's Mental Notes: Initial Psychiatric Evaluation

- Patient seems very upset and apprehensive
- Afraid attending physician is going to prescribe something else
- For the last few years she has not been able to function fully independently, to maintain significant relationships, or to maintain steady and fulfilling employment
- The patient is well-informed and well-read but seems to irrationally overvalue the side effects of medications
  - In particular, she anticipates catastrophic consequences such as death in the middle of the night, problems from

serotonin syndrome, and some of the other most dire potential consequences of psychotropic drugs
- She both readily acknowledges the excessive nature of these fears and yet still has some degree of belief in them and certainly experiences subjective fear about them
    - However, she always has activating side effects, electric shock sensations, headaches, tremors on the inside but not on the outside, hair on her head standing on end, no matter what medication she takes lately
    - Does not understand why these problems were not present with these medications in the past nor why she tolerates and, in fact improves on lorazepam (Ativan)
- She also recognizes that her chronic anxiety is interfering with her life and keeping her from being employed, having relationships, and again becoming independent
- She is therefore highly motivated to find a plan to reduce her symptoms and allow her to resume a normal life with the high level of functioning that she has enjoyed in the past
- She displays a broad affect but a somewhat depressed mood, almost becoming tearful at times while discussing her history
- She is able to respond to humor and paradox and is not currently suicidal

With just the information you have now, what do you think is her diagnosis?

- Hysteria
- Hypochondriasis
- GAD
- Medication phobia
- Panic disorder
- Recurrent major depressive disorder with anxious features
- Bipolar II or bipolar NOS being activated by SSRIs/SNRIs, as suggested by her family history
- Psychological conflicts and dependency issues about separation individuation from parents and gaining full independence
- Other

Considering this patient's history, symptoms, and fear of side effects, would you recommend another trial of a serotonergic antidepressant?

- Yes
- No

In addition to trials of 6 SSRIs/SNRIs, and CBT for several months, only lorazepam is giving any relief. Which of the following strategies would you be most likely to suggest to this patient?

- Discontinue medication treatment and begin cognitive behavioral therapy (CBT) and/or psychotherapy with a new therapist
- Maintain current benzodiazepine dose and add new CBT and/or psychotherapy
- Increase dose of benzodiazepine
- Increase dose of benzodiazepine and add new CBT and/or psychotherapy
- Switch to a serotonergic antidepressant
- Switch to a serotonergic antidepressant and add new CBT and/or psychotherapy
- Add a serotonergic antidepressant
- Add both a serotonergic antidepressant and CBT and/or psychotherapy
- Get plasma drug levels on the next serotonergic antidepressant you try

Attending Physican's Mental Notes: Initial Psychiatric Evaluation, Continued

- She clearly needs some form of treatment beyond her current low-dose benzodiazepine in order to resume her normal life and withstand the associated psychosocial stressors without experiencing symptoms of anxiety and depression from a recurrent anxious depression
- She now has superimposed some legitimate side effects but also seems to exaggerate them
- Does not appear to be conscious exaggeration
- Although her side effects overlap with possible hypomanic activating symptoms in some cases, they are much more consistent with anxiety than with substance-induced hypomania from an SSRI
- Although it seems that some of these side effects may reflect self-fulfilling prophecies, and "all in her head" they are nonetheless real to her and require management
- Although CBT and/or psychotherapy are well-established treatment methods for all of her symptoms, including particularly her phobic symptoms, they are not working here after several months
- It is important to rule out abnormal drug metabolism from a genetic predisposition and unusual cytochrome P450 drug metabolizing system
- She can get genotyping or simply a therapeutic drug level on a normal dose of any SSRI/SNRI
- Blood sent for CY450 2D6, 2C9, 2C19 genotyping
- Agrees to try very low dose venlafaxine again

Case Outcome: First Interim Followup, 3 Weeks

- Predictably, had side effects (nausea) on venlafaxine XR
- Was able to take for one week at 37.5 mg/day and had barely detectable plasma drug levels

- Genotyping comes back with no evidence of being a poor metabolizer
- Thus, abnormally high drug levels due to abnormal drug metabolism cannot explain her side effects
- Showed results to patient and told her that she might very well respond with the same side effects to placebo
- Asked if she would be willing to try a behavioral desensitization approach
- Continuing medication treatment may also be helpful and in fact exposure to medications may be important to overcome her phobia of them
- A useful strategy may be a behavioral desensitization approach involving extremely slow dose titration of a serotonergic antidepressant
- Alternatively, she will have to opt for non medication options
  - Continuing CBT
  - Considering rTMS over the right hemisphere (for anxiety) and over the left hemisphere (for depression)
- Could consider chronic higher dose benzodiazepine treatment
- Escitalopram is selected, as it is generally considered one of the better tolerated selective serotonin reuptake inhibitors
- Escitalopram is also available as a liquid, which allows extra flexibility when developing a slow titration schedule
- The patient is instructed to dilute 10 mg liquid escitalopram in 100 ml of fruit juice and then, using an eye dropper, drink 1 ml and dispose of the rest; this can be done daily for 1–3 days
- She can then increase by 1 ml or so every day as she feels comfortable
- This gives her complete control over the pace of dosing and allows her to defer a dose or back off the dosing if desired
- She should slowly and steadily increase her escitalopram concentration over one or two months, until she is on a full 10 mg/day dose
- In the meantime she should continue to take lorazepam, both to reduce her symptoms and as a rescue medication for her escitalopram
- Once escitalopram has been up-titrated, her dose of lorazepam may also be reevaluated and may need to be increased to allow for full symptom control and return to normal functioning

Case Outcome: Second and Subsequent Interim Followup Visits, Over the Next 6 Months

- Slowly but surely, with some pauses in dose increases and some transient side effects, the escitalopram was increased to 10 mg/day while continuing lorazepam

- She eventually relaxed, was reassured, and her symptoms abated
- Whether this was pharmacologically mediated or was de facto CBT as well as systematic desensitization to medication is not clear
- Referred for psychotherapy to deal with adult development issues

Case Debrief

- A patient with pre existing anxiety disorder and a major depressive episode, developed a recurrent anxious depression and developed a phobia to her medications because she had become sensitized to side effects to them
- Systematic desensitization was successful in getting her to a therapeutic level of drug that was tolerated and she responded
- She was likely avoiding dealing with various adult development issues over many years by concentrating on her drugs and side effects

Take-Home Points

- Many factors can significantly impair adherence, including real or feared side effects; clinicians must do their best to address what factors they can
- This may include using unusual titration schedules, emphasizing behavioral treatments over medication treatments, considering alternative treatments, and other strategies

Posttest Self Assessment Question: Answer

Which of the following is available as a liquid formulation?

A. Citalopram
B. Duloxetine
C. Escitalopram
D. Fluvoxamine
Answer: C

References

1. Mrazek DA, Psychiatric Pharmacogenomics, Oxford University Press, New York, 2010
2. Marangell LB, Martinez M, Jurdi RA et al. Neurostimulation therapies. Acta Psychiatrica Scandinavica 2007: 116: 174–81
3. Berman RM, Narasinhan M, Sanacora G et al., A randomized clinical trial of repetitive transcranial magnetic stimulation in the treatment of major depression. Biol Psychiatry 2000; 47: 332–7
4. Avery DH, Holtzheimer PE, Fawaz W et al. A controlled study of repetitive transcranial magnetic stimulation in medication resistant major depression. Biol Psychiatry 2006; 59: 187–94

5. Herwig U, Lampe Y, Juengling FD et al. Add on rTMS for treatment of depression: a pilot study using stereotaxic coil-navigation according to PET data. J Psychiatry Res 2003: 37: 267–75

6. Lisanby SH, Husain MM, Rosenquist PB et al. Daily left prefrontal repetitive transcranial magnetic stimulation in the acute treatment of major depression: clinical predictors of outcome in a multisite, randomized controlled clinical trial. Neuropsychopharmacol 2009; 34: 522–34

7. Demitrack MA, Thase ME. Clinical significance of Transcranial Magnetic Stimulation (TMS) in the treatment of pharmacoresistant depression: synthesis of recent data. Psychopharm Bull 2009; 42: 5–38

8. George MS, Lisanby SH, Avery D et al. Daily left prefrontal transcranial magnetic stimulation therapy for major depressive disorder: a sham-controlled randomized trial. Arch Gen Psychiat 2010; 67: 507–16

9. Garcia KS, Flynn P, Pierce KJ et al. Repetitive transcranial magnetic stimulation treats postpartum depression. Brain Stim 2010; 3: 36–41

10. Gross M, Nakamura L, Pascual-Leone A et al. Has repetitive transcranial magnetic stimulation treatment for depression improved? A systematic review and meta analysis comparing the recent vs the earlier rTMS studies. Acta Psychiatr Scand 2007; 116: 165–73

11. Lam RW, Chan P, Wilkins-Ho M et al. Repetitive transcranial magnetic stimulation for treatment resistant depression: a systematic review and meta analysis. Can J Psychiatry 2008; 53: 621–31

12. O'Reardon J, Solvason H, Janicak, P et al. Efficacy and safety of transcranial magnetic stimulation therapy in the acute treatment of major depression: a multi site randomized controlled trial. Biol Psychiatry 2007; 62: 1208–16

13. Cohen R, Ferreira M, Ferreira M et al. Use of repetitive transcranial magnetic stimulation for the management of bipolar disorder during the postpartum period. Brain Stim 2008; 1: 224–6

14. Stahl SM, Mood Disorders, in Stahl's Essential Psychopharmacology, 3rd edition, Cambridge University Press, New York, 2008, pp 453–510

15. Stahl SM, Antidepressants, in Stahl's Essential Psychopharmacology, 3rd edition, Cambridge University Press, New York, 2008, pp 511–666

16. Stahl SM, Anxiety Disorders and Anxiolytics, in Stahl's Essential Psychopharmacology, 3rd edition, Cambridge University Press, New York, 2008, pp 721–72

17. Stahl SM, Stahl's Illustrated Anxiety, Stress and PTSD, Cambridge University Press, New York, 2010

18. Stahl SM, Lorazepam, in Stahl's Essential Psychopharmacology The Prescriber's Guide, 3rd edition, Cambridge University Press, New York, 2009, pp 295–9

19. Stahl SM, Escitalopram, in Stahl's Essential Psychopharmacology The Prescriber's Guide, 3rd edition, Cambridge University Press, New York, 2009, pp 171–5

The Case: The psychotic woman with delusions that no medication could fix

The Question: How can you weigh severe side effects with therapeutic benefits of clozapine plus augmentation in a severely ill patient?

The Dilemma: Is it possible for a patient to have better functioning even though treatment does not help her delusions?

Pretest Self Assessment Question (answer at the end of the case)

What do you do when standard doses of clozapine do not work?

A. Get plasma drug levels of clozapine and be sure they are between 400–600 ng/ml
B. Go above 550 mg/day oral dosing of clozapine if necessary
C. Augment with lamotrigine, valproate, topiramate or another anticonvulsant
D. Augment with a second antipsychotic
E. Augment with a benzodiazepine
F. Leave well enough alone and accept the fact that the psychosis cannot be treated

Patient Intake

- 34-year-old woman referred for psychopharmacological evaluation of psychosis resistant to treatment even with clozapine

Psychiatric History

- Developed delusions of persecution, ideas of reference and paranoia at age 21
- Called the local sheriff frequently complaining that someone was trying to harm her
- Then developed delusions of grandiosity, thought control, thought broadcasting, with some racing thoughts
- The mother states that before the patient was ever hospitalized, she was apparently kidnapped and taken to another city during which time she received phencyclidine (PCP, angel dust) and was sexually abused
- This aggravated her pre existing psychotic disorder, but there is no record of her being hospitalized at that time, and she returned home
- Whether this is the full truth of the story is not known but the patient states this is what happened and the mother believes her
- The patient was referred to a psychiatrist who counseled her for post traumatic events and prescribed conventional antipsychotics
- However, the patient then ran away from home, ultimately ended up in another country where she became floridly psychotic, was retained and then brought back to her home for intensive psychiatric care in the hospital

- Since then, for the past 10 years, the patient has had significant treatment with a wide range of antipsychotics
- Examiners at that time were impressed with an affective dimension to her psychotic disorder, and wondered whether she had bipolar disorder, like her father and sister, and whether she also had a superimposed organic disorder of a long lasting or permanent nature caused by phencyclidine use
- Medications tried in the previous 10 years include
  - Conventional antipsychotics including: fluphenazine (Prolixin), thiothixene (Navane), haloperidol (Haldol)
  - Atypical antipsychotics including: risperidone (Risperdal), olanzapine (Zyprexa), quetiapine (Seroquel)
  - clozapine (Clozaril), which seemed to help the most but because of drooling and weight gain, discontinued it after six months
  - Antidepressants somewhat helpful, including nefazodone (Serzone)
  - Mood stabilizer helps with distractability and pressure to talk, but do not help with psychotic symptoms (valproate (Depakote))
  - Currently taking progressively increasing doses of loxapine (Loxitane), now at 250 mg daily, plus topiramate (Topamax) 300 mg and clonazepam (Klonopin) 1 mg three times a day
- The question from the referring physician is whether to send the patient for ECT since her medications are working so poorly

Social and Personal History

- High school graduate, started nursing school and dropped out when kidnapped
- Single, no children
- Lives at home with mother
- No drug or alcohol abuse currently
- On long term disability

Medical History

- The patient had a normal BMI at age 21 but is now obese with a BMI of 31
- Non Smoker
- Elevated triglycerides and total cholesterol
- BP normal
- Glucose normal
- Liver function tests normal
- Complete blood count and differential normal
- Hypothyroidism
- Amenorrhea

Family History

- Both her father and her sister have seriously disabling bipolar disorder
- A second sister is very high functioning

Patient Intake, Continued

- The patient believes that she is the replacement of her mother's daughter, and both she and her mother have both been replaced by doubles
- This was done by her long standing evil "rival," who is her nemesis and the bane of her existence
- This symptom is also known as the Capgras syndrome
- The patient believes she is only 17 years old, and lives on the beach in a castle married to a famous actor
- She states that she herself is a physician and believes others are jealous of her and others think she needs psychiatric care but she is able to turn her medications into placebos with her mind in order to foil their attempts to medicate her
- She has been found on several occasions at a local hospital trying to see her patients there and the police have been called on several occasions to remove her
- She states that she has problems with her neurotransmitters and that she has an EENT machine (no further explanation) which will be implanted into her brain by a professional comedian to prevent future problems
- She believes her neurotransmitters are picking up on other people's messages
- The patient claims that she is able to function by putting herself into a coma five hours a day, flying to France daily and has the assistance of her father who is a mob king and a doctor
- The patient calls the sheriff up to twice daily unless her mother hides the phone
- Her mood is a bit irritable, but not depressed nor euphoric

What do you think is her diagnosis?
- Agree with the previous examiner who thinks it is bipolar like her sister and father
- Agree with the previous examiner who thinks long lasting or permanent organic damage from phencyclidine
- Schizoaffective disorder
- Schizophrenia

Attending Physician's Mental Notes: Initial Psychiatric Evaluation

- Has psychosis when mood is not labile, and seems too unremittingly delusional to be pure bipolar disorder, so the best working diagnosis may be schizoaffective disorder
- Phencyclidine can cause a long lasting psychosis in those without a psychotic disorder and can precipitate a recurrent psychosis in a patient with a psychotic disorder, but not well-documented to cause a permanent psychotic, organic or cognitive condition
- In fact, the drug of abuse most likely to trigger schizophrenia-like illness long after the drug has washed out is not phencyclidine nor amphetamine/stimulants, but marijuana which this patient claims to have never used

How would you treat her?
- Increase her loxapine dose
- Add lamotrigine
- Add valproate
- Restart clozapine
- Send her for ECT
- Increase clonazepam
- Discontinue clonazepam or topiramate

Attending Physician's Mental Notes: Initial Psychiatric Evaluation, Continued

- She seems poorly responsive to anything but clozapine
- ECT is controversial for the treatment of psychosis, especially if not in the presence of a strong affective component, and the mother is not interested anyway
- High doses of conventional antipsychotics alone do not seem to be promising, so she was re-initiated on clozapine with appropriate warnings about weight, dyslipidemia and diabetes
- The patient states she will just turn clozapine into placebo with her mind so it doesn't matter to her what she takes

Case Outcome: First through Third Interim Followup, Months 3, 5 and 6

- Clozapine augmentation at 400 mg per day has no effect at month 3 (added to loxapine 250 mg/day plus topiramate 300 mg/day plus clonazepam 1 mg three times a day)
- Clozapine at 600 mg per day has no effect at month 5
- Clozapine at 900 mg per day at month 6 now seems to be improving

the mother's ability to manage the patient, with the patient having some "good days" when she is more cooperative with the activities of daily living at home, but she remains floridly delusional

- Now claims to be investing at home on the internet (her mother calls it phantom investment) several hours a day, generating a great deal of wealth
- Gaining weight (BMI 34), drooling, spending a lot of time in bed but patient states she is going to bed during the day awaiting a surgeon to operate on her for her weight
- Patient states "I am cured of my PTSD;"
- "I had Thanksgiving dinner with the family clones"
- Mother believes clonazepam is actually the most helpful in keeping her daughter from acting out, such as by arguing, talking about her delusions all day, calling the sheriff, etc.
- Slowly, the dose of clonazepam is increased to 6–8 mg/day and the topiramate is discontinued

Attending Physician's Mental Notes: Third Interim Followup, 6 Months

- Her lack of dramatic response to date is discouraging, but sometimes clozapine has very slow onset of therapeutic effects in refractory patients and, with many months of treatment, improvement can be seen
- Two antipsychotics at very high doses, plus a benzodiazepine at a very high dose, seems heroic and controversial
- However, nothing can dispute the irrefutable logic of results here
- The question is whether this small improvement is all attributable to clozapine
- The question also remains whether the short- and long-term side effects of this combination of medications are worth the small therapeutic gains
- Maybe we can augment with something else and have a chance of lowering the clozapine dose later if we see some improvement

Case Outcome: Fourth and Subsequent Interim Followup, Months 7 through 15

- Still delusional and verbally hostile, on clozapine 900 mg/day, refusing to take showers at month 7
- Continues on loxitane 250 mg, plus clonazepam 2 mg three to four times a day
- Trial of levetiracetam (Keppra) anticonvulsant and potential mood stabilizer for augmentation, no improvement at followup visits, months 8 and 9

- Trial of galantamine (Razodyne) a cholinesterase inhibitor and potential cognitive enhancer for augmentation, with no improvement at followup visits months 10 and 11
- Weight gain continues, BMI now 36
- Still not showering regularly and often extremely verbally abusive and hostile to her mother, unless the patient takes clonazepam
- Severe drooling requiring daily pillowcase changes and carrying a towel around all day
- Lipids elevated but glucose normal
- Trial of quetiapine (Seroquel) augmentation, cross tapering off loxapine, no improvement months 12 and 13
- Trial of ziprasidone (Geodon, Zeldox) augmentation, cross tapering off quetiapine (Seroquel), maybe some improvement in hostility and better cooperation months 14 and 15
- Patient now more active
- Says she is doing commercials at home and selling them
- Mother states patient now gets up, gets ready, is active during the day, cleans the house and cooks for herself although she still sleeps during the day every other day (did this every day during the day on loxapine and on quetiapine augmentation trials)

Attending Physician's Mental Notes: Followup Month 15

- The mother is incredibly supportive despite few signs of improvement with various medication trials for more than a year
- It is as though the augmenting antipsychotics loxapine and quetiapine were only sedating her whereas ziprasidone is not
- Maybe high dose clozapine, with high dose clonazepam augmented with ziprasidone, is the best so far, but far from satisfactory
- Because of some continuing sedation, weight gain and drooling, it seems prudent to lower the clozapine dose since the therapeutic benefits do not seem to justify the observed risks
- Mother and patient agree to a trial of lowering clozapine to 800 mg while continuing ziprasidone 80 mg twice a day and clonazepam 2 mg four times a day

Case Outcome: Followup, Months 17 Through 21

- Month 17, on clozapine 800 mg/day, having some difficulty breathing, saw lung specialist who said it was from her weight and not from pulmonary disease or cardiomyopathy, which can be caused by clozapine
- The patient remains floridly delusional but less argumentative and more cooperative

- BMI has now increased to 39
- Begins to walk and exercise and cooperates with her mother on at least half the days of the week to do this
- Still claims to be making commercials for which she is getting paid in another life
- Continuing very, very slow taper of clozapine
  - Rapid taper of clozapine can precipitate psychosis
- By month 21 is down to 550 mg of clozapine, plus ziprasidone 80 mg twice a day, plus clonazepam 2 mg four times a day
- Lost 10 pounds! BMI 37
- Asked patient: "What's up" and she replies "My libido"
- "I should be cured within a few days"
- Mother says the patient has started talking to herself
- "I go to France every day on a private jet and I walk there so I am losing weight"
- Seems to be "waking up" and now, either more delusional, or her mother thinks, just talking about her long standing delusions more but not really worse
- Also, the patient has a sense of humor again, but watchful for whether this represents incipient mania
- Has taken valproate (Depakote) in the past when thought to be manic
- Has never taken lamotrigine
- At month 21, decided to start lamotrigine while continuing taper of clozapine
- Looks like we need to rate her behavior and not her thought content in assessing her response to medications, and perhaps reduce the clozapine further dose if possible

Case Outcome: Followup, Months 23 Through 27

- At months 23 and 24, patient has regained weight, now BMI 40, becoming more immobile, discussed gastric bypass or lap-band for morbid obesity, but controversial to use this approach for morbid obesity due to clozapine
- "People are taking artificial flesh and putting it on my epidermis and that is why I am gaining weight."
- Says she is 17 when she is actually 37
- Capgras syndrome still active and patient still believes she is a replacement of her mother's daughter and her mother is also a replacement of her original mother
- Began physical therapy month 24
- Month 27 clozapine down to 300 mg per day, no more drooling and towel no longer needed, cooking for herself, but weight still up to BMI 40

- However, has a sense of humor and is exercising
- "My rival hired an axe murderer and he cuts my legs off every night, but I am teleported to France every night where Einstein sews them back on – he has made 5 sets for me and has stashed them away"
- Seems as though the main thing that has happened when going from 900 mg of clozapine to 300 mg, is that the patient has woken up, exposing her delusions, and has stopped drooling
- Mother wants to see how low clozapine can go, and determine if the patient can start to lose weight again
- Mother believes that now patient is more rational in her thinking and talking between the times when she talks about her delusions which have not changed in content that much over recent years
- Agree to further taper of clozapine

Case Outcome: Followup Months 27 to 40

- Patient lost to followup for over a year
- Seeing a local physician, closer to home and less expensive
- Clozapine was steadily decreased and then discontinued, while ziprasidone continued at 160 mg/day and clonazapam continued at 2 mg three times a day
- A few months later, wandered off from home, was rehospitalized and clozapine restarted
- Returns month 40, about 4 years after her initial evaluation, on clozapine 200 mg/day, without drooling, plus ziprasidone 160 mg/day and clonazepam 2 mg four times a day
- "My step mom gave the judicial system 30 million dollars"
- "My cranial nerve got pulled out and it changed my receptors"
- Despite health risks, seems that clozapine is required and necessary
- Mother does not want her to be on a higher dose, but to try aripiprazole augmentation

Attending Physician's Mental Notes: Followup a Year After Last Visit, Now Month 40 Since Original Evaluation

- Seems like clozapine is better than no clozapine. Patient's mother is not satisfied with therapeutic response yet is hesitant to increase dose because of prior experience with side effects
- BMI now 42
- Very little guidance for what to do with a patient like this from the literature or treatment guidelines, but mother is fighting to keep her daughter from being institutionalized
- Agree to try various augmentation strategies, trying to be realistic and optimistic, but not raising false hopes

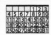

Case Outcome: Followup Months 41 to 48

- Sequential augmentation of clozapine 300 mg plus clonazepam 6 mg with
  - Lamotrigine
  - Aripiprazole
  - Another trial of topiramate
- No improvement over the next 8 months
- Glucose now 111, prediabetic
- High total cholesterol 228
- Normal triglycerides 135
- If anything, delusions getting worse. Mother says one third of her conversation used to be about delusions, now almost all of it is delusional
- Has not showered in two weeks ("devices in the shower") but consents to sponge baths
- "Riley is not dead" so she will not get a haircut

Attending Physician's Mental Notes: Followup, Month 48 a Year After Last Visit, Now Month 40 Since Original Evaluation

- Augmentation is getting us nowhere
- Plan to try dose increases of the three medications she is now taking that have proven somewhat effective

Case Outcome, Months 49 to 72

- Over the next 24 months, sequentially:
  - Ziprasidone increased to 200 mg/day, taken carefully as 100 mg/day with about 400 calories of food to assure maximum absorption
  - Clozapine increased to 400 mg/day
  - Clonazepam increased to 8 mg/day
- Now showering every day, less hostile, some sense of humor but highly delusional
- Walking most days, has lost 30 pounds, getting smaller sizes of clothes now but BMI still 38
- In the office, has a nice smile with good eye contact
- Going to the movies with her mother
- Delusions over these two years wax and wane
  - "I have a bone to pick with you"
  - "I have lost my receptors and need a receptor transplant"
  - "I go parachuting and play basketball"
  - Won't wear certain shirts that are "possessed"
  - Claims that Demons still come into her home
  - Capgras syndrome persists

- Makes some dinners, makes grocery lists, shops appropriately for food with her mother and is helpful, spends less time in bed during the day, and is even beginning to make budgets and run her own personal finances, the best she has been in the 6 years since her initial appointment

Case Debrief

- Treating resistant psychosis is a long journey
- During that journey, there are often many hospitalizations, many clinicians and many medications, often not reaching a good outcome
- In this case, even clozapine had limited efficacy
- Augmentation strategies were eventually useful in boosting the apparent efficacy compared to clozapine alone, but it took a long time, and many trials and errors
- The cost of clozapine in terms of side effects can be high, with obesity and diabetes and possibly premature cardiovascular events and death
- However, this patient's medications mean the difference between living at home with her mother, and either chaotic existence on the street or chronic institutionalization
- It is a quandary why some cases like this fail to respond any better, even with doses so high of more than one antipsychotic, that complete blockade of all D2 dopamine receptors is likely
- Some patients may have delusional systems and psychotic processes that are not improved with D2 receptor blockade, although most psychotic patients do respond to this therapeutic approach
- It can be heart breaking to see the toll that psychosis can take on a patient's life and her family, especially when treatment is so ineffective
- Nevertheless, patience, and iterative trials can lead to satisfactory if partial symptom improvement and be the difference between being able to enjoy a living situation with her mother and something far less adequate

Take-Home Points

- It is easy to give up on these cases
- Side effects can be very severe, but inadequately treated psychosis can be malignant
- Clozapine remains the cornerstone of treatment for such cases, but has its limits and certainly its costs in side effects
- Finding the optimum dose of clozapine may not be the whole answer, since augmentation with a second antipsychotic may be helpful, but only trial and error can determine which one and what dose
- Augmentation with benzodiazepines can be very helpful in these

cases, if done in the absence of drug and alcohol abuse, and without escalating doses or abuse
- The art of psychopharmacology is the only way to tell which error to avoid:
  - Quitting on a patient and either not thinking about another drug trial or referring to another prescriber after having run out of ideas
  - Reckless trials of too many drugs at the same time, creating confusion
  - Constantly implying that there is a solution out there if just the next drug is tried
- It is always good to get lucky, and chance favors the psychopharmacologically-prepared mind

Performance in Practice: Confessions of a Psychopharmacologist

- What could have been done better here?
  - Should clozapine have never been discontinued after the first trial?
  - Should clozapine have never been discontinued after the second trial?
- Possible action items for improvement in practice
  - Getting the mother more community and government support
  - Getting the patient more involved in day treatment or groups of young adults with similar psychotic disorders

Two-Minute Tute: A brief lesson and psychopharmacology tutorial (tute) with relevant background material for this case – D₂ receptor occupancy link to antipsychotic efficacy

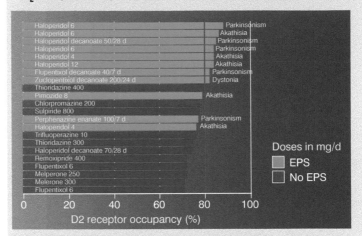

Figure 1: D₂ Receptor Occupancy Induced by Clinical Doses of Antipsychotic Drugs.

D₂ dopamine receptor occupancy for various antipsychotics at various doses was estimated from positron emission tomography studies in adult patients with schizophrenia. Most drugs are not effective until at least 60% of receptors are occupied; however, above that the drugs tend to produce more side effects without more therapeutic effects. Nevertheless, it is possible that in treatment-resistant cases of psychosis, receptor occupancy levels of greater than 80%, attained with higher than normal doses, will show more efficacy

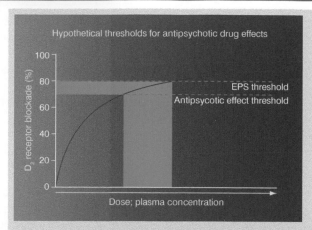

Figure 2: Hypothetical Thresholds for Antipsychotic Drug Effects
Here, about 70% receptor occupancy by second generation atypical antipsychotic drugs may produce antipsychotic actions, but not until 80% receptor occupancy are EPS produced, meaning that in some patients there is window in which they experience therapeutic effects without EPS. However, this is for the routine patient studied in clinical trials. For treatment resistant psychosis, it may be necessary to go above 70% receptor occupancy to get more efficacy even at the expense of more side effects, possibly justified in selected patients

Posttest Self Assessment Question: Answer

What do you do when standard doses of clozapine do not work?

A. Get plasma drug levels of clozapine and be sure they are between 400–600 ng/ml
   – This would be standard practice with clozapine
B. Go above 550 mg/day oral dosing of clozapine if necessary
   – This would be considered aggressive treatment, associated with risk of seizures, more sedation, sialorrhea, weight gain, and only justified if the improvement justifies the side effects and long term potential risks in that individual
C. Augment with lamotrigine, valproate, topiramate or another anticonvulsant
   – There is some evidence for this approach when clozapine alone fails
D. Augment with a second antipsychotic
   – There is some evidence for this when clozapine alone fails
E. Augment with a benzodiazepine
   – There is little evidence for this and in fact during the titration phase of clozapine, concomitant benzodiazepines can be associated with very severe sedation and even respiratory arrest; nevertheless,

when stabilized on clozapine, augmentation with a benzodiazepine can be empirically helpful even though there is scant published evidence for this

F. Leave well enough alone and accept the fact that the psychosis cannot be treated

– At some point, this may need to be the case, but not until all other avenues have been exhausted

Answer: A, B, C, D and E

References

1. Liberman RP. Recovery from Disability: Manual of Psychiatric Rehabilitation. Arlington VA. Amer Psychiatric Publishing Inc; 2008.
2. Stahl SM, Antipsychotics, in Stahl's Essential Psychopharmacology, 3rd edition, Cambridge University Press, New York, 2008, pp 327–452
3. Stahl SM, Clozapine, in Stahl's Essential Psychopharmacology The Prescriber's Guide, 3rd edition, Cambridge University Press, New York, 2009, pp 113–8
4. Stahl SM, Ziprasidone, in Stahl's Essential Psychopharmacology The Prescriber's Guide, 3rd edition, Cambridge University Press, New York, 2009, pp 589–94
5. Stahl SM, Clonazepam, in Stahl's Essential Psychopharmacology The Prescriber's Guide, 3rd edition, Cambridge University Press, New York, 2009, pp 97–101
6. Stahl SM, Grady MM. A critical review of atypical antipsychotic utilization: Comparing monotherapy with polypharmacy and augmentation. Cur Med Chem, 2004; 11: 313–26

The Case: The breast cancer survivor who couldn't remember how to cook

The Question: What is chemobrain?

The Dilemma: Can you treat cognitive dysfunction following chemotherapy for breast cancer?

Pretest Self Assessment Question (answer at the end of the case)

Cancer survivors often report short-term memory loss and difficulty concentrating. What is false about the symptoms that are often bundled under the term "chemobrain"?

A. "Chemobrain" generally resolves with time.
B. "Chemobrain" may be the result of neurotoxic effects of chemotherapeutic drugs.
C. "Chemobrain" can occur with any type of cancer.
D. "Chemobrain" occurs in 17% to 75% of cancer survivors.

Patient Intake

- 49-year-old woman
- Chief complaint: difficulty with problem solving and concentrating

Psychiatric History

- Was well until diagnosed with breast cancer 1 year ago, found to be stage 2 adenocarcinoma with lymph node but no distal metastases, including a normal brain scan
- Given chemotherapy (Adriamycin, Cytoxan, Taxol) and still receiving course of radiation therapy
- As she was recovering from surgery and chemotherapy and adjusting to the diagnosis, she began to notice that she had lost her sense of direction while driving, had problems getting dressed and putting clothes on in the right sequence, and even had problems making coffee; she was completely unable to read a road map
- Could not remember how to cook, find the ingredients in her kitchen, or mix them as she had done before
- She was referred to you for evaluation and treatment of her cognitive complaints

Attending Physician's Mental Notes: Initial Psychiatric Evaluation

- No objective signs of overt memory loss to simple mental status evaluation
- Subjective sense of memory problems

- Actually, a very good historian
- No signs of depression, thought disorder, or other psychiatric signs or symptoms
- Postmenopausal
- Medications: none, considering tamoxifen

Social and Personal History

- Married 20 years, 2 children
- Non smoker
- No drug or alcohol abuse
- Full partner, "high powered" attorney at large, prestigious law firm
- International expert on securities litigation

Medical History

- None prior to diagnosis of breast cancer
- BP normal
- BMI normal
- Normal blood tests

Family History

- Maternal aunt: breast cancer
- No known first degree relatives with cognitive disorders, Alzheimer's dementia, or psychiatric disorders

From the information given, what do you think is her most likely diagnosis?

- Major depression, with mostly cognitive symptoms and "masked" affective symptoms on first interview
- Cognitive symptoms associated with menopause
- Early onset Alzheimer's Disease
- Cognitive impairment secondary to cancer (i.e., metastases or paraneoplastic syndrome)
- Cognitive impairment secondary to chemotherapy
- None of the above

Of the following choices, what would you do?

- Treat her empirically with an antidepressant
- Refer her to a neurologist
- Get neuropsych testing (recent brain MRI is normal)
- Treat her empirically with an Alzheimer drug (cholinesterase inhibitor)
- Treat her empirically with an ADHD drug (stimulant)
- None of the above

PATIENT FILE

Further Investigation:

Is there anything else you would especially like to know about this patient?

- How about a neurological evaluation?
  - Referred for neurological evaluation which found:
    - Normal EEG
    - Normal lumbar puncture
    - No evidence of brain metastases or focal brain lesions
    - No evidence of paraneoplastic syndrome (i.e, remote effects of carcinoma)
- How about a comprehensive neuropsychological evaluation?
  - Referred to internationally renowned experts on dementia and Alzheimer's Disease at a major medical center
  - Evaluation NOT consistent with early onset Alzheimer's Disease
  - Definite cognitive impairment in several domains including
    - Working memory
    - Executive functioning
    - Verbal memory
    - Processing speed
    - Suspicion of unusual/toxic effect of chemotherapy, i.e., "chemobrain"
    - Suggested retesting in 6 months to see if any spontaneous recovery, versus progression, the latter of which would not be consistent with chemobrain

It is now six months since her chemotherapy ended. At this point, what would you do?

- Treat her empirically with an antidepressant
- Treat her empirically with an Alzheimer drug (cholinesterase inhibitor)
- Treat her empirically with an ADHD drug (stimulant)
- Wait for three to six months to observe for spontaneous recovery
- Other

Attending Physician's Mental Notes: Followup Week 12

- Referred back for her first followup appointment to discuss results of now completed neurological and neuropsychological evaluation and to discuss possible treatments
- Symptoms persist, has problems putting things away in her bedroom, can't find things, misplaces things
- Problems parallel parking
- The neurologist who evaluated her reported her to the DMV (department of motor vehicles) as unsafe to drive
- Prescribed bupropion SR, a potentially pro-cognitive antidepressant, 150 mg/day increasing to 300 mg/day

Attending Physician's Mental Notes: Followup Weeks 20 to 60

- No response after two months, 20 weeks after initial psychiatric evaluation
  - Advised to increase dose of bupropion SR to 450 mg XL
  - Referred back to her local neurologist for followup closer to her home
  - Neurologist refuses to increase dose, afraid of seizures
  - Prescription written for the dose increase of bupropion to 450 mg XL/day
- Patient returns in another two months, 28 weeks after initial psychiatric evaluation
  - Symptoms the same or worse
  - "Immobilized" at times, easily distracted, thought blocking
  - Bupropion discontinued
  - Empiric trial of donepezil 5 mg, donepezil is a selective acetylcholinesterase used as first-line treatment for dementia
- Follow-up two months later, 36 weeks after initial psychiatric evalution
  - "Got 10 times as many things done"
  - Felt great, but only for three weeks
  - Now effect seems to have worn off
  - Donepezil increased to 10 mg
- Followup two months later, 44 weeks after initial psychiatric evaluation
  - vomited on first dose of 10 mg donepezil
  - Then another remarkable response
  - Laughing, sense of humor back, quick responses
  - Donepezil continued at 10 mg/day
- Followup two month later, 52 weeks/1 year after initial psychiatric evaluation
  - Now one year since original psychiatric consultation, and no signs of recurrence of breast cancer, and patient seems entirely recovered from surgery, chemotherapy and radiation therapy except for cognitive symptoms
  - "Sporadic confusion creeping back in"
  - Since last visit, had felt improved enough that she felt confident to take an airplane trip on her own to see family out of town
  - Got lost in the airport, flustered at getting directions to the gate, misplaced, then found her ticket, misplaced, then found her cell phone
  - Starting to get depressed and feeling desperate
  - Has been off work for over a year and wants to return, pressure from law partners
  - Reinstituted bupropion at 300 mg and continued donepezil at 10 mg

- Followup two months later, 60 weeks after initial psychiatric evaluation
  - No improvement two months later, problems organizing, cannot put groceries away properly in her own kitchen
  - Advised her to Increase donepezil to 15 mg
  - Lost to followup for one year

Attending Physician's Notes: Followup, One Year Later

- No signs of breast cancer recurrence, brain metastasis or paraneoplastic syndrome
- Was unable to return to work at her law firm yet
- No worsening, but no improvement in cognitive deficits
- Repeat neuropsychological tests one year after first set of tests show no worsening, but continuing cognitive deficits as before, especially in:
  - Verbal memory
  - Processing speed
  - Executive functioning/problem solving
- Believes high dose donepezil 15 mg/day has been effective
- Off donepezil, could not dress herself, could not drive, lost directions, disoriented, word finding difficulties
- On donepezil can drive, dress, groom, but still forgetful of appointments, cannot schedule or follow through with things and still cannot go back to work, cannot remember how to set her own alarm clock and has to read instructions every time
- Has 11- and 13-year-old daughters, emotionally available to them, but cannot organize them and they try to find humor in the situation
- Has stopped bupropion

Of the following choices, what would you do?
  - Increase donepezil dose further
  - Add SSRI/SNRI
  - Add stimulant
  - Add atomoxetine
  - Add modafinil
  - Switch her to a different cholinesterase inhibitor
  - Add memantine
  - Stop medications to see if improvement is spontaneous
  - Other

Attending Physician's Mental Notes: Followup, Week 110

- This is an enduring cognitive deficit that must be related to her chemotherapy, even though the concept of "chemobrain" is controversial and many complaints of breast cancer survivors post chemotherapy are much more subtle and subjective

- This cognitive syndrome is profound, causes a stepoff in her function to a degree almost inconsistent with independent living and certainly not on track to returning to her professional work as a high functioning and top attorney
- Does not appear to be worsening, ruling out likely intercurrent CNS illness such as a dementia
- Also not improving after a year, so the chances of further spontaneous improvement is growing less and less likely
- If any improvement is to occur, it will likely take cognitive restructuring therapies and cognitive enhancing medications
- No medication, however, is approved for "chemobrain"
- Nevertheless, "off label" use of Alzheimer, and ADHD medications may be empirically helpful and worth a try
- Only medication tested in the literature for chemobrain seems to be modafinil
- Thus, suggested a trial of modafinil augmentation (100–400 mg/day split into two doses) of donepezil 15 mg/day

Attending Physician's Notes: Followup, Week 114

- Taking modafinil 100 to 200 mg, once or twice a day
- "I am motoring"
- Husband comes to the appointment and agrees organization around the house is better

Attending Physician's Notes: Followup, Week 126

- Husband and wife agree she is not doing as well as before
- Gets four or five good hours out of 1st dose of modafinil of 300 mg for the day, but the "fidgety" effect outlasts the good cognitive effects
- Feels she does better with conversations and some high intensity cognitive activities on modafinil (plus donepezil)
- Advised a three-day modafinil holiday to determine if any continuing efficacy

Attending Physician's Notes: Followup, Week 138

- Seems to have lost judgment, like "lacking maturity" and less of a filter: "says inappropriate things" and disinhibited
- Also feels mentally slowed down
- On balance, wants to keep treatment the same

Attending Physician's Notes: Followup, Week 142

- "Medicines are not working at all"
- Perception possibly colored by recent job evaluation at her law firm finding her incapable of performing even as a paralegal two years after leaving her job
- "Resigned" and started on permanent disability
- Working with home health care nurse to try to regain more function, including "brain exercises" with vocations rehabilitation specialist
- Wants to stop medications
- All medications are tapered

Attending Physician's Notes: Followup, Week 150

- Felt immediately sleepy off medications
- Has actually gotten worse
- Now cannot order the mess in the kitchen, cannot organize a meal to feed family
- In retrospect, medications were having an effect
- Restarted low dose donepezil and then variable dose modafinil

Attending Physician's Notes: Followup, Week 154

- Restarted donepezil but only 5 mg/day
- Noted improvement in:
  - Organizational skills
  - Putting away dishes
  - Cleaning out a drawer or cleaning a room
- No improvement in driving
- No improvement in concentrating
- Cannot read a recipe and remember the ingredients long enough to find them in the kitchen without re-reading
- Restarted modafinil augmentation to low dose donepezil

Attending Physician's Notes: Followup, Week 158

- "I am motoring" again
- But first daily dose of modafinil improves cognition without the same "kick" she felt the first time she took it – second dose of the day can cause agitation
- Opted for a switch from modafinil to atomoxetine

Attending Physician's Notes: Followup, Week 166

- Two-month trial of atomoxetine, no effect except sleepiness
- Went back to modafinil which had some modest cognitive effects again
- Opted for a trial of switch from modafinil to methylphenidate, increased dose to 20 mg/day

Attending Physician's Notes: Followup, Week 170

- Not liking methylphenidate
  - Only more energy
  - But no help in organizing
  - Feels modafinil is better
  - Also wants to continue donezeil
- Lost to follow-up for four years

Attending Physician's Notes: Followup, Years Later

- Four years later, no cancer recurrence
- However, no further cognitive recovery
- Still disabled, not driving, not cooking for others
- Only on donepezil 15 mg
- Not able to work but can function independently

Case Debrief

- Bad things sometimes happen to nice people
- This patient undoubtedly had a profound cognitive disturbance, causing a marked step-off in function from a high-powered attorney to someone who could not cook or drive and this occurred right after finishing chemotherapy
- The step off in function was not progressive
- However, neither did it improve
- Many pro-cognitive drugs all had some benefit including:
  - Acetylcholinesterase inhibitor donepezil
  - Pro-dopaminergic modafinil
  - Stimulants were too stimulating
  - Atomoxetine not very useful
  - Bupropion not very useful

Take-Home Points

- "Chemobrain" increasingly recognized as long-term survival from cancer increases
- Not well studied, subjectively many breast cancer patients on chemotherapy complain of this and have a more or less spontaneous improvement over several months
- Possibility of neurotoxic effects on central neurotransmitter-containing neurons?
- Patients with long-term symptoms may improve a bit on various agents as shown here, but effects can be only modest, and in these cases are often the best early in treatment and tend to wear off in part
- Much more research is needed on this important and increasingly common problem in cancer chemotherapy survivors (17% to 75% of

cancer survivors report chemotherapy-associated cognitive changes.
Source: http://www.cancer.gov/ncicancerbulletin)

Performance in Practice: Confessions of a Psychopharmacologist

- What could have been done better here?
  - It took a long time to initiate the treatment and then to implement various iterations of treatment, so maybe this could have been done more expeditiously for her
  - However, all treatment is controversial since the notion of chemobrain is not universally accepted and all medication use is off label
- Possible action item for improvement in practice
  - Attending physician did his own literature search but perhaps should have made it available to the patient
  - Attending physician perhaps should make this case available to others in the literature as a case report since very little treatment literature exists for chemobrain

Tips and Pearls

- The same brain areas involved in executive dysfunction in depression, anxiety and ADHD may be involved in patients who have executive dysfunction from chemobrain
- Thus, treatments effective in improving executive dysfunction in depression, anxiety and ADHD may also be helpful in chemobrain
- Other brain areas such as hippocampus and basal forebrain may be involved in chemobrain just as they are early in Alzheimer's disease and thus treatments effective for Alzheimer's disease may also be helpful in chemobrain

Two-Minute Tute: A brief lesson and psychopharmacology tutorial (tute) with relevant background material for this case – Chemobrain

Table 1: What is Chemobrain?

- With more women surviving breast cancer post chemotherapy, more are having cognitive complaints following treatment
- In fact, cognitive complaints are one of the most commonly reported post treatment symptoms by breast cancer survivors
- Studies report up to 75% of participants with cognitive impairment on one or more neuropsychological tests
- Disability seems worst in those with professional positions
- May accelerate cognitive decline seen in unrelated age associated memory impairment as the patient ages
- Hypothetically due to chemotherapy-induced toxicity to the brain
- Some evidence of dose dependent relationship of cognition with chemotherapy dose
- May affect prefrontal cortex since the symptoms are mapped to brain areas in the prefrontal cortex,
- Breast cancer chemotherapy may be toxic to monoaminergic nerve terminals in prefrontal cortex, impairing the proper "tuning" of pyramidal neurons there
- Correlates with anemia/decline in hemoglobin and increased anxiety

Table 2: What Are the Specific Cognitive Deficits in Chemobrain?

- Executive dysfunction
- Difficulties with problem solving
- Slowing of mental processing speed
- Motor slowing
- Divided attention
- Mental flexibility
- Subjective problems with short term memory less documented on formal neuropsychological testing
- Loss of confidence
- Surprisingly low incidence of depression reported, so cognitive symptoms likely to be mediated by a different mechanism than depression

Table 3: Chemobrain is a Controversial Concept

- Is cognitive impairment caused by chemotherapy real?
- Some studies fail to document objective neuropsychological deficits
- Some experts attribute subjective cognitive problems to hormone imbalance
  - Either from menopause
  - Or from ongoing treatment with anti-estrogen therapies which in themselves may interfere with cognition
  - However, this does not explain cognitive problems in patients not taking anti-estrogen hormonal therapies
- Some experts attribute cognitive problems to factors other than chemotherapy toxicity
  - General effects of cancer diagnosis, whatever that means
  - Impact of surgery
  - Impact of anesthesia
  - Anxiety
  - Depression
  - Fatigue
  - Other medications
  - Genetic predisposition
  - Comorbid medical conditions
  - Paraneoplastic

Table 4: Why is Chemobrain Controversial?

- Oncologists do not want to believe that chemotherapy is toxic to the brain and could impair long term outcome and quality of life in breast cancer survivors
- Some studies show cognitive abnormalities, others do not
- Most reported cognitive abnormalities are subjective or have a small objective effect size
- It is hard to believe that the patient discussed in this case had anything other than a profound cognitive abnormality that was real, persistent and remarkably disabling and caused by chemotherapy
- Studies may disagree because of
  - Practice effects (i.e., when cognitive tests are repeated, they may improve because of learning and mask any deterioration that may be present)
  - Different study designs, some being longitudinal, getting baseline cognitive assessment before and after chemotherapy; others cross sectional comparing post chemotherapy patients with controls that may not be well selected

- Effects of different chemotherapies, especially confounded by including or excluding hormone treatments vs other chemotherapies
- Criteria for cognitive deficits
- Premorbid cognitive ability
- Drop outs from the study before completion
- Power and sample size

Posttest Self Assessment Question: Answer

Cancer survivors often report short-term memory loss and difficulty concentrating. What is false about the symptoms that are often bundled under the term "chemobrain?"

A. "Chemobrain" always resolves with time.
B. "Chemobrain" may be the result of neurotoxic effects of chemotherapeutic drugs.
C. "Chemobrain" can occur with any type of cancer.
D. "Chemobrain" occurs in 17% to 75% of cancer survivors.

Answer: A

References

1. Wefel JS, Saleeba AK, Buzdar AU et al. Acute and late onset cognitive dysfunction associated with chemotherapy in women with breast cancer. Cancer 2010; 116(14): 3348–56
2. Muni F, Burrows J, Yarker J et al. Women's perceptions of chemotherapy-induced cognitive side effects on work ability. J Clin Nurs 2010; 19(9–10): 1362–70
3. Debess J, Riis JØ, Engebjerg MC et al. Cognitive function after adjuvant treatment for early breast cancer: a population-based longitudinal study. Breast Cancer Res Treat 2010; 121(1): 91–100
4. Yamada TH, Denburg NL, Beglinger LJ et al. Neuropsychological outcomes of older breast cancer survivors: cognitive features ten or more years after chemotherapy. J Neuropsychiatry Clin Neurosci 2010; 22(1): 48–54
5. Schilder CM, Seynaeve C, Beex LV et al. Effects of tamoxifen and exemestane on cognitive functioning of postmenopausal patients with breast cancer: results from the neuropsychological side study of the tamoxifen and exemestane adjuvant trial. J Clin Oncol 2010; 28(8): 1294–300
6. Tager FA, McKinley PS, Schnabel FR et al. The cognitive effects of chemotherapy in post-menopausal breast cancer patients: a controlled longitudinal study. Breast Cancer Res Treat 2010; 123(1): 25–34

7. Vardy J and Dhillon H. The fog hasn't lifted on "chemobrain" yet: ongoing uncertainty regarding the effects of chemotherapy and breast cancer on cognition. Breast Cancer Res Treat 2010; 123(1): 35–7

8. Boykoff N, Moieni M, and Subramanian, SK. Confronting chemobrain: an in-depth look at survivors' reports of impact on work, social networks, and health care response. J Cancer Surviv 2009; 3(4): 223–32

9. Vearncombe KJ, Rolfe M, Wright M et al. Predictors of cognitive decline after chemotherapy in breast cancer patients. J Int Neuropsychol Soc 2009; 15(6): 951–62

10. Reid-Arndt SA, Hsieh C, and Perry MC. Neuropsychological functioning and quality of life during the first year after completing chemotherapy for breast cancer. Psychooncology 2010; 19(5): 535–44

11. Kohli S, Fisher SG, Tra Y et al. The effect of modafinil on cognitive function in breast cancer survivors. Cancer 2009; 115912): 2605–16

12. Jim HS, Donovan KA, Small BJ et al. Cognitive functioning in breast cancer survivors: a controlled comparison. Cancer 2009; 115(8): 1776–83

13. Weis J, Poppelreuter M, and Bartsch HH. Cognitive deficits as long-term side-effects of adjuvant therapy in breast cancer patients: 'subjective' complaints and 'objective' neuropsychological test results. Psychooncology 2009; 18(7): 775–82

14. Castellon S and Ganz PA. Neuropsychological studies in breast cancer: in search of chemobrain. Breast Cancer Res Treat 2009; 116(1): 125–7

15. Mehlsen M, Pedersen AD, Jensen AB et al. No indications of cognitive side-effects in a prospective study of breast cancer patients receiving adjuvant chemotherapy. Psychooncology 2009; 18(3): 248–57

16. Quesnel C, Savard J, and Ivers H. Cognitive impairments associated with breast cancer treatments: results from a longitudinal study. Breast Cancer Res Treat 2009; 116(1): 113–23

17. Stahl SM, Cognition, in Stahl's Essential Psychopharmacology, 3rd edition, Cambridge University Press, New York, 2008, chapter 19, pp 943–1012

18. Stahl SM, Modafinil, in Stahl's Essential Psychopharmacology The Prescriber's Guide, 3rd edition, Cambridge University Press, New York, 2009, pp 359–63

19. Stahl SM, Donepezil, in Stahl's Essential Psychopharmacology The Prescriber's Guide, 3rd edition, Cambridge University Press, New York, 2009, pp 145–9

20. Stahl SM, Bupropion, in Stahl's Essential Psychopharmacology The Prescriber's Guide, 3rd edition, Cambridge University Press, New York, 2009, pp 57–62

21. Stahl SM, Atomoxetine, in Stahl's Essential Psychopharmacology The Prescriber's Guide, 3rd edition, Cambridge University Press, New York, 2009, pp 51–5

22. Stahl SM, Methylphenidate, in Stahl's Essential Psychopharmacology The Prescriber's Guide, 3rd edition, Cambridge University Press, New York, 2009, pp 329–35

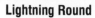
Lightning Round

The Case: The woman who has always been out of control

The Question: How do you treat chaos?

The Dilemma: What can you expect from an antipsychotic in a woman with many problems and diagnoses?

Pretest Self Assessment Question (answer at the end of the case)

How do you approach multiple comorbidities in a chronically mentally ill patient who has essentially never been in good symptomatic control?

A. Empiric trials of antipsychotics

B. Empiric trials of mood stabilizing anticonvulsants

C. The correct combination of medications generally can control most symptoms in most patients at most times

D. Realize that full remission may not be the goal of treatment for some severe longstanding cases, but the goal may be to attain the best level of functioning that the patient has experienced in recent years

E. Aggressive polypharmacy has its limits

Patient Intake

- 30-year-old woman diagnosed with long-standing schizoaffective disorder, bipolar type, polysubstance abuse in remission in a controlled environment and with premorbid childhood onset PTSD, borderline intellectual functions, and antisocial personality disorder with borderline features

- Has carried the diagnosis of PTSD related to childhood sexual and physical abuse by her father

- Juvenile and adult criminal activity and poor school performance, with cognitive testing showing cognitive and memory abilities in the borderline range

- Difficulty managing anger since age 13, longstanding impulsiveness since age 13 with psychotic illness since age 16 associated with irritable and depressed moods, auditory hallucinations (some in her father's voice) command hallucinations to harm herself, ideas of reference and persecutory ideation

- Numerous psychiatric hospitalizations, self mutilatory behavior including cutting and swallowing behaviors (e.g., keys, other objects)

- Convicted of arson and while imprisoned assaulted a prison guard but found not to be criminally responsible by reason of insanity and transferred to a forensic facility

Psychiatric History

- Intermittent violent and self injurious behavior associated with continuing psychotic symptoms, mood lability, and impulsiveness
- Current psychotropic medications:
  - Haloperidol (Haldol) 10 mg at noon and 5 mg at night
  - Ziprasidone (Geodon) 80 mg twice a day
  - Lithium 600 mg at noon and 900 mg at night
  - Modafinil (Provigil) 200 mg at noon
  - Duloxetine (Cymbalta) 60 mg at noon
  - Propranolol (Inderal) 15 mg three times a day
  - Phenytoin (Dilantin) 400 mg twice a day
  - Levothyroxine 225 μg per day
  - Zolpidem (Ambien) 10 mg at night
  - Quetiapine (Seroquel) 200 mg prn

Of the following choices, what would you do?

- Increase the dose of one or more antipsychotics
- Switch one of the antipsychotics to another one
- Increase the dose of duloxetine
- Trials of other anticonvulsants such as topiramate (Topamax), lamotrigine (Lamictal), valproate (Depakote)
- Emphasize nonpharmacological approaches

Case Outcome

- At first, haloperidol was increased to 20 mg a day, and olanzapine was added at 20 mg, increasing to 40 mg a day, while discontinuing ziprasidone with no notable changes
- Topiramate augmentation was tried, and duloxetine was increased to 60 mg twice a day
- Then quetiapine 800 mg a day was substituted for olanzapine
- In the interim, the patient received more nursing attention, more structured time, and occasional intramuscular administration of addition haloperidol or olanzapine or lorazepam (Ativan)
- Although the worst excesses of her behaviors were blunted, the patient continues to have uncontrolled symptoms at times

Case Debrief

- It is important not to expect too much of medication treatment in general and antipsychotic treatment in particular
- Thus, although some patients respond to even higher doses of quetiapine (>800 mg/day) this is not deemed to be likely to be helpful

- Antisocial personality disorder, impulsivity related to borderline intellectual functioning, and long-standing symptoms of PTSD are among the many symptoms that often do not respond to psychopharmacological interventions and have no approved treatments and few well studied treatments
- It is possible that the patient has arrived at the best functioning she can have at the present time

Posttest Self Assessment Question: Answer

How do you approach multiple comorbidities in a chronically mentally ill patient who has essentially never been in good symptomatic control?

A. Empiric trials of antipsychotics
   – Definitely justified
B. Empiric trials of mood stabilizing anticonvulsants
   – Also justified
C. The correct combination of medications generally can control most symptoms in most patients at most times
   – This is unfortunately not true for severe cases, and especially those who end up institutionalized
D. Realize that full remission may not be the goal of treatment for some severe longstanding cases, but the goal may be to attain the best level of functioning that the patient has experienced in recent years
   – Knowing how to lower expectations while remaining in a therapeutic mind set and improving the situation is an important skill in managing severe cases
E. Aggressive polypharmacy has its limits
   – Although clever psychopharmacology and "thinking outside the box" to fashion creative solutions for complex patients is part of the art of psychopharmacology, it is also useful to respect the limits of this approach

Answer: A,B, D and E

References

1. Citrome L, Kantrowitz JT, Olanzapine dosing above the licensed range is more efficacious than lower doses: fact or fiction? Expert Reviews Neurother 2009; 9: 1045–58

2. Citrome L, Quetiapine: dose response relationship to schizophrenia, CNS Drugs 2008; 22: 69–72

3. Lindenmayer J-P, Citrome L, Khan A et al. A randomized double-blind, parallel-grou, fixed dose, clinical trial of quetiapine 600 mg/day vs 1200 mb/day for patients with treatment-resistant schizophrenia or schizoaffective disorder. Abstracts of the Society for Biological Psychiatry, 2010, New Orleans, Louisiana

4. Stahl SM, Antipsychotics, in Stahl's Essential Psychopharmacology, 3rd edition, Cambridge University Press, New York, 2008, pp 327–452

The Case: The young man with alcohol abuse and depression like father, like son; like grandfather, like father; like great grandfather, like grandfather

The Question: How can you help a young man who denies his alcoholism and depression?

The Dilemma: Why do so few psychopharmacologists treat addictive disorders with approved medications?

Pretest Self Assessment Question (see answer at the end of the case)

What is reduced risk drinking?

A. A bad idea
B. A potential stepping stone on the path towards abstinence
C. 5 or fewer drinks a day/35 or fewer drinks a week for a man; 4 or fewer drinks a day/28 or fewer drinks a week for a woman
D. 3–4 drinks per day/maximum or 16 drinks per week for a man; 2–3 drinks per day/maximum or 12 drinks per week for a woman

Patient Intake

- 22-year-old man brought to the office by both parents
- Complains of depression
- Parents complain of his drinking

Psychiatric History

- Feels he has always been depressed
- Denies any periods of feeling better than well, impulsivity, racing thoughts
- Major depressive episode at age 20, while in college
- At that time, insignificant drinking reported and parents confirm
- Symptoms then were poor concentration, lacking energy, lacking motivation, hopeless, helpless
- Did not want to take medication
- Had 6 months of psychotherapy
- Depression never remitted and continues to today
- Willing to take medication now, 2 years later

Social and Personal History

- Single
- College student
- Infrequent use of alcohol
- Tried marijuana a few times, no regular use
- Denies other drugs
- Smokes 5 cigarettes a day
- Somewhat shy and anxious in social settings

Medical History

- Normal blood tests, physical exam

Family History

- Father: depression, alcoholism, attempted suicide, symptoms fairly well controlled with venlafaxine XR (Effexor XR) 225 mg/day
- Paternal grandfather: depression, alcoholism, completed suicide
- Paternal great-grandfather: completed suicide, other details of his history, including depression and alcohol unknown or unclear
- Paternal uncle: depression and alcoholism
- Paternal aunt: depression, alcoholism
- Paternal cousin: bipolar disorder

Further Investigation

- What about more details of his infrequent use of alcohol use?
  - At this time, he reports occasional drinks at fraternity parties, weekends only, never gets intoxicated
  - Parents have no reason to disbelieve him since they have never seen him drink heavily, never seen him intoxicated and no brushes with the law, fights, etc.

Patient Intake, Continued

- Complains of depressed mood
- Hopeless, helpless
- Little pleasure in life
- Denies suicidal ideation but does sometimes feel he'd be better off dead
- Tense and anxious in social situations
- Appears severely depressed and if anything, minimizing his complaints and denying symptoms, so he seems more depressed than he states
- Has felt this way for 6 to 12 months
- Does not want any more psychotherapy
- Diagnosed with major depressive disorder, possible comorbid social anxiety disorder
- Prescribed venlafaxine XR (Effexor XR)

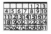

Case Outcome: Followup, Months 1 through 3

- Venlafaxine XR titrated up to 225 mg/day with some mood improvement

Case Outcome: Followup, Month 7

- Lost to followup for 4 months
- Found out he had been arrested for DUI (driving under the influence; drunk driving)
- Hospitalized and then sent to rehab for 39 days
- On the 39th day learned that he would have to serve a 60 day jail sentence for DUI
- Overdosed on propoxyphene (Darvocet) and hydrocodone+acetaminophen (Vicodin), and required medical hospitalization
- During this time he was maintained at the rehab program on venlafaxine 225 mg/day and buporopion SR (Wellbutrin SR) 150 mg was added
- States that his mood brightened with this
- However, he then went to jail after rehab, and they denied him his antidepressants for the past three weeks, now getting worse again
- He only had to serve three weeks of his 60 day sentence and left jail, now returns with his parents for a followup appointment

Have you experienced patients lying about their alcohol use and fooling you into believing them at least initially?

- Yes
- No

Further Investigation

- What about more honest and reliable details of his use of alcohol use?
  - Patient maintains the he drinks "infrequently" (every few weeks)
  - Acknowledges that when he does drink he binges
  - Also acknowledges that when he drinks he would sometimes miss his venlafaxine doses (when he was taking it prior to going to rehab and jail)

Case Outcome: Followup, Month 7, Continued

- Patient willing to take an antidepressant, but not venlafaxine because he does not want anything his dad takes
- Also refused psychotherapy or referral to alcoholics anonymous (AA)
- "I am not an alcoholic"
- "I got drunk once and got caught driving, that's not an alcoholic"
- "I only drink a couple of days a month, so I don't need AA"
- Agrees to take escitalopram (Lexapro)

Case Outcome: Followup, Month 18

- Lost to followup for 12 months
- Found out that three weeks after his last appointment, was arrested again for alcohol-related charges
- Sent to rehab again and then to a recovery home
- Has remained sober for the past 8 months in a structured sober treatment facility
- During this time has received:
  - Paroxetine (Paxil, Seroxat)
  - Bupropion SR
  - Doxepin (Sinequan)
- Little benefit but at least some improvement of mood and socialization
- Patient has resumed college
- In retrospect, the patient fulfills criteria for ADHD since childhood although never diagnosed and never treated previously

What should be treated first?

- Mood disorder
- Alcohol abuse
- ADHD symptoms
- All should be treated at the same time

How would you treat his mood disorder?

- Venlafaxine XR
- Escitalopram
- Bupropion SR
- Other SSRI or SNRI
- TCA (tricyclic antidepressant)
- Lithium
- Mood stabilizing anticonvulsant
- Atypical antipsychotic
- Other medication
- Psychotherapy

Case Outcome: Followup, Month 18, Continued

- Agrees to try a new SSRI, sertraline (Zoloft), 200 mg/day for mood and social anxiety
- Some improvement in these symptoms over the next 2 months, but still has problems with attention

How would you treat his alcohol abuse?

- AA (Alcoholics Anonymous)
- Psychotherapy

- Disulfiram (Antabuse)
- Acamprosate (Camprol)
- Natrexone oral (Revia)
- Naltrexone 30 day injection (Vivitrol)
- Other

Case Outcome: Followup, Month 18, Continued

- Alcohol abuse treatment recommended
- Recommended naltrexone 30 day injection
- Patient argues against it, family believe it is a great idea
- Referred to clinic for injection, and remarkably, he follows through the next week and gets an injection
- However, refuses second and third injections that were recommended
- Still refusing psychotherapy and AA

How would you treat his ADHD symptoms?

- Don't give a stimulant to an alcoholic
- He doesn't have ADHD, he is just lying to get stimulants
- He doesn't have ADHD, just the symptoms of recovery from alcohol abuse plus depression
- Nonstimulant like atomoxetine

Case Outcome: Followup, Month 20

- ADHD treatment recommended
- 2 months after starting antidepressants, patient seems improved slightly, appears not to have drunk in the interim, and going to college but struggling
- To support his tentative recovery and potentially reduce his chances of alcohol relapse, reluctantly prescribed stimulant for ADHD symptoms to see if this would maintain him in college and sober
- Prescribed long acting methylphenidate (Ritalin) LA increasing 20 mg up to three times daily

Case Outcome: Followup, Month 24

- Did not drink again for 9 straight weeks
- Had only ever happened in the past several years in his structured treatment programs
- Finished his college semester with passing grades in all courses
- Does he live happily ever after?
- A few weeks after semester ended, month 25, parents revealed that patient had been hoarding pills, especially methylphenidate and then would binge on them on occasion, as many as 12 pills/day (240 mg of d,l methylphenidate LA)

Have you ever been twice burned by a patient lying about their medications, drugs of abuse, and compromising the trust you extended to them and making you feel foolish?

- Yes
- No

Now, having been fooled at least twice, what would you do now?

- Resign from the case and refer him to someone else
- Discontinue the stimulant
- Discontinue the stimulant and switch to nonstimulant
- Other

Case Outcome: Followup, Month 26

- Feeling gullible and having been fooled again, nevertheless decided to agree to continue to treat, as this is part of the bargain in treating cases like this
- Continued sertraline
- Switched from methylphenidate to atomoxetine (Strattera) 40 mg/day

Case Outcome: Followup, Month 28

- A few weeks after the last appointment, the patient relapsed on alcohol
- Dropped some classes in his current semester of studies
- Stopped his sertraline and atomoxetine
- Began taking methamphetamine from the street (felt like it took the edge off wanting alcohol)
- Parents bring him in yet again, and this time prescribed
  - Olanzapine-fluoxetine combination (Symbyax) for treatment resistant depression 12/50 mg/day
- Restarted atomoxetine 40 mg/day
- Strongly encouraged him to re-start long acting naltrexone injections and go to AA but patient again refuses
- Mention to him that continuing to be a patient will eventually mean resuming naltrexone injections and AA if any further incidents of alcohol abuse (which seems likely)

Case Outcome: Followup, Month 30

- Took medications intermittently and continued to drink
- Got a call from the emergency room, and he and his family agree to check into the psychiatric hospital as he is suicidal and intoxicated
- Despondent, helpless
- "This is no way to live"
- Tired of using drugs to fill the void
- Received 12 electroconvulsive therapy (ECT) sessions

- No adverse effects but no improvement!
- Discharged on duloxetine (Cymbalta) 90 mg/day plus quetiapine (Seroquel) 100 mg at night
- Also discharged on acamprosate (Camprol)

Case Outcome: Followup, Months 30–35

- No notable benefit
- Stopped acamprosate after three days because of nausea
- Trial of aripiprazole (Abilify) augmentation 10 mg/day, no benefit over 2 months
- Trial of bupropion SR augmentation again, 450 mg/day, some benefit on depression and attention but waned
- After another month, relapsed on alcohol
- Switched to venlafaxine XR which has worked in the past when he has taken it and titrated up to 300 mg/day
- Sometimes missed doses
- Actually, his depression improved about 50%
- However, still occasional alcohol binges but has avoided driving or interaction with the law when drinking
- Now is a consistent internet gambler
- Remarkably, however, finished college
- Current status is "only" a couple of 2–3 day binges in the last several months
- Last drink 2 weeks ago
- Internet gambling and continuing symptoms of anxiety and depression
- Discussed AA, long acting injectable naltrexone, MAOIs, TMS, and the case goes on. . . .

Case Debrief

- The patient has a serious, potentially life threatening mood disorder complicated by abuse of alcohol, stimulants and the internet/gambling
- Since he is not a daily drinker, he does not think he is an alcohol abuser or an "alcoholic"
- Rejects the notion that heavy drinking is more than 5 drinks a day or 16 drinks per week; states if you divide the number of drinks in 2 months over the number of days in 2 months, is not a heavy drinker even by the expert definition
- He is poorly compliant, and although his mood disorder tends to respond to antidepressants, his drinking interferes with that, and he is only intermittently compliant with antidepressant treatment
- The patient lacks insight and refuses AA, perhaps the most effective potential treatment for his alcohol abuse

- He has completed college and is functioning at least to some degree, but continues to be symptomatic and to be at high risk for relapse and poor outcome

Take-Home Points

- Denial of alcohol abuse and lack of insight are common in substance abuse/dependence
- Young men commonly binge and their peer group is adamant that this is not alcohol abuse
- A very scary positive history of 4 generations of alcoholism and depression with suicide among men in this family creates a very high-risk situation here
- Being lied to regarding substance use is the rule rather than the exception for treating many cases like this one
- You can lead a horse to water, but . . .

Performance in Practice: Confessions of a Psychopharmacologist

- What could have been done better here?
  - Almost too many to mention
  - A wise person would have perhaps been able to get the true alcohol use at the original appointment
  - In retrospect, it was not a good idea to have prescribed stimulants, since prescribing controlled substances to an active alcohol abuser is usually a ticket to disaster no matter how empathetic and helpful one is trying to be
  - It is probably a mark of failure of the treatment plan that the patient could not be convinced to attend AA or to accept his illness
- Possible action item for improvement in practice
  - Better sources for history of substance use than the patient and his similarly fooled parents, perhaps talking with peers for a true picture
  - Being more proactive in prescribing injectable naltrexone and/or disulfiram

Tips and Pearls

- Treatment with naltrexone can reduce heavy drinking
- Naltrexone injections only require one decision to be compliant every 30 days whereas oral naltrexone requires 30 decisions to be compliant every 30 days
- Use of naltrexone, acamprosate and disulfiram is very low among psychopharmacologists

Two-Minute Tute: A brief lesson and psychopharmacology tutorial (tute) with relevant background material for this case – Definitions of reduced risk drinking and standard drinks

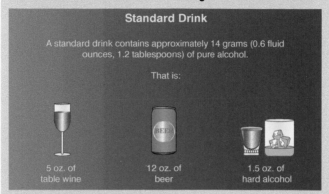

Standard Drink

A standard drink contains approximately 14 grams (0.6 fluid ounces, 1.2 tablespoons) of pure alcohol.

That is:

5 oz. of table wine   12 oz. of beer   1.5 oz. of hard alcohol

Figure 1: Standard Drink.
A standard drink contains approximately 14 grams (0.6 fluid ounces; 1.2 tablespoons) of pure alcohol

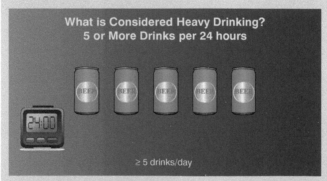

What is Considered Heavy Drinking?
5 or More Drinks per 24 hours

24:00

≥ 5 drinks/day

Figure 2: What is Considered Heavy Drinking?

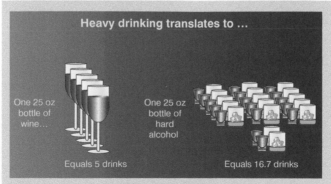

Heavy drinking translates to …

One 25 oz bottle of wine…

One 25 oz bottle of hard alcohol

Equals 5 drinks   Equals 16.7 drinks

Figure 3: Heavy Drinking Also Translates to . . .

Table 1: Reduced Risk Drinking

Men:	3–4 drinks per day; maximum 16 drinks per week
	(heavy drinking is ≥5 drinks/day)
Women:	2–3 drinks per day; maximum 12 drinks per week
	(heavy drinking is ≥4 drinks/day)

Avoid having more than one drink in an hour

Avoid drinking patterns (same people, same location, same time of day)

Avoid drinking to deal with problems

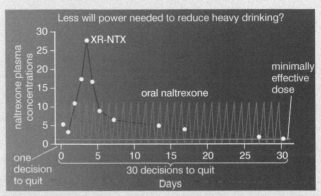

Figure 4: Naltrexone is a mu opiate receptor antagonist that can reduce the pleasurable effects of drinking and thus is used in the treatment of alcohol dependence. It is available in both an oral formulation and as a once-monthly intramuscular injection. One of the complicating factors in treating substance dependence with substances is that one has to renew the decision to quit at each dosing point. Thus with oral naltrexone one must decide daily whether or not to continue the attempt. Because the injection is taken only once a month, this option may require less willpower to refrain from heavy drinking.

Goals of Treatment

- Ideal: abstinence
- Majority of patients do not achieve abstinence, and those who do may require multiple tries
- Abstinence isn't the only possible positive outcome

Moderate Drinking

Problem Drinking

Abstained ¾ days
Reduced alcohol consumption by 87%

Abstinence

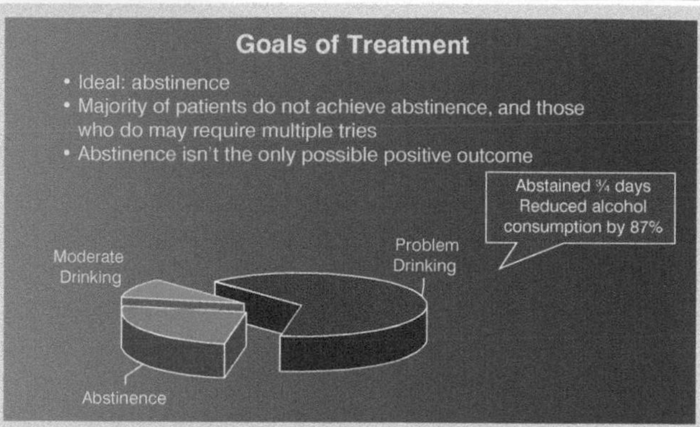

Figure 5: The ideal goal of treatment is abstinence; however, abstinence does not have to be the only positive outcome of treatment. The majority of patients do not achieve abstinence, and those who do may require multiple tries. Even individuals who do not achieve abstinence may exhibit significant and positive changes in drinking behavior. Data shown on slide: findings from seven large multisite studies were combined to derive estimates of the average effectiveness of alcoholism treatment. To provide common outcome measures, conversion equations were used to compute variables not reported in the original studies. During the year after treatment, 1 in 4 clients remained continuously abstinent on average, and an additional 1 in 10 used alcohol moderately and without problems. During this period, mortality averaged less than 2%. The remaining clients, as a group, showed substantial improvement, abstaining on 3 days out of 4 and reducing their overall alcohol consumption by 87%, on average. Alcohol-related problems also decreased by 60%.

Posttest Self Assessment Question: Answer

What is reduced risk drinking?

A. A bad idea
  - According to classical addictionologists, the goal of treatment should be complete abstinence or nothing
B. A potential stepping stone on the path towards abstinence
  - A newer but controversial concept that reduced drinking can be attained by some patients prior to complete abstinence, especially considering the clinical trial results of naltrexone administration
C. 5 or fewer drinks a day/35 or fewer drinks a week for a man; 4 or fewer drinks a day/28 or fewer drinks a week for a woman
  - No
D. 3–4 drinks per day/maximum or 16 drinks per week for a man; 2–3 drinks per day/maximum or 12 drinks per week for a woman
  - Yes

Answer: B and D

References

1. Anton RF, O'Malley SS, Ciraulo DA et al. Combined pharmacotherapies and behavioral interventions for alcohol dependence. The COMBINE Study: a randomized controlled trial. Journal of American Medical Association 2006; 295: 2003–17
2. Brady KT and Sinha R. Co-occurring mental and substance use disorders: the neurobiological effects of chronic stress. American Journal of Psychiatry 2005; 162: 1483–93
3. Dackis CA and Miller NS. Neurobiological effects determine treatment options for alcohol, cocaine, and heroin addiction. Psychiatric Annals 2003; 33: 585–92
4. Dahchour A and DeWitte P. Effects of acamprosate on excitatory amino acids during multiple ethanol withdrawal periods. Alcoholism: Clinical and Experimental Research 2003; 3: 465–70
5. Daoust M, Legrand E, Gewiss M et al. Acamprosate modulates synaptosomal GABA transmission in chronically alcoholised rats. Pharmacology Biochemistry and Behavior 1992; 41: 669–74
6. DeWitte P. Imbalance between neuroexcitatory and neuroinhibitory amino acids causes craving for ethanol. Addictive Behaviors 2004; 29: 1325–39
7. DeWitte P, Littleton J, Parot P et al. Neuroprotective and abstinence-promoting effects of acamprosate. Elucidating the mechanism of action. CNS Drugs 2005; 6: 517–37
8. Fong TW. Why aren't more psychiatrists prescribing buprenorphine? Current Psychiatry 2004; 3: 46–56

9. Galanter M and Kleber HD. (eds.) (2004) Textbook of Substance Abuse Treatment 3rd Edition. American Psychiatric Publishing, Inc., Washington, D.C.

10. Garbutt JC, Kranzler HR, O'Malley SS et al. Efficacy and tolerability of long-acting injectable naltrexone for alcohol dependence. A randomized controlled trial. Journal of American Medical Association 2005; 293: 1617–25

11. Grant JE, Brewer JA and Potenza MN. The neurobiology of substance and behavioral addictions. CNS Spectr 2006; 11: 924–30

12. Heinz A, Reimold M, Wrase J et al. Correlation of stable elevations in striatal μ-opioid receptor availability in detoxified alcoholic patients with alcohol craving. A positron emission tomography study using carbon 11-labeled carfentanil. Arch Gen Psychiatry 2005; 62: 57–64

13. Schreckenberger M, Smolka MN, Rösch F et al. Correlation of alcohol craving with striatal dopamine synthesis capacity and D2/3 receptor availability: a combined [18F]DOPA and [18F]DMFP PET study in detoxified alcoholic patients. American Journal of Psychiatry 2005; 162: 1515–20

14. Hyman SE. Addiction: a disease of learning and memory. American Journal of Psychiatry 2005; 162: 1414–22

15. Ivanov IS, Schulz KP, Palmero RC et al. Neurobiology and evidence-based biological treatments for substance abuse disorders. CNS Spectr 2006; 11: 864–77

16. Johnson BA. New weapon to curb smoking. No more excuses to delay treatment. Archives of Internal Medicine 2006; 166: 1547–50

17. Kalivas PW and Volkow ND. The neural basis of addiction: a pathology of motivation and choice. American Journal of Psychiatry 2005; 162: 1403–13

18. Kessler RC. Impact of substance abuse on the diagnosis, course, and treatment of mood disorders. The epidemiology of dual diagnosis. Biol Psychiatry 2004; 56: 730–7

19. Kiefer F and Wiedemann K. Combined Therapy: What does acamprosate and naltrexone combination tell us? Alcohol & Alcoholism 2004; 39: 542–7

20. Kiefer F, Jahn H, Tarnaske T et al. Comparing and combining naltrexone and acamprosate in relapse prevention of alcoholism. Arch Gen Psychiatry 2003; 60: 92–9

21. Koob G and Moal ML. (eds.) (2006) Neurobiology of addiction. Academic Press, San Diego, CA.

22. Kranzler HR and Ciraulo DA. (eds.) (2005) Clinical manual of addiction psychopharmacology. American Psychiatric Publishing, Inc., Washington, D.C.

23. LeMoal M and Koob GF. Drug addiction: pathways to the disease and pathophysiological perspectives. European Neuropsychopharmacology 2006; 17: 377–93

24. Lobo DSS and Kennedy JL. The genetics of gambling and behavioral addictions. CNS Spectr 2006; 11: 931–9

25. Martinez D, Gil R, Slifstein M et al. Alcohol dependence is associated with blunted dopamine transmission in the ventral striatum. Biol Psychiatry 2005; 58: 779–86

26. Mason BJ, Goodman AM, Chabac S et al. Effect of oral acamprosate on abstinence in patients with alcohol dependence in a double-blind, placebo-controlled trial: the role of patient motivation. Journal of Psychiatric Research 2006; 40: 382–92

27. Mason BJ. Acamprosate and naltrexone treatment for alcohol dependence: an evidence-based risk-benefits assessment. European NeuroPsychopharmacology 2003; 13: 469–75

28. Mason BJ. Acamprosate in the treatment of alcohol dependence. Expert Opin Pharmacother 2005; 6: 2103–15

29. Nestler EJ. Is there a common molecular pathway for addiction? Nature Neuroscience 2005; 11: 1445–9

30. Noël X, Van Der Linden M and Bechara A. The neurocognitive mechanisms of decision-making, impulse control, and loss of willpower to resist drugs. Psychiatry 2006; 30–41

31. O'Brien CP. Anticraving medications for relapse prevention: a possible new class of psychoactive medications. American Journal of Psychiatry 2005; 162: 1423–31

32. Petrakis IL, Poling J, Levinson C et al. Naltrexone and disulfiram in patients with alcohol dependence and comorbid psychiatric disorders. Biol Psychiatry 2005; 57: 1128–37

33. Pettinati HM, O'Brien CP, Rabinowitz AR et al. The status of naltrexone in the treatment of alcohol dependence. Specific effects on heavy drinking. Journal of Clinical Psychopharmacology 26: 610–25

34. Roozen HG, deWaart R, van der Windt DAW et al. A systematic review of the effectiveness of naltrexone in the maintenance treatment of opioid and alcohol dependence. European Neuropsychopharmacology 2005; 16: 311–23

35. Spencer TJ, Biederman J, Ciccone PE et al. PET study examining pharmacokinetics, detection and likeability, and dopamine transporter recepter occupancy of short- and long-acting oral methylphenidate. American Journal of Psychiatry 2006; 163: 387–95

36. Vocci FJ, Acri J and Elkashef A. Medication development for addictive disorders: the state of the science. American Journal of Psychiatry 2005; 162: 1432–40
37. Miller WR, Walters ST, Bennett ME, How effective is alcoholism treatment in the United States? J Studies Alcohol 2001; 62: 211–20

The Case: The woman with psychotic depression responsive to her own TMS machine

The Question: What do you do for TMS responders who need long-term maintenance?

The Dilemma: Finding simultaneous medication treatments to supplement TMS for her psychosis, confusion and mood disorder when ECT and clozapine have failed

Pretest Self Assessment Question (answer at the end of the case)

What is the usual protocol for approved treatment of repetitive transcranial magnetic stimulation (rTMS) in major depression not responding to prior antidepressants?

A. Weekly rTMS sessions of about 30 minutes each for 6 weeks
B. Three times weekly rTMS sessions of about 30 minutes each for about 6 weeks
C. Daily sessions (5 out of 7 days a week) for 4 to 6 weeks followed by antidepressant treatment
D. Daily sessions (5 out of 7 sessions of about 30 minutes each) for 4 to 6 weeks followed by once weekly maintenance treatments weekly indefinitely with or without antidepressant treatment

Patient Intake

- 45-year-old woman with a chief complaint "feeling sick all the time" by which she means being tired, seeing things, hearing things, inability to drive, and problems with daily living
- Her husband states that she has bouts of depression with confusion and that is the main problem
- Her psychiatrist is referring her for recommendations now that many medications including clozapine, as well as ECT have not been adequately effective

Psychiatric History

- Onset of recurrent, severe psychotic depressions with occasional episodes of mania past 12 years
- Onset occurred as a manic episode shortly after taking cimetidine (Tagamet), which some considered to have been the original precipitant of her illness
- Has had other manic episodes in response to antidepressants, but no spontaneous manic episodes
- Multiple hospitalizations for cycling mood disorder, diagnosed at various times and by various examiners as rapid cycling depressive disorder, schizoaffective disorder, bipolar disorder or psychotic depression

- At times she is delusional and hears voices
- However, her mood instability is the biggest factor in her illness with anxiety, agitation, insomnia, depression, occasional suicidal ideation but with a strong element of confusion whenever depressed

What do you think is her diagnosis?
- Bipolar disorder, rapid cycling
- Schizoaffective disorder
- Psychotic depression

Attending Physician's Mental Notes: Initial Psychiatric Evaluation

- Sounds like fundamentally a disorder of very severe, sometimes psychotic depression, with the curious symptom of confusion during such episodes
- Has been manic, perhaps drug-induced, and has been psychotic, but almost always when depressed, never when mood is normal
- Best working diagnosis may be some sort of bipolar illness, probably bipolar II or bipolar spectrum disorder, with cycling and occasional rapid cycling episodes, which are sometimes also psychotic
- She may have mixed episodes with irritability when depressed
- Whatever this is, her depressive episodes are severe and highly disabling

Medication History

- It emerges that for her, haloperidol especially by acute intramuscular injection, has the most efficacy, especially for her depressed states that are accompanied by marked confusion
- Multiple other conventional antipsychotics have been only helpful for transient psychotic or manic symptoms
- Lithium caused a severe tremor and no therapeutic actions
- Valproate (Depakote) made her sedated and had possible efficacy for mood but not continued
- Carbamazepine (Tegretol), possible Stevens Johnson rash
- Fluoxetine (Prozac), made her confused
- Bupropion (Wellbutrin), fair improvement at least briefly at high doses about 6 years ago
- Clozapine (Clozaril) up to 800 mg/day, did fair for a while, then continued to have mood cycles
- Clozapine up to 500 mg/day plus ripseridone (Risperdal) 9 mg/day plus lamotrigine (Lamictal) 200 mg/day, no change
- Olanzapine (Zyprexa) 20 mg, slight help briefly

- olanzapine 15 mg, plus risperidone 6 mg, plus lamotrigine up to 500 mg, no change
- Gabapentin (Neurontin) 2400 mg plus olanzapine 25 mg plus lorazepam (Ativan) 4 mg, more depression
- ECT 2 months ago, 5 treatments, moderate help
- Current medications
  - Olanzapine 20 mg
  - Lorazepam 1 mg at nite for sleep
  - Thyroid for hypothyroidism, testosterone/estrogen for osteoporosis, statin for hypercholesterolemia
  - Haloperidol (Haldol) 5–10 mg IM prn

Social and Personal History

- Married to her second husband for 12 years, no children with him
- First marriage for 14 years, at age 17 with one son, now 26
- Current husband has 2 children from his first marriage
- Patient has intermittently abused alcohol, especially during prolonged depressive episodes
- Sober past 3 years, no other drugs of abuse
- College graduate, RN (registered nurse), currently disabled

Medical History, Continued

- Osteoporosis
- GERD (gastro esophageal reflux disease)
- Hypothyroidism with thyroid replacement
- Normal BP, BMI
- Normal fasting glucose and triglycerides
- Hypercholesterolemia
- Normal EEG and MRI

Family History

- Mother: severe alcoholism

How would you treat her?

- Try to stabilize her without the need for intramuscular injections of haloperidol at home from her physician husband, which she is receiving most weeks
- Try to stabilize her on another second generation atypical antipsychotic
- Try an oral conventional antipsychotic
- Add an antidepressant

Attending Physician's Mental Notes: Initial Psychiatric Evaluation, Continued

- Since haloperidol has unusual and unexplained efficacy for her, and no atypical antipsychotic has been useful yet for her, including clozapine, perhaps the use of another conventional antipsychotic with atypical properties, such as loxapine (Loxitane), may reduce her need for injections and also help stabilize her
- For an antidepressant, perhaps the related compound amoxapine (Asendin), which itself is metabolized into an antipsychotic, may be useful

Case Outcome: First Interim Followup, Month 15

- In the past 15 months, the patient was treated by her local psychiatrist
- She experienced some initial improvement on loxapine 30 mg which has now been increased to 150 mg/day and valproate (Depakote) has been added at 3500 mg/day (blood level 85 ng/ml) with prn oral lorazepam 1–2 mg or intramuscular haloperidol up to 30 mg in a single injection which the husband, a physician, administers when she becomes suicidal or severely depressed and confused
- Seems to have converted from rapid cycling and unstable to unremittingly depressed without any psychotic features
- Since bupropion can be useful in bipolar depression and the patient responded to it previously (several years ago), it is suggested that amoxapine be lowered to 300 mg/day and bupropion be added, first 150 mg and then 300 mg

Case Outcome: Second Interim Followup, Month 19

- 4 months later the patient and her husband report that bupropion made her better than she has been in 12 years, even though she is not fully remitted
- Current medications
  - Bupropion 200 mg bid
  - Topiramate (Topamax) 125 mg (makes her sleepy)
  - Loxapine 150 mg
  - Amoxapine 200 mg
  - Valproate 3000 mg (level 91)
  - Haloperidol IM or lorazepam oral prn
- Also, she developed some dyskinetic mouth movements on bupropion
- Bupropion can unmask dyskinetic movements in some patients, presumably due to its prodopaminergic actions in a vulnerable patient whose dyskinesias are otherwise latent

- Discussed with patient and husband who want to continue bupropion and haloperidol anyway
- Suggested that she discontinue her topiramate and leave the other medications stable in the hope that with time she will get further antidepressant effects

Case Outcome: Followup, Months 24 through 33

- Patient was seen 5 months later, and then every month or two for the next 9 months
- Since her last appointment 5 months ago, she got depressed at first, and then became nearly manic, requiring haloperidol injections of 10–20 mg IM two out of every three days
- Discontinuation of topiramate caused insomnia so it was restarted
- Major symptom is "confusion" responsive whenever she receives a haloperidol injection of 10–20 mg
- Mouth movements have decreased probably secondary to receiving more haloperidol
- Complains now of confusion, but also headache, disorientation, low mood but not hallucinating or signs of any thought disorder
- Current medications
  - Bupropion 375 mg
  - Topiramate 100 mg qhs
  - Valproate 3000 mg
  - Amoxapine 300 mg
  - Loxapine 150 mg
  - Lorazepam 2 mg plus diazepam 5 mg qhs
  - Lorazapam 1 mg three times a day
  - Haloperidol injections 10–20 mg once a day most days
- Reluctantly, given the high amount of haloperidol she is receiving by frequent injection, suggested conversion to haloperidol decanoate, 200 mg every 4 weeks
- This was not fully effective and required augmentation with oral haolperidol 5–10 mg/day, so increased haloperidol decanoate to 300 mg every four weeks
- Results in diminished depression by about 50% according to the patient; husband thinks this is 70% improved; she can exercise some days, go out for dinner, drive on freeway, do some housework
- Patient and husband informed about potential long term concern of tardive dyskinesia
- Rather than leave well enough alone, attempt to cross titrate her onto quetiapine and off at least some of the haloperidol because of worry about tardive dyskinesia with the high dose long term treatment
- Eventually, reaches 1400 mg quetiapine and a low of 75 mg

haloperidol decanoate every 4 weeks while continuing topiramate, loxapine, valproate, bupropion, amoxapine and lorazepam as before
- Unfortunately, at this lower dose of haloperidol, she decompensates with depression, hallucinations

What would you do now?
- Continue high dose haloperidol decanoate
- Continue her other medications
- Slowly discontinue her quetiapine and use haloperidol plus loxapine as her antipsychotics
- Slowly discontinue her loxapine and use haloperidol plus quetiapine as her antipsychotics
- Add an antidepressant
- Refer her back to ECT (patient refuses)
- Refer her to VNS or TMS (not available at the time of this appointment)

Attending Physician's Mental Notes: Followup, Months 24 Through 33, Continued
- Her response seems to prove the unique therapeutic effectiveness of haloperidol for her and so, reluctantly, she was advised to continue high dose haloperidol decanoate
- Also, recommended that she slowly taper her loxapine but keep the other medications stable
- Told she may need to reconsider ECT in the future if relapses not responsive to haloperidol

Case Outcome: Followup 8 Years Later
- The patient returns for advice regarding the long term use of rTMS and input on medications for maintenance
- Over the past 8 years, has been followed locally by a different psychiatrist following the retirement of her original psychiatrist
- She has been maintained on her haloperidol decanoate for the past 8 years, but has had an up and down course over this period of time
- For the first three years after seeing her the last time, she eventually discontinued loxapine and valproate, but needed supplemental haloperidol dosing oral or acute IM injections whenever she worsened
- Maintained on variable doses of quetiapine, amoxapine, bupropion and topiramate as well
- Trials of lamotrigine (Lamictal), venlafaxine XR (Effexor XR) (up to 600 mg/day), duloxetine (Cymbalta) augmentation of venlafaxine, nefazodone (Serzone), aripiprazole (Abilify) augmentation, modafinil (Provigil) augmentation, mirtazapine (Remeron) up to 120 mg, in response to depressive dips or suicidal ideation, never as effective as

giving supplemental acute IM injections of haloperidol of 10–30 mg per injection
- If anything, antidepressants cause transient hypomania and cycling rather than antidepressant effects
- Diagnosed with acoustic neuroma, had neurosurgery, postoperatively had decreased hearing and Bell's palsy on the left, with the Bell's palsy resolving mostly over many months
- Intercurrent health concerns include concussion, diagnosis of benign ependymoma of the spinal cord, nephrolithiasis,
- Trial of bright light curiously helpful
- Medications 2 years ago, when she was doing her best, active and driving for the first time in 4 years
  - Haloperidol decanoate 200 mg every 4 weeks
  - Venlafaxine XR 600 mg/day
  - Lamotrigine 400 mg/day
  - Quetiapine 1400 mg/day
  - Aripiprazole 15 mg/day
  - Bupropion SR 450 mg/day
  - Mirtazapine 120 mg/day
  - Duloxetine 120 mg/day
- When she crashed on these medications after a period of good functioning, decided to travel to Canada to get rTMS treatments, available there but not in the US at the time

Have you seen a patient with depression respond to TMS?
- Yes, someone with major depressive disorder
- Yes, someone with bipolar depression
- Yes, someone with severe treatment resistant depression like this patient

Attending Physician's Mental Notes: Followup, 8 Years Later

- Current FDA approval of rTMS in the USA is for unipolar depression not responding to prior antidepressant treatment, and for 5 days a week treatments for 4 to 6 weeks, followed by antidepressants
- This patient seems far more ill than those in the FDA registration trials and also, she only responded partially to ECT
- Nevertheless, it was worth a try

Case Outcome: Followup Visit 8 Years Later, Continued

- The patient received 30 left sided high frequency treatments at 120% of threshold over the dorsolateral prefrontal cortex (DLPFC) for depression. This is also the approved location for the FDA approved procedure

- She also received 5 right sided treatments for anxiety. This is not an approved use of the FDA approved device and procedure but has been reported to be effective in the literature
- She received these 35 treatments over 21 days, 2 treatments most week days
- FDA approved procedure is for one treatment per day
- She was very much improved by these treatments, but not in full remission
- These improvements were maintained for 60 days after completing her rTMS treatments
- However, improvement began to fade by 90 days so another 2 weeks of left sided treatments, 2 per day were performed again in Canada
- Due to the long-term nature of this treatment, the husband, a physician, decided to purchase one of the TMS machines from Sweden and home TMS was initiated, 2 or 3 treatments per day for 5 consecutive days followed by 2 days of rest.
- After a month of this, the patient became tremulous, sleepless with tachycardia and treatments were discontinued for several days and then re-initiated at 1 per day
- Over the next months, she slowly withdrew from her antidepressants and reduced the dose of her antipsychotics. First was off bupropion, duloxetine and venlafaxine XR
- Stayed on quetiapine, lamotrigine, aripiprazole, haloperidol but lowering the dose of each
- Had a setback due to a family problem and increased her haloperidol again
- Eventually, on only prn haloperidol 5–10 mg orally every 3 days and duloxetine 30 mg
- In an effort to stop smoking, tried varenicline (Chantix, Champix), and had an increase in depression, restarted bupropion, but stopped it after 4 days due to insomnia
- Did well on TMS plus intermittent haloperidol for many months until she had to send the coil to Sweden for maintenance and was without treatment for 5 weeks. She relapsed, but rapidly responded once daily treatments were reinstituted
- One month ago she entered an agitated depressive state and was suicidal despite continued TMS treatments and no change in her medications
- She elected to stop TMS at that time, restarted duloxetine, and after 4 days restarted TMS with improvement of depression
- Today, she is subjectively well, only mildly depressed, about as good as she gets and is accepting this treatment result
- No psychotic features, confusion, or unstable moods
- TMS continues, who knows for how long. . . .

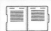

Case Debrief

- A remarkable story of a treatment resistant bipolar depressive disorder, with unusual confusion during depressive relapses with equally unusual response only to heroic doses of haloperidol
- Numerous antidepressants, ECT, numerous antipsychotics including clozapine without robust efficacy
- Prior to FDA approval, the family got TMS treatment outside of the US, and purchased their own TMS machine for home use in maintenance with rather remarkable results
- Thinking outside of the box allowed discovery of the haloperidol effect
- Keeping up hope and trying unproven treatment was rewarded with success
- Why she responds to haloperidol and TMS and not to standard treatments is a mystery that would be interesting to solve

Take-Home Points

- Without a supportive husband and the financial resources to see many psychiatristric experts, including travel out of the country and purchase of a personal TMS machine, this patient may very well not have survived due to the high risk of suicide in cases like this
- Unlikely that many other cases will respond like this one, but the point is that idiosyncratic responses happen all the time, and customizing treatments to the individual patient by paying attention to their unique responses is a good standard for clinical psychopharmacology
- In this case, it was better to get lucky than to be clever

Performance in Practice: Confessions of a Psychopharmacologist

- What could have been done better here?
  - Did it take too long to get to the depot haloperidol recommendation?
  - Should therapeutic drug levels have been sought for more drugs and more often?
- Possible action item for improvement in practice
  - Possibly if patients fail to respond to TMS according to the normal protocol, perhaps twice daily treatments can be suggested
  - This will require liaison with a local expert with a TMS device, and also information to be made available to patients
  - On the other hand, this approach is not likely to be replicated in many patients with treatment-resistant psychosis and depression, so looking at cases with poor treatment responses and trying to find a unique solution, but a different solution from the one that worked in this case, could be justified

Tips and Pearls

- Not all patients respond to all antipsychotic drugs the same
- Some patients get confused when they get depressed in unstable bipolar mood disorders
- Some patients still respond better to conventional antipsychotics than they do to either second generation atypical antipsychotics or even to clozapine
- Trying new treatments in difficult cases can lead to incredible and unexpected results
- Even a new therapy like TMS may need to be tailored with treatment protocols different from those approved for less difficult cases

Two-Minute Tute: A brief lesson and psychopharmacology tutorial (tute) with relevant background material for this case – Explanations of TMS

Table 1: What is Repetitive Transcranial Magnetic Stimulation (rTMS)?

- Rapidly alternating current passes through a small coil placed over the scalp, generating a magnetic field that induces an electrical current in the underlying brain, depolarizing neurons there

- During treatment, the patient is awake and reclining in a chair with a magnetic coil placed snugly against the scalp

- Coil location is usually determined by identifying the motor cortex (stimulation inducing a movement), and then moving the coil 5 cm rostrally (ahead) to approximate the location of the dorsolateral prefrontal cortex

- Treatments last a half hour to an hour

- In general, patients tolerate the treatment well and are able to go back to regular daily activities immediately following treatment

---

Table 2: How Does Repetitive Transcranial Magnetic Stimulation (rTMS) Work?

- Currently, all the stimulus parameters for ideal treatment are not yet known
  - Pulse frequency
  - Pulse intensity
  - Pulse duration
  - Interpulse interval
  - Total number of pulses per treatment session
  - How many treatment sessions over what period of time
  - How long to continue treatment after the initial set of treatments
- Even which side of the brain to stimulate is not known, including whether treatments on the left side are better for all patients with mood disorders, treatments on the right side better for anxiety disorders, and whether bilateral treatment would be useful for some patients
- Presumably, electrical impulses from DLPFC to other brain regions, including monoamine neurotransmitter centers is the mechanism of antidepressant action of rTMS

Table 3: Results of Repetitive Transcranial Magnetic Stimulation (rTMS) in Depression

- Onset of action in controlled studies by second week
- Works about as well as a switch or augmentation with another antidepressant for patients with 1, 2 or 3 prior antidepressant treatment failures
- Not clear if it works as well as ECT or in ECT nonresponders
- Most studies in unipolar depression
- Some studies in bipolar depression
- Some studies in postpartum depression

Table 4: What Are the Side Effects of Repetitive Transcrancial Magnetic Stimulation?

- Most common adverse event is headache or neck pain without observations of cognitive or cardiovascular complications
- The primary safety concern is seizure, which is rare, especially when stimulating dorsolateral prefrontal cortex rather than motor cortex

Posttest Self Assessment Question: Answer

What is the usual protocol for approved treatment of regional transcranial magnetic stimulation (rTMS) in major depression not responding to prior antidepressants?

A. Weekly rTMS sessions of about 30 minutes each for 6 weeks
B. Three times weekly rTMS sessions of about 30 minutes each for about 6 weeks
C. Daily sessions (5 out of 7 days a week) for 4 to 6 weeks followed by antidepressant treatment
D. Daily sessions (5 out of 7 sessions of about 30 minutes each for 4 to 6 weeks followed by one weekly maintenance treatments weekly indefinitely with or without antidepressant treatment

Answer: C

References

1. Stahl SM, Antidepressants, in Stahl's Essential Psychopharmacology, 3rd edition, Cambridge University Press, New York, 2008, pp 511–666
2. Stahl SM, Antipsychotics, in Stahl's Essential Psychopharmacology, 3rd edition, Cambridge University Press, New York, 2008, pp 327–452
3. Stahl SM, Clozapine, in Stahl's Essential Psychopharmacology The Prescriber's Guide, 3rd edition, Cambridge University Press, New York, 2009, pp 113–8
4. Stahl SM, Haloperidol, in Stahl's Essential Psychopharmacology The Prescriber's Guide, 3rd edition, Cambridge University Press, New York, 2009, pp 237–42
5. Marangell LB, Martinez M, Jurdi RA et al. Neurostimulation therapies, Acta Psychiatrica Scandinavica 2007; 116: 174–81
6. Berman RM, Narasinhan M, Sanacora G et al. A randomized clinical trial of repetitive transcranial magnetic stimulation in the treatment of major depression. Biol Psychiatry 2000; 47: 332–7
7. Avery DH, Holtzheimer PE, Fawaz W et al., A controlled study of repetitive transcranial magnetic stimulation in medication resistant major depressin. Biol Psychiatry 2006; 59: 187–94
8. Herwig U, Lampe Y, Juengling FD et al. Add on rTMS for treatment of depression: a pilot study using stereotaxic coil-navigation according to PET data. J Psychiatry Res 2003; 37: 267–75
9. Lisanby SH, Husain MM, Rosenquist PB et al. Daily left prefrontal repetitive transcranial magnetic stimulation in the acute treatment of major depression: clinical predictors of outcome in a multisite, randomized controlled clinical trial. Neuropsychopharmacol 2009; 34: 522–34

10. Demitrack MA, Thase ME, Clinical Significance of Transcranial Magnetic Stimulation (TMS) in the treatment of pharmacoresistant depression: synthesis of recent data, Psychopharm Bull 2009; 42: 5–38

11. George MS, Lisanby SH, Avery D et al. Daily left prefrontal transcranial magnetic stimulation therapy for major depressive disorder: a sham-controlled randomized trial. Arch Gen Psychiat 2010; 67: 507–16

12. Garcia KS, Flynn P, Pierce KJ et al. Repetitive transcranial magnetic stimulation treats postpartum depression. Brain Stim 2010; 3: 36–41

13. Gross M, Nakamura L, Pascual-Leone A et al. Has repetitive transcranial magnetic stimulation treatment for depression improved? A systematic review and meta analysis comparing the recent vs the earlier rTMS studies. Acta Psychiatr Scand 2007; 116: 165–73

14. Lam RW, Chan P, Wilkins-Ho M et al. Repetitive transcranial magnetic stimulation for treatment resistant depression: a systematic review and meta analysis, Can J Psychiatry 2008; 53: 621–31

15. O'Reardon J, Solvason H, Janicak, P et al. Efficacy and safety of transcranial magnetic stimulation therapy in the acute treatment of major depression: a multi site randomized controlled trial. Biol Psychiatry 2007; 62: 1208–16

16. Cohen R, Ferreiraa M, Ferreirra M et al. Use of repetitive transcranial magnetic stimulation for the management of bipolar disorder during the postpartum period. Brain Stim 2008; 1: 224–6

Lightning Round

The Case: The boy getting kicked out of his classroom

The Question: What is pediatric mania?

The Dilemma: What do you do for a little boy with a family history of mania and who is irritable, inattentive, defiant and aggressive?

Pretest Self Assessment Question (answer at the end of the case)

What differentiates pediatric mania from adult onset mania?

A. Elevated, expansive mood is the usual type in pediatric mania
B. Irritable mood is the usual type in pediatric mania
C. Discrete episodes in pediatric mania but last shorter than 4 days
D. Unremitting symptoms lacking discrete episodes is common in pediatric mania

Patient Intake

- 9-year-old boy
- "I am here for new medications to make me behave"

Psychiatric History

- Impulsivity, inattention and hyperactivity since age 3
- By age 5, diagnosed with ADHD and placed on mixed salts of d,l-amphetamine (Adderall) with poor or unclear therapeutic benefits
- OROS d,l-methylphenidate (Concerta) also not very effective
- Has become progressively more oppositional and disruptive in the classroom in the past year
- Teachers and administrators now consider him a threat to other students and maybe to teachers and insist on improved behavior or he will be removed from the mainstream classroom and require special placement
- Neuropsychological testing suggests a bright child intellectually who suffers from ADHD and pediatric mania with oppositional defiant disorder but not conduct disorder, and who also has multiple learning disabilities
- Pediatrician referred the patient to a child psychiatrist who was unwilling to prescribe an antipsychotic or mood stabilizer until the patient was at least 10 years old
- Mother and father are divorced for 3 years
- Has an older sister who lives with him, and parents have joint custody of both children, so the patient and his sister live together but with alternate parents, shuttling back and forth about half the time in each household

Medical History

- None significant

Family History

- Mother: bipolar
- Maternal grandmother: bipolar
- Older sister: bipolar
- Mother's side of the family subtly blamed by the father's side of the family for bipolar disorder and the current problems of the patient (and his sister)

Current medication

- d,l-amphetamine immediate release 30 mg in the morning and 20 mg at 11 am

Attending Physician's Mental Notes: Initial Psychiatric Evaluation

- Seen with his father, his paternal grandmother and a paternal aunt who all sat in on the interview
- Patient was fidgety and squirming in his seat, overactive but not overtly irritable
- Father says his son is on his best behavior and is usually much more grouchy
- The patient actually seemed to feel guilty about his bad behavior and ashamed of not controlling it better
- When asked what behaviors he needed to change in order to improve his situation at school, he stated he needed to stop fighting with kids at school and stop hitting classmates
- When asked what his medication does for him, he says "zilch"
- However, the grandmother, aunt and father all believe that the medication has some effect even though it is inconsistent
- The clearest evidence of its effect is that the patient's concentration and hyperactivity are reportedly better in school but seem to get worse after school is over and he comes home
- The patient meets criteria for pediatric mania in that he has a great deal of irritability most days that does not occur in discrete episodes but appears to be chronic
- However, he does have "rages" where he hits others and attacks property and yells in furor and anger, that are more discrete and periodic, but these never last for 4 days or more
- His tantrums spin out of control for hours at times, and then one of his parents has to come and pick him up from school

- Thoughts fly through his head and he jumps from one idea to the next without adequately expressing the first idea, and he feels powerful and invincible
- He is defiant and aggressive towards both teachers and classmates
- He endorses, and the family agrees, that he meets every one of the diagnostic criteria for ADHD inattentive subtype, almost all of the criteria for hyperactive subtype, and 3 out of 4 for the impulsive subtype
- He meets the criteria for oppositional defiant disorder as well but not enough of the criteria to be diagnosed as having conduct disorder

Based on just what you have learned here, do you agree with any of these diagnoses?
- Pediatric mania
- ADHD
- ODD
- CD
- Developmental reaction to parents' divorce
- Other

How would you treat him?
- Increase his stimulant dose
- Try another stimulant
- Augment with guanfacine XR (Intuniv)
- Augment with an atypical antipsychotic
- Switch to an atypical antipsychotic
- Add or switch to lithium
- Add or switch to carbamazepine or valproate
- Cognitive behavioral therapy
- Family therapy
- Other

Attending Physician's Mental Notes: Initial Psychiatric Evaluation, Continued

- This is obviously a tough situation
- Pediatric mania is a controversial concept
- Cynics believe it was invented in recent years by psychiatrists and pharmaceutical companies to make money off normative and transient events of development
- Few studies in children under 10
- Not clear if prepubertal pediatric mania is linked to adult onset bipolar disorder that runs in his family or if it represents a distinct, but genetically-mediated severe subtype of bipolar disorder
- Atypical antipsychotics probably best studied for prepubertal mania, but only in children older than 10

- Does everybody with pediatric mania also fit the diagnostic criteria for ADHD even though every child with ADHD does not fit the diagnostic criteria for pediatric mania?
- Does everybody with pediatric mania also fit the diagnostic criteria for ODD, CD or both even though every child with ODD or CD does not fit the diagnostic criteria for pediatric mania?
- Is the fad to over-diagnose ADHD in children now being replaced with a new fad of over-diagnosing mania in children?
- Does it matter?
- The question really is, with the child threatened to lose placement in a regular classroom, is an atypical antipsychotic or mood stabilizer justified?
- Also, can you combine an antipsychotic with a stimulant or is that pharmacologically irrational?

Attending Physician's Mental Notes, Initial Psychiatric Evaluation, Continued

- Whatever this is, it seems justified to be more aggressive psychopharmacologically
- Options:
  - increase his stimulant dose
  - try a different long acting stimulant
  - augment the stimulant with guanfacine XR for his hyperactive and oppositional symptoms
  - augment with an anticonvulsant mood stabilizer or even lithium
  - as time is of the essence here, it may be justified to add an atypical antipsychotic to attempt to salvage the patient's placement in his current classroom
- Aripiprazole (Abilify) was recommended
- It may appear to be irrational to give a releaser of dopamine (i.e., a stimulant) with a blocker of dopamine 2 receptors (i.e., an atypical antipsychotic) at the same time
- However, this may be useful in some cases since the antipsychotic will block subcortical D2 receptors in limbic regions while the stimulant will increase dopamine release in prefrontal cortex to stimulate D1 receptors (which many antipsychotics do not block)
- The net result is blockade of D2 receptors in limbic areas and stimulation of D1 receptors in prefrontal cortex, which may be therapeutic in some patients with combinations of ADHD symptoms with mood/mania symptoms
- The case goes on. . . .

Posttest Self Assessment Question: Answer

What differentiates pediatric mania from adult onset mania?

A. Elevated, expansive mood is the usual type in pediatric mania
B. Irritable mood is the usual type in pediatric mania
C. Discrete episodes in pediatric mania but last shorter than 4 days
D. Unremitting symptoms lacking discrete episodes is common in pediatric mania

Answer: B and D

Current experts consider that pediatric mania may be characterized by severe irritability and the absence of discrete episodes of mood disturbance and hyperactivity

References

1.   Biederman J. The evolving face of pediatric mania. Biological Psychiatry 2006; 60 901–2
2.   Baumer FM, Howe M, Gallelli K et al. A pilot study of antidepressant-induced mania in pediatric bipolar disorder: characteristics, risk factors, and the serotonin transporter gene. Biol Psychiatry 2006; 60: 1005–12
3.   Dickstein DP, Milham MP, Nugent AC et al. Frontotemporal alterations in pediatric bipolar disorder. Arch Gen Psychiatry 2005; 62: 734–41
4.   Stahl SM, Mood Disorders, in Stahl's Essential Psychopharmacology, 3rd edition, Cambridge University Press, New York, 2008, pp 453–510
5.   Stahl SM, Antidepressants, in Stahl's Essential Psychopharmacology, 3rd edition, Cambridge University Press, New York, 2008, pp 511–666
6.   Stahl SM, Aripiprazole, in Stahl's Essential Psychopharmacology The Prescriber's Guide, 3rd edition, Cambridge University Press, New York, 2009, pp 45–50

The Case: The young man whose dyskinesia was prompt and not tardive

The Question: What is the cause of a profound and early onset movement disorder in a young man who just started a second generation atypical antipsychotic?

The Dilemma: How can you treat the psychotic illness without making the movement disorder worse?

Pretest Self Assessment Question (answer at the end of the case)

Which of the following has the least risk of causing movement disorders?

A. Clozapine (Clozanil)

B. Olanzapine (Zyprexa)

C. Paliperidone (Invega)

D. Quetiapine (Seroquel)

Patient Intake

- 21-year-old male with a three-year history of psychotic illness arrives with his mother and sister
- Chief complaint: "I've been misdiagnosed as schizophrenia"
- He believes that medications do not help and that they cause movement disorders

Psychiatric History

Premorbid and Prodrome

- According to his mother and sister, premorbidly he was shy, introverted, and bright
- He began behaving strangely at age 17 or so
- He thought that the cable installation man was spying on him
- He would say tangential things in the middle of a conversation and would inappropriately smile
- He began to complain of the inability to sleep yet felt sleep deprived
- Eventually he stopped going to classes and dropped out of school
- He came to believe that his mother and father were evil, and that:
  - His mother commits voodoo with Hillary Clinton, who communicates with her through a voice chip in the mother's brain
  - His mother eats good food with Hillary Clinton and cooks bad food for him and for others
  - His father molested him as a child and communicates with Robert DeNiro via a voice chip in his father's brain
- The patient was told these things via a voice chip in his own head, through which his favorite professor speaks to him

First Psychotic Break

- When he was nearly 19 he had an outburst in which he became violent and was yelling, shoving, pushing, and slapping
- His parents called the police and he was hospitalized for three days, diagnosed with schizophrenia, and prescribed olanzapine (Zyprexa) 12 mg/day, to which he responded
- He attended one semester of college, with good grades and good behavior, while gradually tapering his medication over several months

Second Hospitalization

- Two months after discontinuing medication he relapsed and was rehospitalized after an episode during which he shoved, pushed, and screamed that his food was poisoned
- He initially refused medications but was then court-ordered to take medication for one week, after which he was released but not stabilized
- He immediately stopped his medications upon returning home and became violent with screaming and threatening behavior

Third Hospitaliztion and Onset of Movement Disorder

- He was rehospitalized and initially treated with olanzapine, but seemed not to respond and so was switched to aripiprazole (Abilify) and then to paliperidone (Invega) 12 mg/day
- Over the following several months he did not have overt symptoms of psychosis and was not talking about his delusions or hallucinations, but did have an increasing number of anxiety attacks
- During that time his paliperidone dose was gradually decreased, with the ultimate dose being 3 mg/day
- Despite reduction of paliperidone dose, he experienced noticeable muscle spasms, tremor, leg twitching, abnormal arm posture, neck spasms, and torticollis
- After three months on paliperidone 3 mg/day he stopped his medications, thinking he was fine

What do you think about his movement disorder?

- So far, sounds like drug induced extrapyramidal symptoms (EPS)
- This is already tardive dyskinesia
- Seems like a reaction to high dose paliperidone that has not yet resolved with dosage reduction
- Hysteria
- Bizarre postures of schizophrenia, not caused by antipsychotics

Attending Physician's Mental Notes: Initial Psychiatric Evaluation

- Too early for tardive dyskinesia,
- Very unlikely to be due to hysteria or to bizarre postures of a psychotic illness
- Seems likely to be an EPS in a patient who is very sensitive to high doses of paliperidone, and has not yet resolved with dosage reduction, which can take weeks or months in the vulnerable

Psychiatric History, Continued

Fourth Hospitalization and Worsening of Movements

- Two days after discontinuing his medication he was fully delusional with his usual symptoms, and called the police several times claiming he was being abused
- He also called an ambulance several times because he believed he was having panic attacks, but was not hospitalized
- He reported rush of thoughts, his eyes freezing and moving backwards into his head to stare at the back of his brain, tremor, and feeling that his heart would stop when he breathed
- At this point he was hospitalized, voluntarily, for the fourth time
- He took medication but refused all laboratory testing
- He was discharged on paliperidone 12 mg during the day and quetiapine (Seroquel) 400 mg at night
- Switched as an outpatient to olanzapine 10 mg at night, plus paliperidone 12 mg during the day to reduce psychotic symptoms, but many positive symptoms persist
- Added benztropine (Cogentin) 0.5 mg for movement disorder without any response

Attending Physician's Mental Notes: Initial Psychiatric Evaluation, Continued

- Sounds like he had an old-fashioned oculogyric crisis
- These were described with conventional antipsychotics but rarely if ever with second generation atypical antipsychotics
- Very few EPS likely with quetiapine; also few on this dose of olanzapine, so probably caused by paliperidone
- Why is he so sensitive to paliperidone?
- Is the combination of paliperidone plus quetiapine causing too much dopamine D2 receptor blockade for him?
- Is he a poor metabolizer or does he for some reason have disproportionately high blood levels of his antipsychotics even though paliperidone is not metabolized by CYP450 2D6?

- Seems like a motor reaction well out of proportion to what would be expected for these drugs at these doses
- Does he have an underlying extrapyramidal disorder as well as schizophrenia, or early onset Huntington's disease or similar condition?

Social and Personal History

- Attended one semester of college between his first and second hospitalizations
- Non smoker, denies drug and alcohol abuse including no marijuana
- Lives at home, few friends, no dating
- No notable activities outside the home since dropping out of college before his second hospitalization
- No competitive employment

Medical history

- Thin, low normal BMI
- BP, routine labs including fasting glucose and trigylcerides normal
- Has been refusing venepuncture for over a year

Family history

- Maternal uncle: schizophrenia

Patient Intake

- Patient states, "I have a chip in my brain. It tells me I was starved in Romania before I was age 2 and came to the United States"
- He admits to a three-year history of delusions and hallucinations but believes that medications do not help, yet cause horrible movement disorders
- He has no insight into his illness and is adamant that he does not have schizophrenia; he believes that his current treating doctor is evil because he medicates him
- He wants to live independently but is on social security disability and Medicare
- He is not currently suicidal

Movement Disorder

- He displays torticollis to the right with an abnormal stooped posture with dystonic axial tone
- He also has abnormal bizarre dystonic arm postures and frequent playing finger movements, like playing a piano keyboard constantly
- There are no oral, buccal, lingual, masticatory, or facial dyskinesias noted

Attending Physician's Mental Notes: Initial Psychiatric Evaluation, Continued

- Clearly a psychotic illness, probably schizophrenia as this runs in the family
- However, now his movement disorder presents with signs both of acute EPS (stooped posture), dystonias, and finger dyskinesias more characteristic of long-term treatment and tardive dyskinesia
- Could be due to another illness, but treatment emergent with paliperidone, so most likely drug-induced

Which of the following strategies would be your top priority?
- Send him to a neurologist for a movement disorder evaluation
- Send him for a genetic test for Huntington's Disease
- Do a brain MRI and EEG and lumbar puncture
- Maintain his medications unchanged in order not to jeopardize what response he is having nor worsen his movement disorder
- Adjust his medications in order to try to achieve a greater antipsychotic response as the top priority
- Adjust his medications in order to try to reduce motor side effects even if this jeopardizes his antipsychotic response and risks rehospitalization

Attending Physician's Mental Notes: Initial Psychiatric Evaluation, Continued

- This situation feels like being between a rock and a hard place (i.e., whatever you do for his psychosis may be bad for his movement disorder and vice versa)
- His current medication regimen seems to be causing an unusually disproportionate set of movement disorders; this is most likely attributable to paliperidone as they originated during paliperidone treatment
- Over the long-term he is at risk for tardive dyskinesia or tardive dystonia if he does not have one of these already
- It is therefore best to switch him to a different medication regimen soon or else he risks permanent disfigurement
- So now, how do we have our cake and eat it, too (i.e., improve psychosis as well as current movement disorder while reducing risk for long-term complications of tardive dyskinesia)?

Which of the following would you do?
- Convert him to intramuscular depot paliperidone every 4 weeks
- Discontinue current medications and switch him to risperidone (Risperdal)
- Discontinue paliperidone and maintain olanzapine but at a higher dose
- Discontinue current medications and switch him to another second generation atypical antipsychotic, either quetiapine (Seroquel), ziprasidone (Geodon, Zeldox), aripiprazole (Abilify), asenapine (Saphris), iloperidone (Fanapt), or lurasidone (Latuda)
- Discontinue current medications and switch him to clozapine (Clozaril)
- Discontinue current medications and switch him to a conventional antipsychotic

Attending Physician's Mental Notes: Initial Psychiatric Evaluation, Continued

- Because of the patient's movement disorder, it may not be best to switch him to either a conventional antipsychotic or risperidone (paliperidone, which is causing his movement symptoms, is the active metabolite of risperidone)
- High-dose monotherapy with an agent associated with less risk of movement disorders may be the best option for this patient
- Increasing the dose of olanzapine to as much as 40 mg/day may be efficacious if tolerated
- High-dose quetiapine (800–1000 mg/day) may be efficacious if tolerated
- High-dose aripiprazole (20–30 mg/day) may be efficacious (but previous trials of lower doses of aripiprazole have not been deemed successful for this patient and aripiprazole can be associated with akathisia)
- High doses of asenapine (>20 mg/day) have not been studied and may not be well absorbed due to the need for sublingual administration. Note this agent can cause some EPS
- High doses of iloperidone (>24 mg/day) have been studied somewhat and this agent reportedly has low incidence of EPS and thus might be a consideration if olanzapine fails
- Lurasidone is a new agent just released but has controlled date up to 160 mg/day
- Because he has a history of nonadherence and a somewhat irregular diet, ziprasidone may not be a good choice as a monotherapy (it must be taken twice per day with food and can have erratic absorption), but could be used to augment his current olanzapine dose
- In theory, clozapine may be an excellent choice for this patient as it may help his psychosis more than the other medications and has

least risk of movement disorder; however, this is not a feasible choice unless he becomes compliant with laboratory testing
- Supplementary doses of benzodiazepines for sleep and/or during the day for agitation may be helpful in keeping the doses of any psychotic lower

Case Outcome: First Interim Followup, Week 12

- Family returns for reevaluation
- Patient's doctor angry that family came for the initial evaluation here, and thus refuses to change medications other than to raise olanzapine dose to 20 mg
- Movements persist, and patient is slightly sedated without robust improvement in residual psychotic symptoms
- Family told by treating doctor that changing paliperidone will mean rehospitalization and that the movements cannot be avoided
- Also, treating doctor does not think neurological evaluation or other tests are necessary
- Family told by him that treating the psychosis and avoiding hospitalization is the priority
- Family then asked at the current visit whether this was an acceptable treatment plan for them, or if they wanted to change treating doctors and pursue a plan to treat the movement disorder as well as the psychosis
- Family agrees to change medications and referred to another psychiatrist in their town
- Patient remains without insight, denying psychosis, refusing blood tests, having continued delusions about poisoning but not having aggressive behavior
- Movements continue unabated and unchanged from before
- Recommended trial of high dose olanzapine (if necessary), while discontinuing paliperidone, or high dose quetiapine

Case Outcome: Second Interim Followup, Week 24

- Family returns for another reevaluation
- New physician tried up to 40 mg/day of olanzapine, with improvement in delusions, but worsening of motor restlessness plus new onset of sedation, little or no weight gain
- Did not monitor fasting triglycerides
- Paliperidone reduced to 3 mg/day but lower doses trigger recurrent agitation and acting out
- Now on 600 mg quetiapine XR plus 3 mg paliperidone with benztropine 0.5 mg daily

- Not as well controlled in terms of delusions and occasional aggressive behavior now, compared to high dose paliperidone
- Movements appear slightly better but are still dramatically abnormal, especially the torticollis

What would you do?
- Leave well enough alone
- Increase quetiapine further
- Try to get him to take clozapine
- Trial of iloperidone
- Neuropsychological testing for early dementia, or Huntington's or other disorder
- Neurological evaluation

Attending Physician's Mental Notes: Second Interim Followup, Week 24

- Clozapine, potentially the best option, is not feasible due to lack of patient cooperation with venepuncture
- Although the dose of the possible offending agent paliperidone has been reduced from 12 mg/day to 3 mg/day, it does not seem further dose reduction of this agent can be accomplished unless another agent is added or current dose of quetiapine is increased
- Recommended to slowly increase quetiapine without dose reduction of paliperidone over 4 to 12 weeks, up to 1000 mg/day, and then slowly decrease paliperidone by 0.5 mg per week over 6 weeks
- For now, discontinue benztropine as the dose is too low to be effective and an adequate trial of this agent should await discontinuation of paliperidone
- Neuropsychological evaluation seems prudent for many reasons, both to assess psychosis and cognition, and to get a baseline for the future; family agrees
- Monitor weight and also fasting triglycerides in 8 weeks

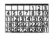

Case Outcome: Third Interim Followup, Week 36

- Now off paliperidone, on quetiapine XR 900 mg qhs
- Some sedation but psychosis better now despite discontinuing paliperidone
- However, no improvement in movements

Case Debrief

- Movement disorders can become permanent and are disfiguring; patients with movement disorders should have their medication regimens adjusted to minimize such side effects if possible

- Long term, movements will impair adherence
- This patient must be extraordinarily sensitive to EPS even from second generation atypical antipsychotics
- Quetiapine is probably the best option other than clozapine, for an antipsychotic that should not exacerbate his movement disorder, assuming that it is a powerful enough antipsychotic for him
- Some patients may require doses above 900 mg/day of quetiapine for adequate control of psychosis although these doses are poorly studied
- Although this patient has been off high doses of paliperidone for several months and off all paliperidone for several weeks, his movements are not improving
- However, this is still a relatively short period of time since it can take many months for the effects of antipsychotics on motor symptoms to wash out and thus there is every possibility that he will improve in the coming months if he can remain off paliperidone
- His dystonias, including his torticollis, are the most worrisome because they may represent tardive dystonia
- Tardive dystonia can be very difficult to treat and can become permanent
- If medication washout of the paliperidone in the next months does not lead to improvement of dystonias, high dose benztropine can be considered
- Local injections of botulinum toxin, especially for neck muscles in torticollis, can be effective in improving this problem as well
- Reconsideration of a neurological condition such as Huntington's disease may be necessary

Take-Home Points
- Although EPS and tardive dyskinesia have remarkably diminished since the introduction of second generation atypical antipsychotics, these conditions have not entirely been eliminated, especially in vulnerable individuals and with certain drugs
- Paliperidone and risperidone may be more likely to cause EPS than some other agents in the class
- No pharmacogenetic test yet exists to predict who is most vulnerable to these complications
- This patient had the rapid onset of movement disorders, including both a probably reversible form of EPS (rigidity and restlessness/akathisia) and also a possibly irreversible form of tardive dyskinesia/tardive dystonia (finger movements, torticollis, arm postures) despite being given second generation atypical antipsychotic agents

- It is nevertheless the duty of the treating psychopharmacologist to attempt to control psychosis while not inducing movement disorders such as this, even though that can be a considerable therapeutic challenge

Performance in Practice: Confessions of a Psychopharmacologist

- What could have been done better here?
  - Would better liaison with the original treating psychiatrist other than just an exchange of a written consultation have led to more rapid implementation of this plan without the delay and disruption of finding another treating psychiatrist?
  - Would more rapid conversion to an antipsychotic other than paliperidone have improved movement disorders?
- Possible action item for improvement in practice
  - Early involvement of movement disorder experts
  - Early neuropsychological evaluation
  - Better support of the family in their heroic efforts to help this patient throughout multiple hospitalizations, medication complications and disruptive changing of physicians

Tips and Pearls

- Movement disorders can still occur with second generation atypical antipsychotics and take a potentially malignant form, such as dystonias, early in treatment
- Quetiapine or clozapine may be the treatments of choice in such patients
- Not only is there evidence that clozapine may not cause EPS, but over long treatment periods, may actually improve tardive dyskinesia
- It can take a long time for the maladaptive effects of an antipsychotic on the motor system to wear off, presumably via potentially reversible re-adaptations of dopamine D2 receptors in the nigrostriatal pathway
- There are theoretical concerns and actual data to suggest that acute EPS may predict chronic tardive dyskinesia; therefore, abolishing acute EPS is a priority and may help reduce the onset of irreversible tardive dyskinesia/dystonia, especially in a patient as seemingly vulnerable as this one to the movement disorder complications of antipsychotics

Two-Minute Tute: A brief lesson and psychopharmacology tutorial (tute) with relevant background material for this case – Tardive dyskinesia and D₂ receptors

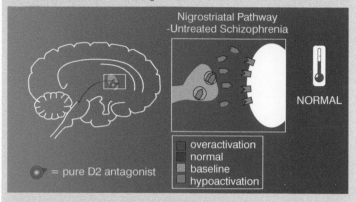

Figure 1: The nigrostriatal pathway is theoretically unaffected in untreated schizophrenia.

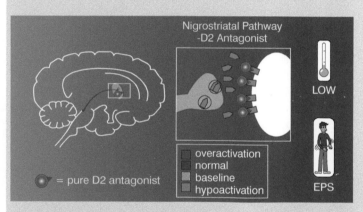

Figure 2: Blockade of D2 receptors in the nigrostriatal pathway by an antipsychotic agent can prevent binding of dopamine to its postsynaptic receptors and thereby cause motor side effects, called extrapyramidal symptoms or EPS. This can include acute dystonias such as torticollis and oculogyric crises, such as this patient experienced.

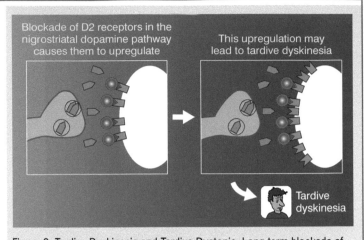

Blockade of D2 receptors in the nigrostriatal dopamine pathway causes them to upregulate

This upregulation may lead to tardive dyskinesia

Tardive dyskinesia

Figure 3: Tardive Dyskinesia and Tardive Dystonia. Long term blockade of D2 receptors in the nigrostriatal pathway(or even shorter term blockade of D2 receptors as in this case) theoretically causes upregulation of those receptors, which may lead to a hyperkinetic motor condition known as tardive dyskinesia, characterized by facial and tongue movements (e.g., tongue protrusions, facial grimaces, chewing) as well as quick, jerky limb movment and distal extremity movements, such as the finger movements this patient experienced. Although this patient did not have classical facial dyskinesias, his acute dystonias were converting into chronic dystonias, with the fear that these represented tardive dystonias and would become potentially irreversible. The upregulation of the D2 receptors may be the consequence of the neuron's futile attempt to overcome drug-induced blockade of its dopamine D2 receptors. In some cases this may lead to classical oro-buccal-facial tardive dyskinesia, and in other cases tardive dystonia in vulnerable individuals.

Posttest Self Assessment Question: Answer

Which of the following has the least risk of causing movement disorders?

A. Clozapine
B. Olanzapine
C. Paliperidone
D. Quetiapine

Answer: A

References

1. Stahl SM, Psychosis and Schizophrenia, in Stahl's Essential Psychopharmacology, 3rd edition, Cambridge University Press, New York, 2008, pp 247–326
2. Stahl SM, Antipsychotic Agents, in Stahl's Essential Psychopharmacology, Cambridge University Press, New York, 2008, pp 327–452
3. Stahl SM, Clozapine, in Stahl's Essential Psychopharmacology The Prescriber's Guide, 3rd edition, Cambridge University Press, New York, 2009, pp 113–8
4. Stahl SM, Quetiapine, in Stahl's Essential Psychopharmacology The Prescriber's Guide, 3rd edition, Cambridge University Press, New York, 2009, pp 459–64
5. Stahl SM, Paliperidone, in Stahl's Essential Psychopharmacology The Prescriber's Guide, 3rd edition, Cambridge University Press, New York, 2009, pp 403–7
6. Dessler RM, Ansari MS, Riccardi P et al. Occupancy of striatal and extrastriatal dopamine D2 receptors by clozapine and quetiapine, Neuropsychopharmacol 2006; 31: 1991–2001
7. Tenback DE, van Harten PN, Sloof CJ et al. Evidence that early extrapyramidal symptoms predict later tardive dyskinesia: a prospective analysis of 10,000 patients in the European schizophrenia outpatient health outcomes (SOHO) study. Am J Psychiatry 2003; 163: 1438–40

The Case: The patient whose daughter wouldn't give up

The Question: Is medication treatment of recurrent depression in an elderly woman worth the risks?

The Dilemma: Should remission still be the goal of antidepressant treatment if it means high doses and combinations of antidepressants in a frail patient with two forms of cancer and two hip replacements?

Pretest Self Assessment Question (answer at the end of the case)

Parkinsonism may be antipsychotic-induced in the elderly, but will generally reverse within a week or two.

A. True
B. False

Patient Intake

- 72-year-old female
- Chief complaint: anxiety

Psychiatric History

- Was well until age 32, first major depressive episode
  - Characterized by depressed mood and loss of appetite but not anxiety
  - Treated with tricyclic antidepressant
  - Recovered fully
- Second episode age 45
  - After her husband died prematurely
  - Lasted about a year
  - May have been a prolonged grief episode
  - Not treated
  - Recovered fully
- Third episode age 69
  - Severe anxiety as well as depression
  - Paroxetine (Paxil, Seroxat) treatment
  - Recovered fully
  - Discontinued paroxetine after a few months
  - Relapsed
- Fourth episode age 69
  - Re-treated with paroxetine
  - Full recovery again
  - Discontinued paroxetine again after several weeks
  - Relapsed again
- Fifth episode age 70
  - Re-treated with paroxetine

Current Medications

- Because of severe anxiety, given olanzapine (Zyprexa) 5 mg, which helped anxiety but not depression
- No response to nefazodone (Serzone)
- No response to desipramine (Norpramin)
- Venlafaxine XR (Effexor XR) made her more anxious
- Given seven ECT treatments and depression not improved but memory worse
- Lithium, T3 (Cytomel) and perphenazine (Trilafon) not very helpful
- Now on loxapine (Loxitane) and alprazolam (Xanax) with marginal improvement
- Referred to you for a consultation from her psychiatrist in a city a few hours drive away

Social and Personal History

- Married once, two children, several grandchildren
- Widowed 25 years ago
- Lives alone but visited frequently by a daughter who lives nearby
- Non smoker
- No drug or alcohol abuse

Medical History

- Postmenopausal on estrogen/progestin replacement therapy
- BMI, BP, lipids normal

Family History

- No first degree relatives with depression or other psychiatric disorders

Patient Intake

- Brought to the office by her daughter who sits in on the interview
- Walked into office with shuffling gait, masked facies, rigidity and tremor
- Parsimonious in speech, appears flat and apathetic yet complains of severe anxiety
- Not suicidal, memory intact
- Complains of anhedonia, lack of energy and motivation and interest while also experiencing anxiety and disruptive sleep

From the information given, what do you think her primary diagnosis is?

- Unipolar major depression with anxiety
- Nonresponsiveness to antidepressant treatment suggests mixed-state bipolar disorder rather than anxious depression

- Motor symptoms suggest the depression subtype that is associated with Parkinson's Disease
- Nonresponsiveness to antidepressant treatment with prominent apathy suggests early dementia

Attending Physician's Mental Notes: Initial Psychiatric Evaluation

- Certainly her parksinonism is prominent, but might be due to loxapine, not Parkinson's disease
- Not enough information to diagnose dementia or to rule it out
- However, seems mentally sharp in terms of cognition but quite depressed and anxious
- Wonder why her antidepressant medications have been stopped so often when she has had good responses to them until the last episode
- Wonder also whether had she maintained antidepressant treatment indefinitely following her third episode of depression would her fourth and fifth episodes have been prevented and would her fifth episode not have become treatment resistant?
- At this point the diagnosis made was major depression, recurrent, with drug-induced parkinsonism, not Parkinson's Disease

Of the following choices, what would you do?

- Discontinue loxapine
- Switch to another antipsychotic
- Add antidepressant
- Add mood stabilizer
- Switch antipsychotic plus add antidepressant
- Add mood stabilizer plus antidepressant
- None of the above

If you would give an antidepressant, which would you add?

- SSRI (serotonin selective reuptake inhibitor)
- SNRI (serotonin norepinephrine reuptake inhibitor)
- NDRI (bupropion; norepinephrine dopamine reuptake inhibitor)
- Mirtazapine
- Trazodone
- Tricyclic antidepressant
- MAO inhibitor
- I would not give an antidepressant

If you would give an antipsychotic, which would you add?

- Clozapine
- Risperidone

- Paliperidone
- Olanzapine
- Quetiapine
- Ziprasidone
- Aripiprazole
- Asenapine
- Iloperidone
- Lurasidone
- Conventional antipsychotic
- Depot antipsychotic
- I would not add an antipsychotic

If you would give a mood stabilizer/anticonvulsant, which would you add?

- Lithium
- Divalproex
- Lamotrigine
- Carbamazepine
- Oxcarbazepine
- Topiramate
- Levetiracetam
- Zonisamide
- Gabapentin/pregabalin
- I would not add a mood stabilizer/anticonvulsant

Attending Physicians Mental Notes: Initial Psychiatric Evaluation, Continued

- Obviously the loxapine should be discontinued and no new antipsychotic given to see if the parkinsonism reverses
- Continued alprazolam 0.25 mg three times a day
- Because of anxiety with depression, initiated mirtazapine (Remeron) 15 mg qhs, increasing to 30 mg in a few days if well tolerated
- Mirtazapine often well tolerated in the elderly
- See no need for a mood stabilizer at this time

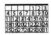

Case Outcome: First Interim Followup, Week 4

- Daughter drives her mother back for a follow up consultation
- Four weeks after stopping loxapine, still parkinsonian
- Daughter is concerned her mother has Parkinson's disease since the medication has been stopped a long time now
- Somewhat sleepy during the day but wakes up anxious and nervous; decreased appetite continues; if anything, anxiety is worse
- Increased mirtazapine to 45 mg and alprazolam to 0.5 mg three times a day

Are you beginning to get worried like the daughter that the patient has Parkinson's disease because her motor symptoms are not improving a month after the last dose of loxitane which has a 24 hour half life and should now have been entirely out of her system for weeks?

- Yes
- No

Attending Physician's Mental Notes: First Interim Followup, Week 4

- Although it is certainly possible the patient has Parkinson's Disease, four weeks is often insufficient time for dopamine receptors to readapt to normal following antipsychotic washout even though all antipsychotic should have been out of her system 5 half lives, or five days, following the last dose
- Patient and daughter reassured and told that 2 to 6 months washout is necessary to be sure that the movements are not due to loxapine
- It is possible that loxapine unmasked underlying and previously clinically silent Parkinson's disease
- Waitful watching is encouraged for a few months while giving no antipsychotic

Case Outcome: Second Interim Followup, Week 16

Patient Lost to Followup for 3 months

- Eight weeks after stopping loxapine, parkinsonism had largely resolved
- Now, 16 weeks after stopping loxapine, no parkinsonism evident at all
- Also, the patient has less depression and worry, less sedation
- However, discovered that about a month after her last appointment here, she had fallen and broken her hip and had a hip replacement
- Still problems coping and with activities of daily living following recent hip replacement, so living with daughter in her home
- Has continued mirtazapine 45 mg and alprazolam 0.5 mg three times a day since previous appointment 3 months ago, as tolerating it well and responding to it but not in full remission, perhaps 50% better

Do you think her fall causing the hip fracture could have been related to sedative mediations such as mirtazapine and alprazolam, or to sedation in combination with incompletely resolved drug-induced parkinsonism?

- Yes
- No

Attending Physician's Mental Notes: Second Interim Followup, Week 16

- Indeed, her fall could have been due to sedative medications, especially alprazolam, as benzodiazepines as well as sedating antidepressants have been reported in some, but not all studies, to increase the risk of falls
- Parkinsonism, whether drug-induced or Parkinson's Disease is also associated with falls in the elderly
- Nevertheless, this patient is not sedated by her medications, is thin and frail, and if anything, her lack of energy from her depression may also have been contributors and it is not clear that in her particular case that her medications led to her fall
- Thus, on balance, felt that continuing prior medications was still indicated
- Furthermore, to attempt to reach remission of her depressive symptoms, initiated venlafaxine 37.5 mg increasing to 75 mg

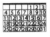

Case Outcome: Fourth Interim Followup, Week 24

- Eight weeks after previous appointment, a total of 24 weeks since her initial evaluation, daughter drove her back for a followup appointment
- Patient "not as nervous"
- Looks lively, spontaneous, feels basically well except gets very anxious under stress
- Playing bridge – daughter thinks she is improving and able to run errands on her own; more confidence; coping better
- Planning to move back to her own home soon
- Continued same meds

Case Outcome: Fifth Interim Followup, Week 36

- Three months later, continued improvement
- Essentially in complete remission from her depression
- Driving again
- Shopping on her own but still living with daughter

Case Outcome: Sixth Interim Followup, Week 48

- A few months later, full remission and lost to follow-up

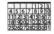

Case Outcome: Seventh Interim Followup, Year 6

Years Later, a Total of 6 Years Since Initial Psychiatric Evaluation

- Four years later, patient is now age 77, daughter calls
- Patient has no depression, no anxiety and no insomnia
- However, BUN (blood urea nitrogen) and creatinine rising and

creatinine clearance falling for past several months, and her family physician thinks renal changes may be due to venlafaxine and/or mirtazapine, so decreases these medications to half dose

- Patient is about to undergo hip surgery on her other hip for bursectomy, and family physician actually considering stopping meds altogether for surgery and not reinstituting them afterwards
- Daughter is alarmed by this
- Patient is also status post colon resection from colon carcinoma, presumed cured, and also repair of abdominal hernia which have occurred since the previous appointment two years ago
- Advised them to get therapeutic drug levels before deciding to discontinue meds entirely

Do you think her rising BUN and creatinine, and falling creatinine clearance were likely caused by her venlafaxine, mirtazapine or both?

- Yes
- No

Attending Physician's Mental Notes: Seventh Interim Followup, Year 6

- Although anything is theoretically possible, venlafaxine and mirtazapine are not noted for their ability to cause renal failure/ complications
- However, for patients with renal impairment from any cause, venlafaxine and mirtazapine doses may need to be lowered by 25%–50%
- This patient only has borderline to normal renal functioning and not any clear renal impairment
- Any necessary dosing alterations in her venlafaxine and/or mirtazapine can be determined by getting therapeutic drug levels, and if high, oral doses can be reduced

Attending Physician's Mental Notes: Eighth Interim Followup, Year 7.5

- 6th episode of major depression
- 16 months after the last phone call, daughter brings patient in for re-evaluation
- Her now 79-year-old mother relapsed on the reduced doses of 37.5 mg of venlafaxine and 15 mg of mirtazapine which the family physician prescribed since the last call
- Renal function now normal
- No blood levels of venlafaxine or mirtazapine were ever obtained

- In the meantime had lung resection for Stage I lung cancer, presumed cured
- Depressed again – "nothing makes me happy" – no enthusiasm, loss of appetite, pain in hip replacement not satisfactorily relieved by Vicodin (hydrocodone-acetaminophen)
- Moved back in with daughter
- Family physician has increased doses to venlafaxine 75 mg and mirtazapine 45 mg in response to her depressive relapse, but no response past two months
- Continues alprazolam 0.5 mg three times a day
- What is going on here?
- Why was a depressive relapse risked by reducing her antidepressant doses in the absence of any renal failure and without getting any therapeutic blood levels?
- Advised to increase venlafaxine to 150 mg

Attending Physician's Mental Notes: Week 4 After Reestablishing Contact

- Daughter brings her mother back 4 weeks later
- Reports that her mother's primary care physician very uncomfortable with increasing venlafaxine to 150 mg, but complied
- Now, however, it looks like yet another increase in venlafaxine dosing will be required
- Letter sent to primary care physician trying to reassure and justify dose increase, and venlafaxine increased to 225 mg/day

Attending Physician's Mental Notes: Week 8 After Reestablishing Contact

- One month later, daughter dutifully brings mother back for reevaluation since therapeutic results not yet satisfactory
- Less daytime sleeping, better sleep at night
- Better appetite and mood
- Maybe 50% better but not back to normal self
- Some fluctuations in level of improvement as well from day to day
- Facing second hip replacement in the next month
- Advised to await until after hip replacement to change medications from current level
- Also advised to stop medications only shortly before surgery, and to reinstitute them as soon as possible postoperatively, and to return four weeks after surgery

Attending Physician's Mental Notes: Week 16 After Reestablishing Contact

- Four months following reestablishment of contact for treatment of her sixth episode of depression, daughter drives her mother back for another appointment
- Patient did well with surgery
- However, mood still only about 50% better
- Advised to increase venlafaxine to 300 mg and monitor BP
- Family physician called and reluctantly agrees to increase dose of venlafaxine
- Family physician forewarned that failure to respond to 300 mg/day of venlafaxine may lead to recommendation to dose even higher

Attending Physician's Mental Notes: Week 20 After Reestablishing Contact

- Four weeks later, no further improvement, on 300 mg/day so increase venlafaxine to 375 mg

Attending Physician's Mental Notes: Week 24 After Reestablishing Contact

- Four weeks later, BP 129/84 and patient in remission
- Current meds:
  - Venlafaxine 375 mg
  - Mirtazapine 45 mg
  - Alprazolam 0.5 Mg three times a day
  - Hydrocodone q 4–6 hr prn pain

Case Debrief

- A lifetime of recurrent episodes of major depression was managed here despite intercurrent medical illnesses
- Taking medications until symptom remission and then stopping them is not adequate long term maintenance since this patient recurred many times after stopping medications or reducing her dose
- Aggressive treatment options with antidepressant combinations can be justified if the goal is sustained remission from depression
- Treating depression may be one of the most powerful ways to improve quality of life in an elderly patient with multiple medical complications, since remission is often still possible from depression, even in a patient with several other illnesses that may be difficult to treat, including two cancers, and two hip replacements and chronic related pain

Take-Home Points

- Many elderly patients respond well to mirtazapine, especially agitated depression with reduced appetite and weight loss
- Antipsychotic-induced parkinsonism may not reverse completely for a few months after discontinuation of drugs, especially in the elderly
- Sedative antidepressants and benzodiazepines may increase the incidence of falls and hip fractures in the elderly
- Therapeutic drug levels are available for many drugs and can help determine their absorption and dosing; using them here may have prevented an unnecessary dose reduction and consequent relapse
- Aggressive antidepressant therapy (such as "California rocket fuel," i.e., venlafaxine plus mirtazapine) may be necessary even in elderly patients with multiple medical complications
- This patient had several relapses induced by discontinuation or reduction of antidepressants on the advice of her physicians
- In retrospect, it may be that many relapses may lead to more difficult-to-treat relapses requiring more aggressive treatment than may have worked in the past for that patient
- Antidepressant treatment may be necessary for a lifetime and without interruption, as seems to be for this patient with mood disorder who continues to need treatment and respond to it well for over 47 years

Performance in Practice: Confessions of a Psychopharmacologist

- What could have been done better here?
  - Clearly, this patient should have been advised to continue her antidepressant maintenance indefinitely following her third episode of major depression
  - Therapeutic drug monitoring when dose reduction was implemented could have led to no dose reduction of her antidepressants and this could have prevented her sixth major depressive episode which took many months of treatment before she attained remission
- Possible action item for improvement in practice
  - More pro-active advice and monitoring to make sure patients like this do not stop their medications
  - More pro-active monitoring of actions of referring physicians to make sure they implement rational treatment recommendations
  - Better support of the daughter's efforts to help her mother, with information, reassurance and possible evalutation for her own stress related illnesses and possible need for short term supportive psychotherapy

Tips and Pearls

- Aggressive treatment strategies, including medication combinations and high dosing that are often utilized for treatment resistant depression in younger patients without medical complications can nevertheless be helpful even in elderly patients with multiple medical complications
- Complete remission of depression is still possible for elderly medically ill patients with many reasons to be depressed
- It is good to have a loyal daughter who does not give up on you and acts as your advocate to steer you through a complex and confusing medical care delivery system

Two-Minute Tute: A brief lesson and psychopharmacology tutorial (tute) with relevant background material for this case
– Brain changes in depression
– Chances of recovering from depression

Table 1: Are brain changes progressive in depression?

- A frontal-limbic functional disconnection is present in depression and correlates with the duration of the current depressive episode
- Hippocampal volume loss is greater with longer periods of untreated depression
- The likelihood that a life stress precipitates a depressive episode is greatest for the first episode of depression and declines with each subsequent episode, although the risk of subsequent episodes increase as though prior episodes of depression as well as life stressors are causing subsequent episodes of depression
- More episodes of depression as well as residual symptoms both predict poorer outcome in terms of more relapses
- Antidepressants may boost trophic factors, normalize brain activity, suggesting that successful and early treatment may attenuate progressive maladaptive brain changes and improve the clinical course of the illness
- Symptomatic remission may be the clinician's benchmark for enhancing the probability of arresting disease progression
- Sustained remission may be a clinician's benchmark for reversing the underlying pathophysiology of major depression

---

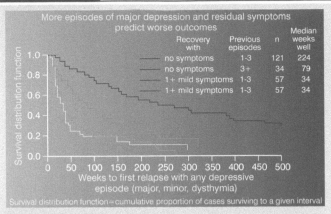

More episodes of major depression and residual symptoms predict worse outcomes

Recovery with	Previous episodes	n	Median weeks well
no symptoms	1-3	121	224
no symptoms	3+	34	79
1+ mild symptoms	1-3	57	34
1+ mild symptoms	1-3	57	34

Weeks to first relapse with any depressive episode (major, minor, dysthymia)

Survival distribution function=cumulative proportion of cases surviving to a given interval

Figure 1: More Episodes of Major Depression and Residual Symptoms Predict Worse Outcomes. In other words, the more depression you have, the more depression you get. Depression begets depression. Lack of remission begets relapse. This shows the importance of doing everything possible to reduce the number of episodes of depression, and also to treat every symptom to the point of remission when there is an episode of depression. The name of the game is sustained remission in the modern conceptualization of the treatment of depression.

Residual symptoms and episode count thus add to the complexity of diagnosing and treating depression and can lead to worse outcomes.
- The main finding of this study was that depressed patients who experienced recovery with no symptoms remained well for a median of 4.3 years (224 weeks) before depression recurrence, compared to approximately six months for patients who recovered with residual symptoms. Therefore, recovery with residual symptoms from depression was an important clinical marker associated with rapid episode relapse in depression
- Asymptomatic recovery included those patients with at least 80% of well interval weeks rated as the following: "Subject is returned to 'usual self' without any residual symptoms of the major depressive disorder, although significant symptomatology from underlying conditions may continue."
- Even the mildest residual symptoms, however, can negatively impact outcomes. Patients with residual subthreshold depressive symptoms (recovery with 1+ mild symptoms – one or more mild residual depressive symptoms – experienced on average a faster time to relapse than did asymptomatic patients.
- Episode count, too, was a negative prognosticator. Patients with more than three major depressive episodes (MDEs) tended to relapse

earlier than those with histories of three or fewer episodes, although this did not reach significance.

- **BACKGROUND**
  - Patients with MDD (as diagnosed using Research Diagnostic Criteria, or RDC) were followed naturalistically for 10 years or longer.
  - Patients were divided on the basis of intake MDE recovery into recovery with residual subthreshold depressive symptoms (recovery with 1+ mild symptoms; N=82) and asymptomatic recovery (N=155) groups. Trained raters interviewed patients every six months for the first five years and every year thereafter.
  - Depressive symptomatology was rated using the Longitudinal Interval Follow-up Evaluation (LIFE) Psychiatric Status Rating (PSR) scales.
  - Recovery with 1+ mild symptoms as defined by the PSR includes those experiencing one or more depressive symptoms but of no more than a mild degree.
  - P values (given according to color of lines on slide graphic): Orange vs green, $P < .0001$; orange vs blue, $P < .0001$; orange vs red, $P < .0001$; green vs blue, $P = .013$; green vs red, $P = .004$; blue vs red, $P = .283$.

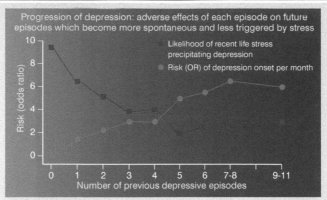

Figure 2: Progression of Depression: Adverse Effects of Each Episode on Future Episodes Which Become More Spontaneous and Less Triggered by Stress. These data are consistent with the notion that symptoms of depression and episodes of depression "kindle" subsequent episodes of depression.

- The kindling hypothesis states that previous episodes of depression change the brain, making patients more likely to experience subsequent episodes of depression
- After 4 to 5 episodes, the best predictor of subsequent episodes of depression is the number of previous depressive episodes, not stress
- Does this suggest that recurrent depression is a progressive disease?
- **BACKGROUND:**
  - Female twins from a population-based registry (N=2,395) were interviewed 4 times during a period of 9 years, forming a study group that contained 97,515 person-months and 1380 onsets of MDD
  - To assess the interaction between life-event exposure and the number of previous episodes of MDD in predicting future MDD episodes, discrete-time survival, a proportional hazards model, and piece-wise regression analyses were used
  - This pattern of results was unchanged by the addition of measures of event severity and genetic risk, as well as the restriction to "independent stressful life events"
  - The same pattern of results emerged when within-person changes in the number of episodes were examined

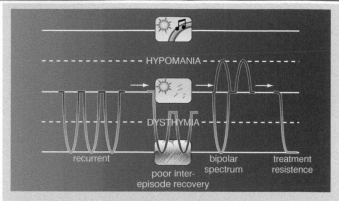

Figure 3: Is Major Depressive Disorder Progressive? Studies as well as direct observations of cases over long periods of time suggest that one episode of major depression may not only increase the chances of having another, but that subsequent recurrences may not be followed by remission and only by partial treatment responses, ultimately with episodes recurring that may become treatment-resistant.

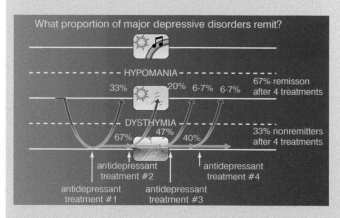

Figure 4: What Proportion of Major Depressive Disorder Remit? Approximately one-third of depressed patients will remit during treatment with any antidepressant initially. Unfortunately, for those who fail to remit the likelihood of remission with another antidepressant monotherapy goes down with each successive trial. Thus, after a year of treatment with four sequential antidepressants taken for twelve weeks each, only two-thirds of patients will have achieved remission.

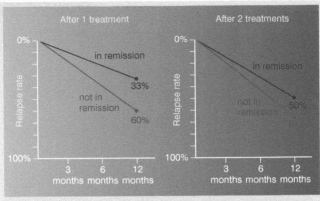

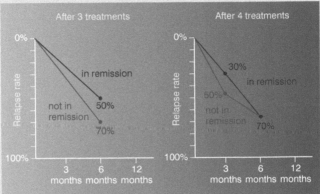

Figure 5: What Proportion of Major Depressive Disorders Relapse? The rate of relapse of major depression is significantly less for patients who achieve remission. However, there is still risk of relapse even in remitters, and the likelihood increases with the number of treatments it takes to get the patient to remit. Thus, the relapse rate for patients who do not remit ranges from 60% at twelve months after one treatment to 70% at six months after four treatments, but for those who do remit it ranges from only 33% at twelve months after one treatment all the way to 70% at six months after four treatments. In other words, the protective nature of remission virtually disappears once it takes four treatments to achieve remission.

Posttest: Self Assessment Question: Answer

Parkinsonism may be antipsychotic-induced in the elderly, but will generally reverse within a week or two.

A. True

B. False

Answer: B. False

References

1. Stahl SM, Mood Disorders, in Stahl's Essential Psychopharmacology, 3rd edition, Cambridge University Press, New York, 2008, pp 453–510
2. Stahl SM, Antidepressants, in Stahl's Essential Psychopharmacology, 3rd edition, Cambridge University Press, New York, 2008, pp 511–666
3. Stahl SM, Mirtazapine, in Stahl's Essential Psychopharmacology The Prescriber's Guide, 3rd edition, Cambridge University Press, New York, 2009, pp 347–51
4. Stahl SM, Venlafaxine, in Stahl's Essential Psychopharmacology The Prescriber's Guide, 3rd edition, Cambridge University Press, New York, 2009, pp 579–84
5. Trivedi MH, Rush AJ, Wisniewski SR et al. Evaluation of outcomes with citalopram for depression using measurement-based care in STAR*D: implications for clinical practice. Am J Psychiatry 2006; 163: 28–40
6. Rush AJ, Trivedi MH, Wisniewski SR et al. Bupropion-SR, sertraline, or venlafaxine-XR after failure of SSRIs for depression. N Engl J Med 2006; 354(12): 1231–42
7. Rush AJ, Trivedi MH, Wisniewski SR et al. Acute and longer-term outcomes in depressed outpatients requiring one or several treatment steps: a STAR*D report. Am J Psychiatry 2006; 163: 1905–17
8. Warden D, Rush AJ, Trivedi MH et al. The STAR*D Project results: a comprehensive review of findings. Curr Psychiatry Rep 2007; 9(6): 449–59
9. Judd LL, Akiskal HS, Maser JD et al. Major depressive disorder: a prospective study of residual subthreshold depressive symptoms as predictor of rapid relapse. J Affect Disord 1998; 50(2–3): 97–108
10. Kendler, KS, Thornton, LM, Gardner, CO. Stressful life events and previous episodes in the etiology of major depression in women: an evaluation of the "kindling" hypothesis. Am J Psychiatry 2000; 157: 1243–51

Lightning Round

The Case: The psychotic arsonist who burned his house and tried to burn himself

The Question: How to keep an uncooperative 48-year-old psychotic man with menacing behavior under behavioral control

The Dilemma: What can you do after you think you have blocked every dopamine receptor and cannot give clozapine?

Pretest Self Assessment Question (answer at the end of the case)

Which of the following is a reasonable approach to treatment resistant psychosis when clozapine is not an option?

A. Augment depot risperidone (Consta) with aripiprazole (Abilify)

B. Dose olanzapine (Zyprexa) >40 mg/day

C. Dose olanzapine to attain plasma drug levels between 5–75 ng/ml

D. Dose olanzapine to attain plasma drug levels >120 ng/ml but lower than 700–800 ng/ml which are associated with QTc prolongation

E. Use olanzapine with risperidone

F. Augment with lamotrigine (Lamictal)

G. Augment with high dose benzodiazepines

H. Use nonpharmacologic interventions

Patient Intake

- 48-year-old man diagnosed with paranoid schizophrenia and alcohol dependence (now in a controlled environment) with a 23-year history of alcohol abuse and relapse, and a 16-year history of psychotic illness
- Referred by his treating psychiatrist for expert psychopharmacological consultation because the patient continues to have symptoms despite heroic treatment with antipsychotics
- Multiple prior psychiatric hospitalizations with history of poor compliance
- Predominant symptoms are persecutory ideation, ideas of reference, auditory hallucinations, and disorganized thinking with history of suicide attempts
- History of thrombocytopenia, considered a contraindication for clozapine by medical consultants
- History of alcohol and marijuana abuse
- At least one first degree relative with a psychotic illness
- Current hospitalization resulted from an incident in which the patient believed that his family was being abused via the internet and thus he needed to burn down his house to stop it, which he did, plus dousing himself with gasoline intending to commit suicide but was unable to successfully light himself on fire

- Arrested and convicted of the acts but found not criminally responsible by reason of insanity and admitted to a forensic facility

Psychiatric History

- Patient continues to have irritability, low frustration tolerance and bizarre, violent, and sexual delusions
- Has persecutory delusions that the CIA is after him, has labile and inappropriate affect, pacing, laughing to himself
- He believes the staff have glued braces on his arms and legs
- Has threatened to strangle staff and has grabbed a female staff member
- Believes that local police raped his family and are projecting images onto the outside of a glass building of him and his wife having sex

Treatment History

- Many previous antipsychotics given with unclear efficacy, unclear compliance, but had a dystonic reaction to haloperidol previously
- Seems to have responded to a combination of aripiprazole 30 mg plus quetiapine (Seroquel) 200 mg qhs prior to this hospitalization when he was compliant for a short period of time
- During this hospitalization, has been partially responsive to depot risperidone 37.5 mg every 2 weeks, so the dose was increased to 75 mg every 2 weeks with further improvement of symptoms but not adequate remission
- Now on depot risperidone 50 mg every 2 weeks plus aripiprazole 30 mg with continuing inadequate control

Of the following choices, what would you do?
- Increase the risperidone dose
- Increase the aripiprazole dose
- Stop the aripiprazole
- Add a second antipsychotic
- Add lamotrigine
- Add benzodiazepine

Case Outcome: First Interim Followup

- Recommended increase of depot risperidone to 37.5 mg every week, as it is theoretically possible that further blockade of dopamine D2 receptors could be helpful

- Recommended discontinuation of aripiprazole because this can interfere with risperidone actions, since aripiprazole has a higher affinity at the D2 receptor than risperidone, but is only a partial agonist, thus potentially mitigating the therapeutic actions of risperidone
- This was done, but after 1 month, was ineffective
- Recommended augmentation with lamotrigine, also ineffective
- Although quetiapine was helpful in the past, for some reason the patient is refusing this at the present time

Of the following choices, what would you do?
- Switch to another antipsychotic
- Add another antipsychotic to depot risperidone
- Give prn injections of haloperidol (lorazepam, diphenhydramine)
- Give a daily benzodiazepine

Case Outcome: Second Interim Followup

- Added olanzapine 5 mg daily, going up 5 to 10 mg per week to 40 mg/day
- Behavior necessitates use of concomitant haloperidol, lorazepam, diphenhydramine prn IM or olanzapine IM prn
- Patient not sedated, nor orthostatic, with olanzapine plasma drug level 46 ng/ml, so cautiously increased dose of olanzapine to 30 mg twice a day
- Plasma olanzapine level 94 (target range supposedly 5–75 ng/ml for routine cases; 125 ng/ml for refractory cases, avoiding levels seen in overdose with QTc prolongation such as 700–800 ng/ml)
- EKG normal, with QTc 384
- Increased olanzapine transiently to 30 mg three times daily, but patient became sedated
- Lowered dose of olanzapine to 30 mg twice daily, and augmented with clonazepam titrating up to 2 mg twice daily
- Patient now under relative control without needing prn injections and not sedated
- Patient is gaining weight and lipids are elevated

Case Debrief

- It appears as though this patient does have an improved response to eye-popping doses of two antipsychotics
- Almost no written documentation in the literature for treating cases at these doses

- The dilemma is whether to risk the danger to the staff and to the patient by treating with ineffective but evidence-based doses, or to risk medical complications of heroic (or desperate) off-label use
- A treatment committee with a patient advocate reluctantly approved this treatment approach, with quarterly reviews and the patient and family agree to this extraordinary treatment approach in writing

Posttest Self Assessment Question: Answer

Which of the following is a reasonable approach to treatment resistant psychosis when clozapine is not an option?

A. Augment depot risperidone with aripiprazole
 - Aripiprazole can interfere with risperidone actions so is not a totally rational combination
B. Dose olanzapine >40 mg/day
 - Almost no published data on this approach, but some anecdotal experience in institutional settings in extremely unusual and well selected cases
C. Dose olanzapine to attain plasma drug levels between 5–75 ng/ml
 - These are standard levels for standard doses, and probably will be inadequate for this case
D. Dose olanzapine to attain plasma drug levels >120 ng/ml but lower than 700–800 ng/ml which are associated with QTc prolongation
 - Many are uncomfortable with this approach, and almost no published data on this approach, but these are the plasma levels associated with olanzapine treatment above 40 mg/day and might be helpful in extremely unusual cases
E. Use olanzapine with risperidone
 - Generally better to give one drug at a high dose rather than two drugs at regular doses and this is also very expensive in practice, with almost no experience to guide long term use, yet some anecdoates from heroic cases suggest it may be occasionally justified
F. Augment with lamotrigine
 - This is fairly standard
G. Augment with high dose benzodiazepines
 - Although this can be helpful, one has to think twice in an alcoholic patient; however, in an institutional setting without access to alcohol, it may be a viable if reluctant option
H. Use nonpharmacologic interventions
 - This is obvious, but seclusion, restraint, isolation or disciplinary housing are not long term options and often are instituted after an assault, and may not prevent assaults to others or self harm

Answer: B, D, E, F, G and H

References

1. Stahl SM, Lamotrigine, in Stahl's Essential Psychopharmacology The Prescriber's Guide, 3rd edition, Cambridge University Press, New York, 2009, pp 259–65
2. Stahl SM, Clozapine, in Stahl's Essential Psychopharmacology The Prescriber's Guide, 3rd edition, Cambridge University Press, New York, 2009, pp 113–8
3. Stahl SM, Risperidone, in Stahl's Essential Psychopharmacology The Prescriber's Guide, 3rd edition, Cambridge University Press, New York, 2009, pp 475–81
4. Stahl SM, Olanzapine, in Stahl's Essential Psychopharmacology The Prescriber's Guide, 3rd edition, Cambridge University Press, New York, 2009, pp 387–92
5. Citrome L, Kantrowitz JT, Olanzapine dosing above the licensed range is more efficacious than lower doses: fact or fiction? Expert Reviews Neurother 2009; 9: 1045–58
6. Stahl SM, Antipsychotics, in Stahl's Essential Psychopharmacology, 3rd edition, Cambridge University Press, New York, 2008, pp 327–452
7. Goff DC, Keefe R, Citrome L et al. Lamotrigine as add-on therapy in schizophrenia. J Clin Psychopharmacol 2007; 27: 582–9
8. Stahl SM, Grady MM. A critical review of atypical antipsychotic utilization: comparing monotherapy with polypharmacy and augmentation. Cur Med Chem 11: 313–26

The Case: The woman with depression whose Parkinson's disease vanished

The Question: Can state dependent parkinsonism be part of major depressive disorder?

The Dilemma: How to diagnose and treat with simultaneous antidepressants and anti-parkinsonian drugs?

Pretest Self Assessment Question (answer at the end of the case)

The severity of depression associated with Parkinson's disease usually correlates with the severity of the movement disorder

A. True
B. False

Patient Intake

- 53-year-old female
- Chief complaint: "I'm always tired"

Psychiatric History

- States she was well until about three years ago
- Eventually felt she "needed bedrest" and finally stayed in bed for eight months!
- Medical workup negative
- Felt better spontaneously, went back to work, and then "relapsed" four months later
- Previous trials of nortriptyline (Pamelor) and paroxetine (Paxil, Seroxat) worsened fatigue and she discontinued after a few doses
- Felt somewhat better on low dose amitriptyline (Elavil) when she was staying in bed

Medical History

- Normal BMI, BP, blood tests
- Extensive recent medical evaluation within normal limits

Social and Personal History

- Middle East origin, English is her second language
- Emigrated to the US 20 years ago
- Married for 30 years
- 2 children
- Non smoker, non drinker, no drugs of abuse
- Works in her husband's business

Family History

- No psychiatric, neurologic or medical illnesses known in relatives

Current medications

- Zolpidem (Ambien)
- Alprazolam (Xanax)
- Estrogen/progestin

Patient Intake

- States she doesn't like to look at faces because she has a hard time turning to look at them
- States her "feet are tired"
- She always wants to stay at home
- Also describes a sort of restless movements in her legs
- Upon closer questioning it is clear that she is depressed with insomnia, but what is striking is her neurological examination
  - She sits with a stooped posture
  - Masked face and "reptilian stare,"
  - Walking with a rigid manner and much decreased arm swing bilaterally, turning "en bloc" with obvious axial rigidity about the neck
  - Positive Myerson's sign
  - Cogwheeling bilaterally
  - States she has akathisia
  - States she has problems turning over in bed

Attending Physician's Mental Notes: Initial Psychiatric Evaluation

- Some current symptomatic relief from alprazolam for agitation, but not dramatic
- Diagnosed with primary Parkinson's disease with secondary depression and insomnia, not necessarily a major depressive episode, pending neurological evaluation
- Because of the prior good response to amitriptyline, given 50–75 mg/day at night for sleep, and for its anticholinergic effects that might improve parkinsonism while she is awaiting neurological evaluation, although the dose is probably too low for robust antidepressant action
- She is referred to a neurologist for evaluation
- Lost to follow-up for three years

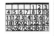

Case Outcome: Three Years Later

- Returned three years later with the following interim history
- First neurological consultation shortly after her initial psychiatric evaluation

- While awaiting her first neurological consult for a few weeks on amitriptyline, she became much more animated, with improved facial expression and less rigidity
- Speech still hard to initiate at times
- Remained apathetic but now was able to sleep well
- Neurologist saw her shortly thereafter and diagnosed Parkinson's disease and started levodopa/carbidopa
  - Not helpful
- Neurologist then added a dopamine agonist
  - Patient began to experience "mood swings" with increased pressure of speech and was somewhat inappropriately talkative on an airplane trip and was referred to a local psychiatrist
- Neurologist then discontinued the dopamine agonist and reduced the dose of levodopa/carbidopa
  - Patient had no more mood swings and movements seemed to be better
- Neurologist referred her to a local psychiatrist for evaluation of mood swings
- New psychiatrist
  - Patient saw the psychiatrist to whom the neurologist had referred her, and he increased amitriptyline to 150 mg at night and also started clonazepam
  - Parkinsonism again improved along with depression, but patient had weight gain and increased fatigue from amitriptyline so stopped it
- Third psychiatrist
  - Then went to another psychiatrist in a nearby city who spoke her native language and was prescribed mirtazapine (Remeron) and risperidone (Risperdal) !!
  - Predictably worsened and patient stopped all meds, resulting in her looking more parkinsonian and more depressed
- Second neurological consultation
  - Referred to second neurologist at a major medical center where she seemed somewhat parkinsonian
  - Was a nonresponder to dopaminergic treatments
  - A PET scan failed to confirm Parkinson's disease
  - Led to a diagnosis of "atypical parkinsonism"
  - No antiparkinson treatment
  - Referral to psychiatry at that center
- Fourth psychiatrist
  - Patient had several short term trials
    - Various SSRIs
    - Trazodone
    - Venlafaxine (Effexor XR)

- Every drug and every combination caused some therapeutic effects for both depression and parkinsonism, but unacceptable side effects for the first few doses of each and stopped every one each time she got an early side effect
- Third neurological consultation
  - Referred to a third neurologist at yet another major medical center who diagnosed Parkinson's disease and depression
  - Tried amantadine (Symmetrel) and other dopamine agonists without positive effects, so all antiparkinson treatment stopped
- Patient returns now to you, the original psychiatrist, for a re-evaluation three years after your first and only visit
  - Has moderate parkinsonism and moderate depression
  - Taking low dose amitriptyline

From the information given, what do you think her primary diagnosis is?

- Recurrent major depression and Parkinson's disease
- Depression secondary to early Parkinson's disease
- Recurrent major depression and severe psychomotor retardation masquerading as Parkinson's disease
- Other

Of the following choices, what would you do?

- Add antidepressant alone
- Refer to a fourth neurologist for antiparkinsonian treatment first
- Coordinate addition of antiparkinsonian treatment by a neurologist with your addition of an antidepressant
- None of the above

If you would give an antidepressant, which would you add?

- SSRI (selective serotonin reuptake inhibitor)
- SNRI (serotonin-norepinephrine reuptake inhibitor)
- NDRI (bupropion; norepinephrine-dopamine reuptake inhibitor)
- NRI (norepinephrine reuptake inhibitor)
- Mirtazapine
- Trazodone
- Tricyclic antidepressant
- MAO inhibitor
- I would not give an antidepressant.

Attending Physician's Mental Notes: First Followup, 3 Years Later

- This poor women has been running in circles between neurologists and psychiatrists, including this attending physician, without resolution of the problem

- Seems like parkinsonian symptoms are curiously linked to depressive symptoms, and both seem coupled together, rising together when one gets worse and falling together when one gets better
- Parkinson's disease does not behave like this
- Also, the PET scan does not confirm actual loss of dopaminergic neurons consistent with the diagnosis of Parkinson's disease
- Could this be profound psychomotor retardation that rises and falls as the patient's depression gets worse, and better, respectively?
- The way to tell is to closely track psychomotor symptoms and depressive mood status as antidepressants are given
- If this formulation is correct, her so-called parkinsonian symptoms should not require direct treatment, only improvement of the depression
- Her hypomanic episode clearly suggests a mood disorder as well
- She thought she was an angel in first class cabin flying on an international trip and kept taking the slippers off other passengers as they slept
- She herself did not sleep at all on the trip, shortly after starting a dopamine agonist, and was talkative, intrusive to sleeping passengers, and embarrassed her husband who witnessed this
- Since her symptoms seem linked to dopamine, a trial of a pro-dopaminergic agent, perhaps bupropion, an effective antidepressant often well tolerated in bipolar spectrum patients, might be worth a try
- Given a trial of bupropion SR 150 mg increasing to 300 mg per day

Case Outcome: Second Followup, 4 Weeks Later

- Bupropion causes tongue dyskinesias

Attending Physician's Mental Notes: Second Followup, 4 Weeks Later

- Well, I guess this was not such a brilliant idea to try bupropion
- This patient seems to be extraordinarily sensitive to dopamine actions, looking very parkinsonian when her depression is bad and her psychomotor retardation is poor, and with prodopaminergic drugs causing either hypomania or dyskinesias
- Better avoid drugs with direct actions on dopamine for now
- At this first followup visit, discontinued the bupropion and switched her to citalopram (Celexa)
- Continued amitriptyline 50 mg at night
- Continued clonazepam 0.5 mg prn

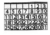

Case Outcome: 8 Weeks Later and for the Next 5 Years

- Amazingly, the citalopram was robustly effective for her depression over the next few months
- She completely resolved her parkinsonism
- She has had intermittent anxiety treatable by varying doses of supplemental clonazapam over the years but has had essentially no recurrence of depression and no signs of parkinsonism again

Case Debrief

- In retrospect, the patient's parkinsonism has always fluctuated in direct proportion to the severity of her depression
- The patient may indeed have some kind of presymptomatic movement disorder underlying her depression, or such severe psychomotor retardation that it looks parkinsonian even to international neurological experts at more than one major medical center, and that remits not with parkinsonian treatment but with only those antidepressants that improve her mood
- Cultural and language problems can make analyzing and managing a complex case even more complicated
- This case is unusual in that the severity of depression associated with Parkinson's disease does NOT usually correlate with the severity of the movement disorder
- This case is also unusual in that what now seems to be simply very severe psychomotor retardation presented as parkinsonism and led to a complicated set of failed treatments by both neurologists and psychiatrists at first

Take-Home Points

- Reversible parkinsonism is not Parkinson's disease
- Specialists in both neurology and psychiatry can tend to see a case through the prism of their own specialty's perspective when a patient with neurological and psychiatric symptoms may require a dual and simultaneous perspective
- This patient has more prominent parkinsonism than depression and fooled all of us that this was a primary motor disorder and not a primary mood disorder, as was ultimately shown to be the case
- The patient wasted years in back and forth consultations and ineffective treatments awaiting a good outcome

Performance in Practice: Confessions of a Psychopharmacologist

- What could have been done better here?
  - Should the depression have been treated more aggressively from the beginning, and while the original neurological consultation was taking place?
  - Should the normal PET scan have signaled that this was a mood disorder and not a primary motor disorder?
  - Better coordination between neurology and psychiatry may have led to the discovery of her diagnosis and her treatment much more quickly
- Possible action item for improvement in practice
  - Learn more about Parkinson's disease and its treatments
  - Do not be hesitant to treat depression in an undiagnosed motor disorder, but start treatment while motor disorder is being evaluated

Tips and Pearls

- Dopamine agonists and prodopaminergic agents that do not improve parkinsonism or depression, but instead cause dyskinesias and hypomania should suggest a case that is out of the ordinary
- When levodopa/carbidopa is not effective and the PET scan does not confirm degeneration of striatal dopamine nerve terminals, the patient does not have Parkinson's disease no matter how convincing the motor examination
- None of the neurologists had ever seen such a convincing case of clinical parkinsonism, state dependent upon mood
- Nor had any of the psychiatrists
- In the end, this case turned out to have a remarkably simple therapeutic solution that was robust and long lasting

Posttest Self Assessment Question: Answer

The severity of depression associated with Parkinson's disease usually correlates with the severity of the movement disorder?

A. True
B. False

Answer: B. False

References

1. Stahl SM, Antidepressants, in Stahl's Essential Psychopharmacology, 3rd edition, Cambridge University Press, New York, 2008, pp 511–666

2. Stahl SM, Citalopram, in Stahl's Essential Psychopharmacology The Prescriber's Guide, 3rd edition, Cambridge University Press, New York, 2009, pp 83–8

3. Stahl SM, Bupropion, in Stahl's Essential Psychopharmacology The Prescriber's Guide, 3rd edition, Cambridge University Press, New York, 2009, pp 57–62

4. Silberstein, S, Marmura M, Stahl SM (Ed), Carbidopa/Levodopa, in Essential Neuropharmacology: The Prescribers Guide, Cambridge University Press, 2010, pp 55–8

5. Silberstein, S, Marmura M, Stahl SM (Ed), Pramipexole, in Essential Neuropharmacology: The Prescriber's Guide, Cambridge University Press, 2010 pp 262–5

6. Silberstein, S, Marmura M, Stahl SM (Ed), Amantadine, in Essential Neuropharmacology: The Prescribers Guide, Cambridge University Press, 2010, pp 11–13

7. Dalley ,IW, Mar AC, Economidou D, Robins TW. Neurobehavioral mechanisms of impulsivity, fronto-striatal systems and functional neurochemistry. Pharmacol Biochem Behav 2008; 90: 250–60

8. Groenwegen HJ. The ventral striatum as an interface between the limbic and motor systems. CNS Spectrums 2007; 12: 887–92

9. Meridith GE, Baldo BA, Andrezjewski ME et al. The structural basis for mapping behaviour onto the ventral striatum and its subdivisions. Brain Struct Funct 2008; 213: 17–20

The Case: The depressed man who thought he was out of options

The Question: Are some episodes of depression untreatable?

The Dilemma: What do you do when even ECT and MAOIs do not work?

Pretest Self Assessment Question (answer at the end of the case)

If a patient has low blood levels of an antidepressant at standard doses, what could this mean?

A. Pharmacokinetic failure
B. Genetic variant causing pharmacokinetic failure
C. Pharmacodynamic failure
D. Genetic variant causing pharmacodynamic failure
E. Noncompliance

Patient Intake

- 69-year-old man
- Chief complaint: unremitting, chronic depression

Psychiatric History

- Recurrent, unipolar major depressive episodes for the past 40 years, with good response to treatment and good inter-episode recovery until five years ago
- Onset then of one long, waxing and waning major depressive episode ever since
- Five years ago, relapsed on venlafaxine 225 mg after having had a good response to it
- Two years ago had nine electroconvulsive therapy (ECT) treatments with a partial response
- In the past few years since relapse on venlafaxine has tried (adequate trials, no severe side effects) essentially every known antidepressant and augmentation combination known or reported in the literature, from many capable psychiatrists and numerous consultations from local, regional, and national psychiatrists, and distinguished medical centers
  - 5 SSRIs
  - Duloxetine
  - Mitazapine
  - 2 TCAs
  - Augmentation with 5 different atypical antipsychotics
  - Augmentation with
    - Lithium
    - Thyroid
    - Buspirone

- L-methylfolate
- Others
- Following ECT, given the MAOI phenelzine (Nardil) up to 105 mg/day with some orthostasis, some antidepressant response, wearing off despite increasing doses, and then all response to phenelzine wore off
- Trials even included the controversial and heroic combination of an monoamine oxidase inhibitor (MAOI) and a tricyclic antidepressant (TCA) phenelzine plus nortriptyline, all ineffective
- Came to you on phenelzine 90 mg, nortriptyline 50 mg, and occasional lorazepam, for your treatment recommendations

Medical History

- Not contributory
- Other medications:
  - Boniva for osteoporosis
  - Avapro for hypertension
  - Lipitor for hypercholesterolemia
  - Flomax for enlarged prostate
  - Melloxicam for arthritis

Social and Personal History

- Married, 3 children, 8 grandchildren
- Retired engineer
- Non smoker, no drug or alcohol abuse

Family History

- Several first degree relatives: depression
- No family history of suicide

Patient Intake

- Severely depressed and demoralized
- No joy or pleasure; sad, feeling helpless, hopeless, worthless, problems concentrating
- Past two years rates himself 9/10 in severity (10 worst)
- Wife states he is letting go and giving up

Of the following choices, what would you do?

- Add one of the new antipsychotics, asenapine, iloperidone or lurasidone that he has not taken yet
- Augment the MAOI with a stimulant, which is one of the few combinations he has not tried yet

- Discontinue the nortriptyline and augment the MAOI
- Discontinue the MAOI and augment the nortriptyline
- Discontinue both the TCA and the MAOI and prescribe something else
- Send to another psychopharmacologist; this patient is too sick and the prognosis is poor
- Do a complete medical and endocrine and neurological evaluation to see if any underlying condition has developed that has been missed
- Look into personal and family dynamics to see if this is really a resistant depression disguising other problems
- None of the above

Further Investigation

Is there anything else you would especially like to know about this patient?

- What about details concerning his medical and neurological status?
  - During the past year the patient has had extensive medical, endocrine and cancer workups, all negative
  - During the past year has also had neurological evaluation, with normal EEG, MRI
  - Neuropsychological tests consistent with severe depression but without signs of an early dementia
- What about personal and family dynamics?
  - Patient and family are indeed quite concerned about his depression, fearing he will die before he recovers
  - Patient has a long standing supportive marriage and supportive children and no major financial problems
  - Has coped with recurrent episodes of depression his whole life, bouncing back after each setback, but now has given up, frightening his family
  - No obvious reason to suspect family or personal dynamics as the source of his depression
  - However, he does have extreme negativity and a cognitive approach may be useful if he begins to get enough motivation to participate in this approach

If you would give or refer him for an experimental or "off label" protocol, test or treatment, which would you choose?

- Intravenous single injection of ketamine (NMDA N-methyl-d-aspartate antagonist) in an experimental protocol
- Send him for experimental DBS (deep brain stimulation)
- Oral riluzole (putative inhibitor of glutamate release)
- Acetylcholinesterase inhibitor in case this is really early dementia
- Send him for a quantitative EEG

- Send him for pharmacogenomics testing
- Send him for therapeutic drug monitoring
- I would not prescribe experimental treatments off label, nor send him for an experimental protocol

Attending Physician's Mental Notes: Initial Psychiatric Evaluation

- There are very few remaining treatment options

Acetylcholinesterase inhibitor
- No evidence of dementia
- Treatment seems a long shot for his depression

TMS
- The patient may be a candidate for TMS
- However, TMS is not well documented to work in a case this severe, especially in a case with less than robust responses to ECT

DBS
- DBS is a possibility, but only a research protocol, even though it might save his life
- Only a few centers offer this procedure in the US and Canada
- Unclear how this will be paid as insurance probably does not cover
- However, some promising early results in treatment resistant depression
- Will tell patient and family and referring psychiatrist about this and provide literature but not advise action yet

Ketamine
- Intravenous single injection of ketamine is an experimental protocol
- Available as a research test at the NIMH (National Institute of Mental Health) and a few universities
- A number of studies confirm efficacy in treatment resistant major depression
- However, it only works for a few hours and then wears off and not practical to repeat it
- Not only ketamine, but several NMDA 2B subtype selective antagonists (NR2B selective antagonists) are in clinical testing, some of which are orally administered
- Too early to tell whether this will pan out and not available for open label administration, only double blind trials

Referenced EEG
- A new type of EEG protocol, referenced EEG reports promising results, but not in patients this severe and still considered a research tool
- Only available in a limited number of research centers and not proven to predict clinical response to specific antidepressants, especially in a case like this

SPECT scans

- Some commercial clinics offer older imaging technology (SPECT is Single Photon Emission Computed Tomography) as brain scans for sale
- They do generate color pictures of brain activity that can be impressive looking to patients
- Scans are accompanied with an algorithm claiming to predict which drug to use
- Although this looks has a high-tech, scientific appearance, and raises hope, it is not well accepted in the scientific community and costs several thousand dollars not covered by insurance

Genotyping

- This approach may be useful in vulnerable populations of patients such as children or elderly and those who do not respond to many medications
- Genetic variants of cytochrome P450 (CYP45) drug metabolizing enzymes can in some cases explain unusually high or unusually low blood and brain concentrations of drugs:
  - 2D6
  - 2C19
  - 2D9
  - Others
  - This might be useful here since this patient seems not to respond to a wide number of medications now, and also has no notable side effects from them
  - Is it possible that his drug levels are low due to a drug metabolizing enzyme variant, some variant of drug absorption, or possibly noncompliance?
- Genetic variants of multiple neurotransmitter based genes, upon which many antidepressants act, may help explain both who responds to what antidepressant, and who gets side effects from what antidepressant

Phenotyping

- Determining whether a patient has high or low blood levels of a drug establishes the phenotypes of:
  - Poor metabolizers
  - Extensive metabolizers
  - Compliance/adherence
  - Pharmacokinetic variants can explain how he absorbs and metabolizes his antidepressants and thus measurement of genetic variants of CYP450 drug metabolizing enzymes may be helpful in explaining why the patient is not responding, especially if he does not generate adequate plasma and brain drug levels (pharmacokinetic)
- Advised his local treating psychiatrist to augment phenelzine with stimulant

Attending Physician's Notes: First Interim Followup, Week 20

- Local/referring psychiatrist declined to augment MAOI with stimulant as recommended
- Decided instead to give ECT again
- Local/referring psychiatrist thought eleven ECT treatments improved him 60%
- Stopped MAOI prior to ECT and then started venlafaxine 225 mg/mirtazapine 30 mg ("California rocket fuel") as ECT began
- Post ECT, severe subjective memory problems, patient very discouraged
- Nevertheless, given maintenance ECT; venlafaxine increased to 375 mg and mirtazapine increased to 45 mg
- After ninth maintenance ECT (20th overall), developed an expressive aphasia, question of a stroke versus a complication of ECT; cardiac catheterization was normal except for a possible patent foramen ovale of unknown significance
- Consulting neurologist thought patient's aphasia was a complication of ECT
- However, referring psychiatrist thought the patient's aphasia was due to a stroke so lowered venlafaxine to 225 mg, being afraid of potential elevated BP, pulse and further cardiovascular/cerebrovascular complications
- BP remained normal and under control; aspirin added to treatment

Case Outcome: First Interim Followup, Week 20

- Phone consultation one month after the post-ECT "event" and 20 weeks since initial evaluation in the office
- Patient was still having memory problems, speech problems, and worsening depression
- Taking venlafaxine 225 mg, plus mirtazapine 45 mg, plus alprazolam prn, now augmented with aripiprazole 10 mg
- Before chasing after exotic testing and treatments considered in the mental notes during the initial psychiatric evaluation 20 weeks ago (listed above), perhaps it would be a good idea simply to send off blood for therapeutic drug monitoring to see how well he is absorbing his venlafaxine and whether there is any room for a rational and safe dose increase
- Unclear why he is no longer responding to doses of venlafaxine that have occurred would in the past, but this is frequently observed in the progression of major depressive episodes over many years
- Specifically recommended getting drug levels of venlafaxine and its active metabolite O-desmethyl-venlafaxine, and consider increasing dose of venlafaxine XR to 300 mg or 375 mg while monitoring BP and mood

Case Outcome: Second Interim Followup, Week 24

- Phone consultation in another month showed patient's aphasia had resolved and memory improving, but mood still low; mood as bad as it was prior to ECT
- Seems more clear that aphasia was due to ECT and not to a stroke
- Venlafaxine blood levels not obtained and dose stayed at 225 mg
- Aripiprazole was increased to 15 mg
- Requested blood levels of venlafaxine/O-desmethylvenlafaxine again, and then to raise venlafaxine dose to 300 mg, as advised 4 weeks ago

Case Outcome: Third Interim Followup, Week 28

- Phone consult in another month, referring psychiatrist did get venlafaxine/O-desmethylvenlafzine blood levels, both of which were found to be low while taking a dose of 225 mg of venlafaxine XR
- Referring psychiatrist now agrees to increase venlafaxineXR to 300 mg and to discontinue aripiprazole

Case Outcome: Fourth Interim Followup, Week 32

- No improvement in depression
- Advised getting repeat venlafaxine/O-desmethylvenlafaxine blood levels again at 300 mg and then raising the dose to 375 mg if still low

Case Outcome: Fifth Interim Followup, Week 36

- Phone consultation in another month
- Venlafaxine/O-desmethylvenlafaxine levels still low at a dose of 300 mg of venlafaxine XR, so raised the dose to 375 mg
- "A pretty good few weeks" then followed but then patient relapsed a bit
- No increase of BP and no apparent side effects from venlafaxine
- Given that the blood levels of venlafaxine/O-desmethylvenlafaxine were so low on a dose of 300 mg/day, advised them to increase venlafaxine to 450 mg/day and to get another set of therapeutic drug levels

Case Outcome: Sixth Interim Followup, Week 40

- Increased venlafaxine XR dose to 450 mg/day, then got blood levels on this dose, which are only in the low normal range of the very broad therapeutic range suggested by the laboratory of venlafaxine/O-desmethylvenlafaxine
- Aphasia and memory better, mood definitely improved enough so that patient was no longer completely demoralized and was beginning to have hope
- Suggested raising the dose by 75 mg, getting levels again and if necessary, raising the dose again to 600 mg

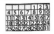

Case Outcome: Seventh Interim Followup, Week 52

- Dose increased to 600 mg, with full remission of depression
- However, at 600 mg dose, began to have some irritability, insomnia and 5–10 mm BP elevation, so reduced to 525 mg, and then to 450 mg of venlafaxine XR
- Tolerated it well at this dose
- BP normal by report
- Still in remission, now finally a year after the original consultation
- The case continues. . . .

Case Debrief

- A highly recurrent but readily treatable major depressive disorder suddenly turned treatment-resistant in this patient's 60s
- Not clear but hypothetically possible that this represents disease progression secondary to changes in brain functioning
- This case was looking very complicated due to nonresponse to standard and aggressive therapies at standard doses. Major depressive disorder can be treatable even in the seemingly most treatment-resistant cases
- In retrospect, this patient's transient aphasia without evidence of stroke was probably a rare complication of ECT
- Aggressive treatment does not have to be reckless but does have its risks
- It is possible for experts to augment MAOIs with a stimulant, while monitoring BP in heroic cases where the possible benefit (which has been reported with this combination) outweighs the risk (elevated BP, cardio and cerebrovascular events)
- However, this did not happen here
- Another heroic if old-fashioned option is the combination of MAOI with a TCA, well tolerated here but not effective
- Plasma drug level-guided heroic dosing of venlafaxine (or more recently desvenlafaxine) can be useful for resistant cases as it was here
- This may lead to venlafaxine dosing higher than 375 mg or desvenlafaxine dosing up to 200 mg

Take-Home Points

- Never give up
- Consider therapeutic drug monitoring before exotic research options
- Therapeutic drug levels of antidepressants such as venlafaxine are not well quantified, but if absorption is low or metabolism is high (or compliance is low), the blood levels of drug and active metabolites can still guide dosage above the normal approved therapeutic range

Performance in Practice: Confessions of a Psychopharmacologist

- What could have been done better here?
  - Did it take too long to get to therapeutic drug monitoring?
  - Was the second set of ECT treatments not a good idea?
- Possible action item for improvement in practice
  - Consider therapeutic drug monitoring earlier in the treatment algorithm for cases where there are inadequate therapeutic actions and low side effects
  - Consider genetic testing, especially in treatment resistant cases, the elderly and children

Tips and Pearls

- High doses of drugs taken orally sometimes deliver normal doses of drug to the brain because of various pharmacokinetic or genetic factors
- The point is how much drug is getting into the brain, not how much is taken by mouth
- The future promises better guidance of drug and dose selection by genetic tests and neuroimaging

Two-Minute Tute: A brief lesson and psychopharmacology
tutorial (tute) with relevant background material for this case
- Genotyping in depression
- Ketamine treatment of resistant depression
- Brain changes in chronic depression
- Development of treatment resistant depression

Table 1: Genotyping Neurotransmitter-Related Enzymes and Receptors in Patients with Treatment Resistant Depression?

- Still considered research tools by many
- However, beginning to be available for clinical practice applications
- Published results are not always consistently replicated
- Include variants of genes for many candidates:
  - Serotonin related receptors
    - SERT (the serotonin transporter)
    - 5HT1A receptor
    - 5HT2A receptor
    - 5HT2C receptor
  - Various glutamate receptors
  - Dopamine regulating enzymes and receptors
    - COMT (catechol-O-methyl-transferase)
    - MTHFR (methylene tetrahydrofolate reductase)
    - D2 receptor (dopamine)
  - Hypothalamic-pituitary-adrenal (HPA) axis
    - CRH1 receptor (corticotrophin releasing hormone)
    - CRH binding protein
    - Cortisol binding protein regulators (FKBP5)
  - Measuring cytochrome P450 enzyme genotypes
  - Ion channels
    - KCNK2
    - CACNA1
  - Growth factors
    - BDNF (brain derived neurotrophic factor)
    - Many others

Table 2: Glutamate, Ketamine and the Future of Treatments for Resistant Depression

- Ketamine, like PCP/phencyclidine, is an antagonist at NMDA (N-methyl-d-aspartate) receptors
- Several groups have reported that ketamine can at least transiently improve symptoms in patients with treatment resistant depression
- Ketamine blocks NMDA receptors, and some experimental treatments target a subtype of these receptors, the NR2B receptor, hypothesizing that this is the receptor through which ketamine acts
- A novel hypothesis has been proposed for ketamine that it activates the mammalian target of rapamycin (mTOR) pathway
- This leads to increased synaptic signaling proteins
- It also increases the number and the function of new spine synapses, at least in the prefrontal cortex of rats
- These effects of ketamine are the opposite to the synaptic deficits that result from exposure to stress and thus could be the hypothetical mechanism of any therapeutic action of ketamine in treatment resistant depression, where the effects of stress upon the brain may render standard antidepressants ineffective

Table 3: Are Brain Changes Progressive in Depression?

- A frontal-limbic functional disconnection is present in depression and correlates with the duration of the current depressive episode
- Hippocampal volume loss is greater with longer periods of untreated depression
- The likelihood that a life stress precipitates a depressive episode is greatest for the first episode of depression and declines with each subsequent episode, although the risk of subsequent episodes increase as though prior episodes of depression as well as life stressors are causing subsequent episodes of depression
- More episodes of depression as well as residual symptoms both predict poorer outcome in terms of more relapses
- Antidepressants may boost trophic factors, normalize brain activity, suggesting that successful and early treatment may attenuate progressive maladaptive brain changes and improve the clinical course of the illness
- Symptomatic remission may be the clinician's benchmark for enhancing the probability of arresting disease progression
- Sustained remission may be a clinician's benchmark for reversing the underlying pathophysiology of major depression

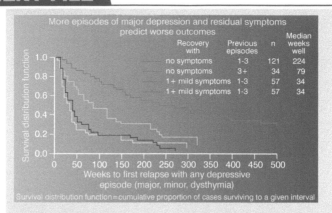

Figure 1: More Episodes of Major Depression and Residual Symptoms Predict Worse Outcomes. In other words, the depression you have, the more depression you get. Depression begets depression. Lack of remission begets relapse. This shows the importance of doing everything possible to reduce the number of episodes of depression, and also to treat every symptom to the point of remission when there is an episode of depression. The name of the game is sustained remission in the modern conceptualization of the treatment of depression.

Residual symptoms and episode count thus add to the complexity of diagnosing and treating depression and can lead to worse outcomes.

- The main finding of this study was that depressed patients who experienced recovery with no symptoms remained well for a median of 4.3 years (224 weeks) before depression recurrence, compared to approximately six months for patients who recovered with residual symptoms. Therefore, recovery with residual symptoms from depression was an important clinical marker associated with rapid episode relapse in depression

- Asymptomatic recovery included those patients with at least 80% of well interval weeks rated as the following: "Subject is returned to 'usual self' without any residual symptoms of the major depressive disorder, although significant symptomatology from underlying conditions may continue."

- **Even the mildest residual symptoms, however, can negatively impact outcomes**. Patients with residual subthreshold depressive symptoms (recovery with 1+ mild symptoms)—one or more mild residual depressive symptoms—experienced on average a faster time to relapse than did asymptomatic patients.

- **Episode count, too, was a negative prognosticator**. Patients with more than three major depressive episodes (MDEs) tended to relapse earlier than those with histories of three or fewer episodes, although this did not reach significance.

BACKGROUND

- Patients with MDD (as diagnosed using Research Diagnostic Criteria, or RDC) were followed naturalistically for 10 years or longer.
- Patients were divided on the basis of intake MDE recovery into recovery with residual subthreshold depressive symptoms (recovery with 1+ mild symptoms; N=82) and asymptomatic recovery (N=155) groups. Trained raters interviewed patients every six months for the first five years and every year thereafter.
- Depressive symptomatology was rated using the Longitudinal Interval Follow-up Evaluation (LIFE) Psychiatric Status Rating (PSR) scales.
- Recovery with 1+ mild symptoms as defined by the PSR includes those experiencing one or more depressive symptoms but of no more than a mild degree.
- P values (given according to color of lines on slide graphic): Orange vs green, P<.0001; orange vs blue, P<.0001; orange vs red, P<.0001; green vs blue, P=.013; green vs red, P=.004; blue vs red, P=.283.

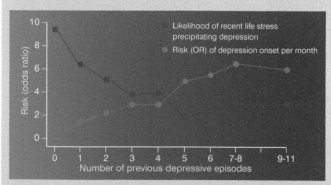

Figure 2: Progression of Depression: Adverse Effects of Each Episode on Future Episodes Which Become More Spontaneous and Less Triggered by Stress. These data are consistent with the notion that symptoms of depression and episodes of depression "kindle" subsequent episodes of depression.

- The kindling hypothesis states that previous episodes of depression change the brain, making patients more likely to experience subsequent episodes of depression
- After 4 to 5 episodes, the best predictor of subsequent episodes of depression is the number of previous depressive episodes, not stress
- Does this suggest that recurrent depression is a progressive disease?

BACKGROUND:

- Female twins from a population-based registry (N=2,395) were interviewed 4 times during a period of 9 years, forming a study group that contained 97,515 person-months and 1380 onsets of MDD

- To assess the interaction between life-event exposure and the number of previous episodes of MDD in predicting future MDD episodes, discrete-time survival, a proportional hazards model, and piece-wise regression analyses were used
- This pattern of results was unchanged by the addition of measures of event severity and genetic risk, as well as the restriction to "independent stressful life events"
- The same pattern of results emerged when within-person changes in the number of episodes were examined

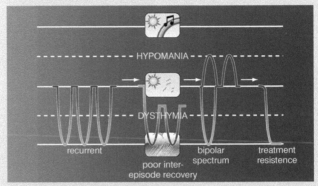

Figure 3: is Major Depressive Disorder Progressive? Studies as well as direct observations of cases over long periods of time suggest that one episode of major depression may not only increase the chances of having another, but that subsequent recurrences may not be followed by remission and only by partial treatment responses, ultimately with episodes recurring that may become treatment resistant.

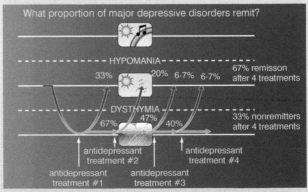

Figure 4: What proportion of major depressive disorder remit? Approximately one-third of depressed patients will remit during treatment

with any antidepressant initially. Unfortunately, for those who fail to remit the likelihood of remission with another antidepressant monotherapy goes down with each successive trial. Thus, after a year of treatment with four sequential antidepressants taken for twelve weeks each, only two-thirds of patients will have achieved remission.

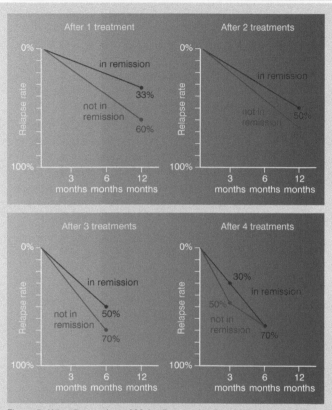

Figure 5: What Proportion of Major Depressive Disorders Relapse? The rate of relapse of major depression is significantly less for patients who achieve remission. However, there is still risk of relapse even in remitters, and the likelihood increases with the number of treatments it takes to get the patient to remit. Thus, the relapse rate for patients who do not remit ranges from 60% at twelve months after one treatment to 70% at six months after four treatments, but for those who do remit it ranges from only 33% at twelve months after one treatment all the way to 70% at six months after four treatments. In other words, the protective nature of remission virtually disappears once it takes four treatments to achieve remission.

Posttest Self Assessment Question: Answer

If a patient has low blood levels of an antidepressant at standard doses, what could this mean?

A. Pharmacokinetic failure
   – Pharmacokinetics is the body acting upon a drug; so, if the body does not absorb or metabolize a drug in a way that normal therapeutic levels are delivered to the brain via the blood, a low blood level at standard doses can mean a pharmacokinetic failure
B. Genetic variant causing pharmacokinetic failure
   – Genetic variants of CYP450 enzymes can cause excessive metabolism of a drug and thus pharmacokinetic failure
C. Pharmacodynamic failure
   – Pharmacodynamics is the drug acting upon the body, in this case, transporters in the brain; so, if a patient has low blood levels of an antidepressant, there is not adequate opportunity to see if the drug will work, and this is not considered a pharmacodynamic failure; a pharmacodynamic failure occurs when the brain does not respond to normal levels of drug
D. Genetic variant causing pharmacodynamic failure
   Genetic variants are considered to cause pharmacodynamic failures when despite adequate levels of drug, there is no therapeutic response
E. Noncompliance
   – low blood levels are more often caused by noncompliance/ nonadherence than they are by pharmacokinetic failures

Answer: A, B and E

References

1. Stahl SM, Mood Disorders, in Stahl's Essential Psychopharmacology, 3rd edition, Cambridge University Press, New York, 2008, pp 453–510
2. Stahl SM, Antidepressants, in Stahl's Essential Psychopharmacology, 3rd edition, Cambridge University Press, New York, 2008, pp 511–666
3. Stahl SM, Venlafaxine, in Stahl's Essential Psychopharmacology The Prescriber's Guide, 3rd edition, Cambridge University Press, New York, 2009, pp 579–84
4. Stahl SM, Phenelzine, in Stahl's Essential Psychopharmacology The Prescriber's Guide, 3rd edition, Cambridge University Press, New York, 2009, pp 427–32
5. Stahl SM, How to dose a psychotropic drug: beyond therapeutic drug monitoring to genotyping the patient. Acta Psychiatrica Scand, in press

6. Mrazek DA, Psychiatric Pharmacogenomics, Oxford, New York, 2010

7. Marangell LB, Martinez M, Jurdi RA et al. Neurostimulation therapies. Acta Psychiatrica Scandinavica 2007; 116: 174–81

8. Andrade P, Noblesse LHM, Temel Y et al. Neurostimulatory and ablative treatment options in major depressive disorder: a systematic review. Acta Neurochir 2010; 152: 565–77

9. Goodman WK, Insel TR, Deep brain stimulation in psychiatry: concentrating on the road ahead. Biol Psychiatry 2009; 65: 262–6

10. Bewernick BH, Hurlemann R, Matusch A et al. Nucleus accumbens deep brain stimulation decreases ratings of depression and anxiety in treatment-resistant depression. Biol Psychiatry 2010; 67: 110–6

11. Nahas Z, Anderson BS, Borchardt J et al. Biolateral epidural prefrontal cortical stimulation for treatment resistant depression, Biol Psychiatry 2010; 67: 101–9

12. Sartorius A, Kiening KL, Kirsch P et al. Remission of major depression under deep brain stimulation of the lateral habenula in a therapy refractory patient. Biol Psychiatry 2010; 67:e9-e11

13. Lakhan SE, Callaway E, Deep brain stimulation for obsessive compulsive disorder and treatment resistant depression: a systematic review. BMC Research Notes 2010; 3(60): 1–9

14. Ward HE, Hwynn N, Okun MS, Update on deep brain stimulation for neuropsychiatric disorders. Neurobiol of Disease 2010; 38: 346–53

15. Rabins P, Appleby BS, Brandt J et al. Scientific and ethical issue related to deep brain stimulation for disorders of mood, behavior and thought. Arch Gen Psychiat 2009; 66: 931–7

16. Schlaepfer TE, George MS, Mayberg H, WFSBP Guidelines on Brain stimulation treatments in psychiatry. World J Biol Psychiat 2010; 11: 2–18

17. DeBattista C, Kinrys G, Hoffman D et al. The use of referenced EEG in assisting medication selection for the treatment of depression. J Psychiatr Res 2010; 45(1): 64–75

18. Salvadore G, Cornwell BR, Sambataro F, et al. Anterior cingulate desynchronization and functional connectivity with the amygdala during a working memory task predict rapid antidepressant response to ketamine. Neuropsychopharmacology 2010; 35(7): 1415–22

19. Salvadore G, Cornwell BR, Colon-Rosario V, et al. Increased anterior cingulate cortical activity in response to fearful faces: a neurophysiological biomarker that predicts rapid antidepressant response to ketamine. Biol Psychiatry., 2009; 65: 289–95

20. Stahl SM. Psychiatric stress testing: novel strategy for translational psychopharmacology. Neuropsychopharmacology 2010; 35: 6, p.1413–4

21. Price RB, Knock MK, Charney DS et al. Effects of intravenous ketamine on explicit and implicit measures of suicidality in treatment-resistant depression. Biol Psychiatry 2009; 66: 522–6

22. Zarate CA, Jr., Singh JB, Carlson PJ, et al. A randomized trial of an N-methyl-D-aspartate antagonist in treatment-resistant major depression. Arch Gen Psychiatry 2006; 63: 856–64

23. Mathew SJ, Manji HK, Charney DS. Novel drugs and therapeutic targets for severe mood disorders. Neuropsychopharmacology 2008; 33: 2080–92

24. Li N, Lee B, Liu R-J, Banasr M, Dwyer JM, Iwata M, Li X-Y, Aghajanian G, Duman RS, mTOR-dependent synapse formation underlies the rapid antidepressant effects of NMDA antagonists, Science 2010; 329: 959–64

The Case: The woman who was either manic or fat

The Question: Will patients be compliant with effective mood stabilizers that cause major weight gain?

The Dilemma: Can you find a mood stabilizer that does not cause weight gain or a medication that blocks the weight gain of the mood stabilizer?

Pretest Self Assessment Question (answer at the end of the case)

Which of the following most accurately describes asenapine?

A. Has a high risk of metabolic side effects
B. Is available as a sublingual formulation
C. Works primarily as a very potent dopamine D3 receptor agonist

Patient Intake

- 32-year-old woman diagnosed with bipolar 1 disorder
- Current chief complaint
  - Patient's mania has been relatively stable for four months but she experienced 50 pounds of weight gain on olanzapine (Zyprexa) just before getting pregnant and is now 60 pounds overweight 2 months into her pregnancy
  - Uncertain about whether the weight gain is unsafe or if stopping her olanzapine would be unsafe

Psychiatric History

- She was diagnosed with bipolar disorder almost seven years ago
- Since then has had fairly resistant and chronic mania with intermittent mixed or depressive states less commonly
- No medication other than olanzapine seems effective for her mania, including many other antipsychotics, anticonvulsant mood stabilizers, and lithium
- Unfortunately, she has incredible weight gain (at least 40 pounds) associated with massive hunger every time she takes olanzapine to attain remission of mania, and then discontinues it because of the weight gain and relapses
- This is the third time she has tried olanzapine, failing each time to find an effective alternate medication, with olanzapine being highly effective as a mood stabilizer every time she has taken it
- She takes olanzapine about 10 mg/day for mania as higher doses seem to induce depression (above 12.5 mg/day)
- Without olanzapine she becomes "catatonic," crying, numb, and apathetic, a state of irritable mixed mania and depression, mostly irritable mania with lesser depression
- She also became angry and bitter against psychiatry due to the toll

her bipolar illness and its treatment have taken on her and the inability of others to help her get back to work, have no symptoms, and also normal weight
- She is also bitter around home and is having domestic conflict with her husband and wants to divorce him after she delivers her baby

Treatment History

- Previous medication trials
  - Lithium: discontinued when it became toxic at 900 mg/day (level 1.7) and ineffective
  - Ziprasidone (Geodon): not effective for mania and mood cycling at doses as high as 240 mg/day; it may also have uncovered allergies leading to vomiting and sneezing
  - Oxcarbazepine (Trileptal): made patient feel "catatonic" at 150 mg twice per day
  - Aripiprazole (Abilify): not effective for mania at 15–30 mg/day and caused akathisia
  - Risperidone: not as effective as olanzapine at 2 mg twice per day and also caused weight gain
  - Divalproex (Depakote): not effective and caused "moon face" due to weight gain in the face as well as liver problems
- Patient also had 27 electroconvulsive therapy (ECT) treatments two years ago that were effective for her depression but left her with significant cognitive impairment
- She has tried numerous antidepressants in the past, including sertraline, paroxetine, venlafaxine XR, and bupropion XL without robust results and with possible worsening of mixed states
- She has not tried asenapine, carbamazepine, clozapine, iloperidone, paliperidone, quetiapine, or lurasidone

Social and Personal History

- Married 4 years, pregnant with first child
- Non smoker
- No drug or alcohol abuse
- College educated
- Teacher, but had to resign due to disability from her mania several years ago

Medical History

- BP normal
- Normal fasting glucose
- Triglycerides elevated when overweight and when taking olanzapine
- Normalize when she stops olanzapine (but becomes manic)

Family History

- Mother: with depression
- Maternal uncle: alcohol abuse
- Maternal grandmother: "manic depressive"

Current Medications

- Fluoxetine 40 mg/day
- Olanzapine 10 mg/day
- Lamotrigine 400 mg/day

Considering her history and current pregnancy, would you make any of the following adjustments to her medication regimen?

- Discontinue/switch olanzapine
- Discontinue/switch fluoxetine
- Discontinue/switch lamotrigine

Attending Physician's Mental Notes, Initial Psychiatric Evaluation

- Manic symptoms may worsen during pregnancy, necessitating some form of treatment
- The risk of treatment during pregnancy must be weighed against the risk of no treatment
- Atypical antipsychotics may be preferable to anticonvulsant mood stabilizers during pregnancy
- Olanzapine is a risk category C drug (some animal studies show risk, no controlled studies in humans)
  - Early findings suggest no adverse consequences to infants exposed in utero
- Fluoxetine is a risk category C drug (some animal studies show risk, no controlled studies in humans)
  - May not be recommended for use during pregnancy, especially in the first trimester
  - Longitudinal studies suggest that continuous treatment during pregnancy is not harmful to the fetus or developing child
  - There may be increased bleeding in the mother at delivery and of sedation in the newborn
- Lamotrigine is a risk category C drug (some animal studies show risk, no controlled studies in humans)
  - Has been associated with increased incidence of cleft palate/lip deformity if exposure occurs during first trimester
  - If lamotrigine is used during pregnancy it may be necessary to check plasma levels as they can be reduced during pregnancy, possibly requiring increased doses with dose reduction following delivery

- Patient is currently asymptomatic in terms of mood
- Distressed over weight gain on olanzapine
- Considering the patient's history of fairly chronic mania, especially whenever she stops olanzapine, and the risks versus the benefits to the fetus, including the implications to the fetus and newborn in terms of a mother with mania versus a mother in remission, the decision is made to maintain her medications

Case Outcome: First Interim Followup, Month 6

- The patient returns at eight months pregnant reporting that her mood is stable but that she has gained a substantial amount of weight during her pregnancy (>100 pounds)
- Wants to know if she can stop her medications as soon as she delivers so she can get the weight off
- Current medications
  - Fluoxetine 40 mg/day
  - Olanzapine 10 mg/day
  - Lamotrigine 400 mg/day

Which of the following would you most likely choose for this patient?

- Maintain her current medication regimen post-partum
- Switch olanzapine to an agent with less propensity to cause weight gain postpartum
- Augment with an agent that may mitigate weight gain

If you were to switch, which of the following antimanic medications (i.e., those she has not yet tried) would you most likely choose for this patient?

- Asenapine
- Carbamazepine
- Clozapine
- Iloperidone
- Lurasidone
- Paliperidone
- Quetiapine

If you were to augment, which of the following would you most likely choose for this patient?

- Metformin
- Pramlintide
- Topiramate
- Zonisamide
- Naltrexone
- Bupropion
- Phentermine

Attending Physician's Mental Notes: First Interim Followup, Month 6

- Because her symptoms are stable, it would not be prudent to switch from olanzapine during the high risk period for mania recurrence postpartum (i.e., until at least 3–6 months postpartum)
- After the patient is past the vulnerable postpartum period, could consider giving an agent that could possibly reduce weight along with olanzapine
  - An anticonvulsant such as topiramate or zonisamide, which have been associated with weight loss
  - The antidepressant bupropion has been associated with weight loss
  - The opiate antagonist naltrexone has been associated with weight loss
  - Experimental treatment with antidiabetic agents have been reported to cause weight loss caused by antipsychotics
    - Metformin
    - Pramlintide
- A number of weight loss agents combining known weight loss agents are in testing, as are some novel compounds
  - Lorcaserin, a 5HT2C agonist
  - Combination of the weight loss agent phentermine plus topiramate in sustained release formulations aimed at lowering the dose, reducing the side effects and increasing weight loss
  - Combination of bupropion SR with naltrexone SR
  - Combination of zonisaminde with bupropion SR
- For now, these are not practical considerations until more research is completed on these agents, but she could try several agents after she delivers including metformin, bupropion, naltrexone, or zonisamide
- Probably best to avoid phentermine, a stimulant, so as not to activate her mania and destabilize her
- Advised her to continue psychotropic medications for at least six months following delivery of her baby and to consider one of the weight loss medications as augmentation after she delivers

Case Outcome: Second Interim Followup, Month 22

- Patient delivered a healthy baby boy, and her mood stayed stable throughout pregnancy and delivery
- She did not want to add another medication to address the weight gain post partum
- Plus she wanted to breast feed and she was advised not to do so while taking the recommended psychotropic medications and weight loss medications

- Instead, she insisted on stopping olanzapine for the fourth time, starting three months after the birth of her son
- A few months later, relapses, developing depression and mixed/rapid cycling states off all medications
- However, she lost over 60 pounds of the 100 pounds she had gained during pregnancy
- She refused re-treatment with olanzapine
- To treat her relapse, was given
  - Lithium 750 mg/day
  - Quetiapine extended release 600 mg/day
  - Lamotrigine 400 mg/day
  - Fluoxetine 10 mg/day
  - Temazepam 60 mg/day for insomnia
- She experiences hypomanic/manic and mixed dysphoric states (no pure major depressive episodes)
  - She reports that she feels manic most days and that the mania worsens diurnally as the day proceeds, characterized by "my pupils being huge," agitation and anger towards her husband, racing thoughts, and impulsivity
- This continuous state of instability persists over the course of a year despite many medication adjustments
  - Increased quetiapine dose (seemed to exacerbate mania)
  - Added olanzapine 15 mg/day while decreasing quetiapine dose (to 500 mg/day)
  - Discontinued lithium (did not think it was helping)
  - Discontinued fluoxetine (possibility it might exacerbate mania)
  - Added carbamazepine 200 mg/day in divided doses (worked well for helping the patient sleep but she discontinued after 10 days when she researched the drug and "freaked out" about potential side effects)
  - Added oxcarbazepine because of inadequate prior trial and titrated to 1200 mg in split doses (was well tolerated and patient liked it – "mood enhancer . . . makes me feel good, my attitude is better")
- Patient abruptly stopped quetiapine during oxcarbazepine titration
  - Oxcarbazepine exacerbated her migraines and despite apparent therapeutic effects it had to be stopped
  - Due to continuing weight problems, another attempt was made with ziprasidone 60 mg twice per day, but it destabilized her and was discontinued
  - Added topiramate 25 mg/day but she felt "wacko" and cut her wrists so topiramate was discontinued
  - During this time, she lost all of the 100 pounds she had gained on olanzapine

- Reluctantly, restarts olanzapine
  - Olanzapine 15 mg/day
  - Lamotrigine 400 mg/day
  - Temazepam 60 mg/day for insomnia
  - Propranolol 10 mg twice per day for akathisia
  - Has already gained 30 pounds in 2 months and still only an incomplete recovery although a clear therapeutic effect since starting olanzapine

Of the following options (i.e., those she has not yet tried or had an adequate trial), which would you most likely choose for this patient?

- Add/switch to asenapine
- Add/switch to carbamazepine
- Add/switch to clozapine
- Add/switch to iloperidone
- Add/switch to lurasidone
- Add/switch to paliperidone
- Add/switch to zonisamide
- Add/switch to a conventional antipsychotic

Attending Physician's Mental Notes: Second Interim Followup, Month 22

- Asenapine may be beneficial as it has a pharmacological profile that is similar to olanzapine's but seems to carry less risk of weight gain
- Carbamazepine may also be useful as it was effective previously for sleep (but without an adequate trial); in addition, oxcarbazepine, which is the 10-keto analog of carbamazepine, was previously effective for her mood symptoms
- Although clozapine is generally the most effective of the antipsychotics, it carries as much if not more weight gain risk as olanzapine
- Iloperidone may be beneficial as it seems to carry less risk of weight gain than olanzapine
- Paliperidone is the active metabolite of risperidone, which was previously ineffective and caused weight gain
- Lurasidone (Latuda) not available at the time of this appointment, is now available and associated with a low risk of weight gain
- Zonisamide may be useful as augmentation for weight issues, but is not well studied in bipolar disorder
- A conventional antipsychotic may be helpful, but as she already has akathisia it may be preferable to avoid agents with higher risk of movement disorder

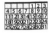

Case Outcome: Third Interim Followup, Month 26

- Asenapine 5 mg twice per day is added
- After a few weeks she reports improvement in mania and also a surprising and welcome reduction in appetite
- Her insomnia continues and the dose of temazepam is increased to 60 mg in split doses
- Her current regimen includes
  - Olanzapine 5 mg three times per day
  - Asenapine 5 mg twice per day
  - Lamotrigine 400 mg/day
  - Temazepam 15 mg four times per day
  - Propranolol 10 mg three times per day
- She appears to have an irritable edge of a hypomanic state but no overt depression or mania and is relatively stable
- She starts losing weight as soon as asenapine is started despite continuing olanzapine
- Asenapine increased to 10 mg twice a day and other medications unchanged
- Lost all weight she had gained on olanzapine
- Has become stable

What would you do now?

- Taper olanzapine
- Increase asenapine above the recommended dose range of 10 mg twice a day
- Leave well enough alone for now
- Other

Case Debrief

- This patient with bipolar disorder has chronic treatment-resistant mania and mixed, rapid cyclic states
- These seem to be inadequately controlled when not taking olanzapine; however, olanzapine causes unacceptable weight gain
- Addition of asenapine seems to have ameliorated the metabolic side effects associated with olanzapine, though it is not clear why
- She is relatively stable on a complicated regimen of medications including at the moment antipsychotic polypharmacy which is not only expensive but poorly studied
- Because she is taking large doses of medications, it remains a possibility that she does not absorb them well and it may be beneficial to take plasma levels
- Further options for this patient include:

- – Increasing doses of both asenapine and olanzapine while monitoring blood plasma levels
- Adding carbamazepine (previously beneficial but not tried for adequate trial)
- Switching asenapine and olanzapine to lurasidone
- For now, left well enough alone
- The case continues. . . .

Posttest Self Assessment Question: answer

Which of the following most accurately describes the recently approved drug asenapine?

A. Has a high risk of metabolic side effects
  - – Experience so far does not suggest a high risk of metabolic side effects, but some patients do gain weight
B. Is available as a sublingual formulation
  - – This is true
C. Works primarily as a very potent dopamine D3 receptor agonist
  - – Thought to work primarily as a D2 and 5HT2A antagonist

Answer: B

References

1. Stahl SM, Mood Disorders, in Stahl's Essential Psychopharmacology, 3rd edition, Cambridge University Press, New York, 2008, pp 453–510
2. Stahl SM, Antidepressants, in Stahl's Essential Psychopharmacology, 3rd edition, Cambridge University Press, New York, 2008, pp 511–666
3. Stahl SM, Mood Stabilizers, in Stahl's Essential Psychopharmacology, 3rd edition, Cambridge University Press, New York, 2008, pp 667–720
4. Stahl SM, Olanzapine, in Stahl's Essential Psychopharmacology The Prescriber's Guide, 3rd edition, Cambridge University Press, New York, 2009, pp 387–92
5. Stahl SM, Asenapine, in Stahl's Essential Psychopharmacology The Prescriber's Guide, 4th edition, Cambridge University Press, New York, 2011 in press
6. Stahl, SM, Lurasidone, in Stahl's Essential Psychopharmacology Prescriber's Guide, 4th edition, Cambridge University Press, New York, 2011 in press
7. Einarson A. Risks/safety of psychotropic medication use during pregnancy. Can J Clin Pharmacol 2009; 16(1): e58–65
8. Sharma V. Management of bipolar II disorder during pregnancy and the postpartum period. Can J Clin Pharmacol 2009; 16(1): e33–41

The Case: The girl who couldn't find a doctor

The Question: How aggressive should medication treatment be in a child with an anxiety disorder?

The Dilemma: Can you justify giving high dose benzodiazepines plus SSRIs to a 12-year-old?

Pretest Self Assessment Question (answer at the end of the case)

A dose of 3 mg lorazepam is too high for a thin twelve-year-old girl.

A. True
B. False

Patient Intake

- 12-year-old girl
- Chief complaint: "fear"

Psychiatric History

- Symptoms of generalized fear and anxiety started at age seven, but then got better; returned at age eleven; no identifiable stressors
- Currently prepubescent
- Denies panic attacks; currently tearful, depressed
- One year ago began "getting an overactive mind"
- Rituals and obsessions also began a year ago
- So distressed by these that withdraws from friends, cannot be in a classroom with others, so pulled out of the classroom and home schooled for the past year

Family History

- Mother, a physician: with generalized anxiety
- Maternal grandmother: bipolar
- Maternal great-grandmother: committed suicide
- Maternal aunt: has schizophrenia
- Paternal cousin: committed suicide

Social and Personal History

- Was an excellent student prior to dropping out for home schooling
- No drug or alcohol abuse
- Has a younger brother

Medical History and Medications

- None

Patient Intake

- Patient admits to have compelling thoughts; almost, but not clearly, a voice making her sense that something horrible was about to happen, something or somebody would die
- She has to clean the cage of her rabbit perfectly or he will die
- She has some counting rituals in which she walks a certain number of steps and needs to end on a certain number to prevent something horrible, like the brutal death of her parents
- Has to have items facing her squarely and not at an angle, and has to move certain objects, like the remote control, so it does not face her at home, or even objects on the attending physician's desk so that they are "straight"
- These thoughts and rituals take most of the day every day and distract her from school work

Given just the information you have here, what do you think is her diagnosis?

- Behavioral inhibition (a temperament at risk for developing an anxiety disorder)
- Separation anxiety disorder
- Generalized anxiety disorder
- Obsessive compulsive disorder
- Major depressive disorder
- An overly involved mother
- Other

Attending Physician's Mental Notes: Initial Psychiatric Evaluation

- Looks like OCD with comorbid GAD, possibly in a patient who had premorbid behavioral inhibition, although no clear history of separation anxiety
- If anything, she has separation anxiety now
- Characteristic of anxiety disorders in children, it appears as though this patient has an ever evolving polymorphic anxiety disorder that morphs from GAD to OCD and beyond
- So far, does not admit to panic attacks, and does not have major depression
- Social anxiety may play a role in her avoidance of school as well
- Advised treatment with SSRI
- The mother, a physician, had already anticipated this, and had gone to their pediatrician who will not prescribe SSRIs to children anymore because of the risk of suicide and suicidality
- Told them only a child psychiatrist should do this now

- The mother is at a distance from the attending physician, and so with the written consultation sent to the pediatrician recommending an SSRI fom this consultation, will go back to the pediatrician and see if she will prescribe the SSRI
- Also referred to a local child psychiatrist

Would you be willing to prescribe an SSRI to this twelve-year-old child, presenting with OCD and anxiety?

- Yes
- No

If you would give an SSRI, which one would you prescribe to her?

- Fluoxetine (Prozac)
- Paroxetine (Paxil)
- Sertraline (Zoloft)
- Fluvoxamine (Levrox)
- Citalopram (Celexa)
- Escitalopram (Lexapro)
- Any of the above
- I would not give an SSRI.

Given the FDA warning and recommendations of caution prescribing antidepressants to children six to twelve, do you think that this patient, with a very positive family history of bipolar disorder, must be seen weekly if you prescribe an SSRI?

- Yes
- No

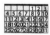

Case Outcome: First Interim Followup, Week 8

- Pediatrician still will not prescribe SSRIs
- After waiting for four weeks, the child psychiatrist was not available to see patient weekly for FDA-advised monitoring, so referred her back to her pediatrician with the recommendation to use an SSRI
- Pediatrician continues to refuse to do so
- Refers patient back to you
- In desperation, mother gives her daughter an intermittent dose of lorazepam from her own prescription, with very robust but short-lasting relief of intense anxiety

Would you be willing to prescribe a benzodiazepine to this twelve-year-old child, presenting with OCD and anxiety?

- Yes
- No

Case Outcome: First Interim Followup, Week 8

- Recommended escitalopram 10 mg and lorazepam 0.5 mg once or twice a day as needed in consultation letter to referring physician/pediatrician as well as to another child psychiatrist
- Recommended weekly follow-ups locally as suggested by the FDA and some experts and some treatment guidelines
- Called a second child psychiatrist in the patient's area who agreed to see the patient within a week and then weekly

Case Outcome: Second Interim Followup, Week 12

- Followup phone call
- When patient finally seen 4 weeks later and not immediately as promised, child psychiatrist had to cancel and had partner see child; partner recommended cognitive behavioral therapy and refused to follow recommendations to prescribe meds
- Mother calls, desperate
- Immediate phone consultation of attending physician with local pediatrician, who agrees to see patient briefly, weekly, and to monitor for activation and suicidality, as long as she does not have to write prescriptions
- Mother is medically sophisticated, understands risks and benefits, and agrees to monitor child closely as well
- Prescriptions are phoned in by the attending physician, and patient begins escitalopram and lorazepam
- Agrees to return for a face-to-face appointment in 4 weeks

Case Outcome: Third Interim Followup, Week 14

- Seen after two weeks, because mother runs out of lorazepam, having given twice as much as was prescribed so 30 day supply lasted only 2 weeks
- Lorazepam has robust, but short lived, effects, so mother gives 0.5 mg three or four times a day and shortly runs out
- Pediatrician monitoring patient weekly
- No side effects, no activation or suicidality
- "A little better, but on summer break, so who knows"
- Not crying, still anxious, sleeps very well at night now
- Advised to continue escitalopram 10 mg and prescribed an increase of lorazepam to 0.5 mg four times a day

Even if you would have been willing to prescribe a benzodiazepine previously, do you agree with giving an increased dose of benzodiazepine in this situation?

- Yes
- No

Attending Physician's Mental Notes: Third Interim Followup, Week 14

- It is already controversial in the minds of some mental health experts to prescribe benzodiazepines at all, more controversial to prescribe for a child, even more controversial to prescribe at high doses, especially if the mother is escalating the dose before getting prior approval from the attending physician
- Is this headed for disaster?
- Is this too aggressive and not justified?

Case Outcome: Fourth Interim Followup, Week 18

- Scheduled to be seen two months later, with pediatrician monitoring weekly for a few more weeks, then every other week for a few weeks, then monthly
- However, seen after one month because runs out of lorazepam again; no sedation, no suicidality
- "Has kicked in a bit" meaning decreases in compelling thoughts, less general worry about symmetry, contamination, and religious themes
- In fact, now that she is a bit better, she is able to disclose many more obsessions and thoughts she had been too concerned about to express previously
- "Maybe my OCD is 33% better"
- Worst time is during the day, and mother gives her two or three tabs of 0.5 mg lorazepam on some days, in the middle of the day, with dramatic results

Attending Physician's Mental Notes: Fourth Interim Followup, Week 18

- Now a dilemma
- Here we finally have a patient who is responding but due to a second dose increase in lorazepam by the physician-mother taking things into her own hands without prior approval again
- Many would stop the benzodiazepine or refuse to continue to treat this situation, referring to another psychiatrist
- Nevertheless, nothing disputes the irrefutable logic of results
- Looked at objectively, if anything, the benzodiazepine dose may be still too low

- Lorazepam may have also been useful in masking potentially activating side effects of escitalpram if taken alone
- Mother is honest about what she is doing with the lorazepam
- If mother is willing to have her child take strictly as prescribed, will actually increase dose of lorazepam, realizing this is controversial and may generate criticism by other physicians involved in the case
- Now 6 weeks on the SSRI, could recommend increasing the dose of that too; if the escitatopram becomes more efficacious, lorazepam may be tapered.

Attending Physician's Mental Notes: First Interim Followup, Week 18, Continued

- Advised to increase escitalpram to 20 mg/day
- Increased lorazepam strictly to 0.5 mg in the morning/1.0 mg late morning or early afternoon/1.0 mg late afternoon or early evening for homework/0.5 mg at night (3 mg total daily dose)
- Patient weighs 80 pounds

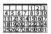

Case Outcome: Fifth Interim Followup, Week 22

- Seen one month later, situation improving
- Seeming compliance to dosing as prescribed

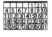

Case Outcome: Sixth Interim Followup, Week 26

- Seen in another month, "doing well"
- Rating herself 85% better
- At this point only taking 2 mg lorazepam per day
- Only a few obsessive thoughts in the background
- Only occasional "down" days in terms of mood
- Lorazepam is still very helpful
- Sleep is good

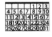

Case Outcome: Seventh Interim Followup, Week 38

- Three months later: tired, on spring break, but otherwise doing well
- Still on escitalopram 20 mg and lorazepam 2 mg/day

Case Outcome: Eighth Interim Followup, Week 50

- Three months later, about a year since the initial psychiatric evaluation
- A bit nervous, some peer problems
- Now age 13, still no menstrual periods
- Worried about school in general, but no depression
- Obsessive thoughts still in the background
- Meds continued unchanged

Case Outcome: Ninth Interim Followup, Week 62

- Patient and her mother decide cautiously to return to public school
- Has been anxiety provoking
- Has increased lorazepam back to 3 mg/day
- Worried about whether she will make the transition

Case Outcome: Tenth Interim Followup, Week 74

- Attending high school
- Highly strung, anxious
- Afraid that her homework is not perfect
- Has some friends but not boyfriends
- Thinks some of her peers are "pure jerks"
- Wants to become a pediatric intensive care nurse
- Planning to go to college and taking college prep courses
- Actually, looks and acts and functions the closest to normal ever

Case Debrief

- This adolescent had the onset of a polymorphic and disabling anxiety disorder
- These conditions are often trivialized as being less disabling than other psychiatric conditions such as psychosis and thus not warranting aggressive psychopharmacological treatment
- It is difficult to get even standard approved treatments to children and adolescents given the lack of experts and the fear of prescribers in giving SSRIs and benzodiazepines to children and adolescents
- Aggressive treatment with a benzodiazepine and an SSRI were ultimately quite successful
- Treatment did not require an atypical antipsychotic which could be justified here if the SSRI and benzodiazepine were ineffective
- Treatment did not involve CBT which the daughter refused and the mother felt was not credible given her problems with child psychiatrists whom she felt did not help her or her daughter

Take-Home Points

- FDA warnings of suicidality in children on SSRIs has sent a chill through prescribers, making it difficult sometimes to find someone willing to prescribe them
- Also it is controversial to many clinicians to prescribe daily high doses of a benzodiazepine to any child
- Paradoxically, atypical antipsychotic prescribing in children has skyrocketed and seems to be less controversial
- Treating children can feel like "damned if you do, damned if you don't"
- Psychopharmacologists comfortable with risks and benefits can

prescribe with confidence as experts realize the FDA regulates the sale of medicine by pharma, not the practice of medicine by licensed prescribers
- The flurry of warnings of suicidality now for antidepressants, antipsychotics approved as antidepressants, all anticonvulsants, varenicline for smoking cessation, and others, is producing "label fatigue" among prescribers who look to medical standards and common sense, not to the package insert and product label alone for practice guidelines

Performance in Practice: Confessions of a Psychopharmacologist

- What could have been done better here?
  - Should SSRIs have been started earlier and not worry about the need to set up close monitoring since that caused a great delay in initiating treatment?
  - Should a bigger push have been made for CBT despite the mother's lack of confidence both in the CBT and in the child psychiatrists or child therapists who would have administered it?
  - Should an anxiolytic/sedating atypical antipsychotic such as quetiapine been prescribed rather than the benzodiazepine lorazepam?
- Possible action item for improvement in practice
  - Make a concerted effort to find psychopharmacologists comfortable in treating children and adolescents
  - Make a more concerted effort to find CBT therapists who are experts in treating OCD and GAD in children and adolescents

Tips and Pearls

- SSRIs and benzodiazepines are effective in children and adults alike
- Good documentation of efficacy of SSRIs in children and adolescents for OCD
- Controversy exists for treating children with SSRIs, less controversy exists for treating adolescents and young adults under 25 with SSRIs
- Controversy exists for treating children and adolescents with benzodiazepines as few if any studies of them in various anxiety disorders in children
- Off-label prescribing, or nonpharmaceutical approaches may be the only rational choices in cases as disabled as this one
- Anxiety disorders also deserve to be treated and to have symptoms go into sustained remission so that normal development of the child and adolescent can proceed, even at the cost of taking controversial medications

Two-Minute Tute: A brief lesson and psychopharmacology tutorial (tute) with relevant background material for this case – Anxiety disorders in children

Table 1: What is Generalized Anxiety Disorder in a Child?

- Called overanxious disorder in the past
- Is a generalized and persistent anxiety that is not the result of separation or recent stress
- Characterized by self-consciousness
- Obsessive concern over past behavior, future events, personal health, and competence in athletics, social, or academic arenas but not obsessions or compulsions per se

Table 2: What is Behavioral Inhibition?

- An early temperamental trait characterized by the tendency to withdraw when exposed to unfamiliar situations
- Longitudinal studies of behaviorally inhibited children indicate that it tends to be an enduring temperamental trait
- Children classified as behaviorally inhibited at age 21 months continue to be shy, timid, and fearful in unfamiliar settings at the ages of 4 and 7
- Children who are inhibited may have a lower threshold of responsivity in the limbic and hypothalamic circuits and, as a result, they react with greater sympathetic activation when exposed to novel situations
- Children of parents with panic disorder with agoraphobia have a higher rate of behavioral inhibition than children of parents without panic disorder with agoraphobia
- Multiple anxiety disorders are found at increased rates in children classified as behaviorally inhibited
- Thus, behavioral inhibition may indicate increased vulnerability for anxiety disorders
- Behavioral inhibition is linked to a familial predisposition to anxiety disorders, because behavioral inhibition in children is associated with increased rates anxiety disorders in their first-degree relatives

Table 3: What is Separation Anxiety Disorder (SAD)?

- One of the most common childhood anxiety disorders
- Reported prevalence ranging from 3.5% to 5.4%
- The defining feature is developmentally inappropriate, excessive, and unrealistic anxiety regarding separation from home or from major attachment figures, usually a parent
- Children with SAD become extremely distressed when separated from a parent
- This distress can reach panic proportions, with accompanying autonomic symptoms of anxiety
- Often these children actively resist or refuse to be separated from important attachment figures
- For example, they may follow a parent around the house and refuse to sleep alone
- Children with SAD worry excessively that their parents will die or suddenly disappear, or that they will be abducted, causing permanent separation
- When these children are separated from their parents, even for a brief period of time, they spend much of this time worrying about the safety of their parents and anxiously await the parents' return
- Because these children avoid situations involving separation, school refusal frequently accompanies SAD
- Separation anxiety disorder and "school refusal" or "school phobia" are terms that have been used interchangeably, even though they are not necessarily the same thing
- For example, not all children with "school refusal" have SAD, and not all children with SAD have "school refusal"
- In fact, "school refusal" can be due to social phobia, anxiety about competence or performance in school, and other disorders, such as conduct disorder (truancy) or depression (social withdrawal)
- Furthermore, depression and overanxious disorder are frequent comorbid conditions of SAD
- Unfortunately, no firm conclusions about the usefulness of psychotropic medications for separation anxiety disorder can be drawn from treatment studies because of problems with:
  - diagnostic heterogeneity
  - small sample size
  - brief duration of treatment
  - inclusion of cases of "school refusal" secondary to truancy or depression
- If pharmacotherapy is used, it should be in the context of a multimodal treatment plan that includes behavioral interventions

Posttest Self Assessment Question: Answer

A dose of 3mg lorazepam is too high for a twelve-year old girl.

A. True

B. False

In psychopharmacology, you never say "never" – even though this is not standard treatment, and would be controversial to many, the risks and benefits in this case and the obvious good outcome, justified the use of this agent at this dose here.

Answer: B

References

1. Nardi AE and Perna G. Clonazepam in the treatment of psychiatric disorders: an update. Int Clin Psychopharmacol 2006; 21(3): 131–42

2. Rosenbaum JF. The development of clonazepam as a psychotropic: the Massachusetts General Hospital Experience. J Clin Psychiatry 2004; 65(suppl5): 3–6

3. Rosenblaum JF, Moroz G, and Bowden CL. Clonazepam in the treatment of panic disorder with or without agoraphobia: a dose-response study of efficacy, safety, and discontinuance. Clonazepam Panic Disorder Dose-Response Study Group. J Clin Psychopharmacol 1997; 17(5): 390–400

4. Susman J and Klee B. The role of high-potency benzodiazepines in the treatment of panic diosorder. Prim Care Companion J Clin Psychiatry 2005; 7(1): 5–11

5. Pollack MH, Otto MW, Tesar GE et al. Long-term outcome after acute treatment with alprazolam or clonazepam for panic disorder. J Clin Psychopharmacol 1993; 13(4): 257–63

6. Stahl SM, Mood Disorders, in Stahl's Essential Psychopharmacology, 3rd edition, Cambridge University Press, New York, 2008, pp 453–510

7. Stahl SM, Anxiety Disorders and Anxiolytics, in Stahl's Essential Psychopharmacology, 3rd edition, Cambridge University Press, New York, 2008, pp 453–510

8. Stahl SM, Antidepressants, in Stahl's Essential Psychopharmacology, 3rd edition, Cambridge University Press, New York, 2008, pp 511–666

9. Stahl SM, Stahl's Illustrated Anxiety, Stress and PTSD, Cambridge University Press, New York, 2010

10. Stahl SM, Escitalopram, in Stahl's Essential Psychopharmacology The Prescriber's Guide, 3rd edition, Cambridge University Press, New York, 2009; pp 171–5

11. Stahl SM, Lorazepam, in Stahl's Essential Psychopharmacology The Prescriber's Guide, 3rd edition, Cambridge University Press, New York, 2009, pp 295–9

12. Bridge JA, Iyengar S, Salary CB et al. Clinical response and risk for reported suicidal ideation and suicide attempts in pediatric antidepressant treatment. JAMA 2007; 297: 15, 1683–96

13. Gibbons RD, Hur K, Bhumik DK et al. The relationship between antidepressant prescription rates and rate of early adolescent suicide. Am J Psychiatry 2006; 163: 1898–1904

14. Birmaher B, Brent D, AACAP Work Group on Quality Issues et al. Practice parameter for the assessment and treatment of children and adolescents with depressive disorders. J Am Acad Child Adolesc Psychiatry 2007; 46: 1503–26

15. Cheung A, Ewigman B, Zuckerbrot RA et al. Adolescent depression: is your young patient suffering in silence? J Fam Pract 2009; 58(4): 187–92

16. Goren JL. Antidepressant use in pediatric populations. Expert Opin Drug Saf 2008; 7(3): 223–5

17. Zuckerbrot RA, Cheung AH, Jensen PS et al. Guidelines for adolescent depression in primary care (GLAD-PC): I. identification, assessment, and initial management. Pediatrics 2007; 120; e1299–312

18. Witek MW, Rojas V, Alonso C et al. Review of benzodiazepine use in children and adolescents. Psychiatr Q 2005; 76(3): 283–96

19. Graae F, Milner J, Rizzotto L et al. Clonazepam in childhood anxiety disorders. J Am Acad Child Adolesc Psychiatry 1994; 33(3): 372–6

20. Simeon JG, Ferguson HB, Knott V et al. Clinical, cognitive, and neuropsychological effects of alpazolam in children and adolescents with overanxious and avoidant disorders. J Am Acad Child Adolesc Psychiatry 1992; 31(1): 29–33

21. Kutcher SP and MacKenzie S. Successful clonazepam treatment of adolescents with panic disorder. J Clin Psychopharmacol 1988; 8(4): 299–301

22. Popoviciu L and Corfariu O. Efficacy and safety of midazolam in the treatment of night terrors in children. Br J Clin Pharmacol 1983; 16(suppl1): 97S–102S

The Case: The man who wondered if once a bipolar, always a bipolar?

The Question: Is antidepressant induced mania real bipolar disorder?

The Dilemma: Can you stop mood stabilizers after 7 years of stability following one episode of antidepressant induced mania without boarding a 2-year roller coaster of mood instability?

Pretest Self Assessment Question (answer at the end of the case)

Precipitous discontinuation of mood stabilizers has been reported to induce manic relapse, so discontinuation of mood stabilizer when indicated should be tapered over several months.

A. True
B. False

Patient Intake

- 62-year-old male
- Chief complaint: "feeling drugged and lethargic"

Psychiatric History

- Psychoanalysis in early 20s for family of origin issues
- Psychotherapy for career indecision in 30s, anxiety and insomnia also treated with hypnotics but not antidepressants
- Seven years ago: first major depressive episode, onset after diagnosed with bladder carcinoma; also not happy with job plus financial problems
- Bladder carcinoma treated and presumed cured but the patient remained depressed so begun on an SSRI
- Five weeks after starting antidepressant, tried to buy four cars in four days including a Ferrari and Mercedes and three expensive condominiums
- Hospitalized for acute manic episode, diagnosed as substance-induced mood disorder since no previous history of mania or hypomania
- Given lithium without good results, then divalproex plus bupropion with good results
- Continues meds for seven years
- However, is tired of feeling "drugged" and also feels his normal mood modulation is very compressed, feeling flat at the top and unable to cry
- No manic, hypomanic or depressive episodes in seven years
- Also, significant weight gain and development of diabetes since starting valproate
- Wants to have a trial off meds, but several physicians have refused
- "Once a bipolar, always a bipolar"

Social and Personal History

- Married 33 years, 2 children
- Non smoker
- No drug or alcohol abuse
- From a wealthy family
- Retired early from sales role while residing in another state and moved to California to retire
- Now considering going back to work because money is running out especially since losing substantial money in stock market down turn over the past 8 years since retiring

Medical History

- Bladder carcinoma 8 years ago, removed and assumed cured
- Diabetes mellitus
- Obesity

Family History

- No family history of psychiatric disorder

Current Medications

- Oral hypoglycemic
- Valproate 500 mg four times a day with therapeutic blood levels documented consistently
- Bupropion SR 150 mg bid
- Clonazepam 0.5 mg, usually 2 tab qhs

Given his unequivocal manic episode and robust response to mood stabilizer treatment, would you treat him indefinitely with mood stabilizers?

- Yes
- No

If you are willing to attempt a trial at discontinuation of his valproate because of the patient's sedation and metabolic risks, how would you do it?

- Taper divalproex, continue bupropion
- Taper bupropion, continue divalproex, then taper divalproex after bupropion discontinued
- Taper both simultaneously
- I am not willing to discontinue these meds

Attending Physician's Mental Notes: Initial Psychiatric Evaluation

- Issues in favor of a trial off mood stabilizers:
  - Patient has never experienced a spontaneous manic episode

- No family history of bipolar disorder
- Has had only a single episode of depression, and a single episode of substance-induced (i.e. antidepressant-induced) mania a long time ago
- Patient believes his long term risks of cardiovascular complications from valproate are greater than the theoretical risk that valproate is preventing recurrent mania in him
- Also, is 7 years stable on antidepressant treatment for his one episode of depression
- Could be unipolar depression with substance induced mania, resolved, single episode of each
- Becoming frustrated at his medications and his doctors, so is ready to discontinue his medications on his own if necessary
- Wife is supportive of a trial off medications to see if his sedation and daytime energy will improve and if he can lose weight
- Issues against a trial off mood stabilizers:
  - It is possible that he has more history of symptoms consistent with bipolar disorder than he is describing because he might lack insight into those symptoms
  - It is possible that antidepressant-induced mania only occurs in those who have bipolar disorder or actually is a form of bipolar disorder and thus warrants life-long treatment with mood stabilizers to prevent relapse
  - If he relapses, it may be difficult to restablize him
- Risks, benefits and alternatives explained to the patient and his wife and they consented to a cautious taper of his medications under medical supervision over several months, rather than stopping medications on his own
- Agreed to taper both medications, starting with bupropion first
- Made a contingency plan to restart bupropion if signs of relapse into depression
- Made a contingency plan for psychiatric hospitalization if necessary
- Reduced bupropion SR by half to 150 mg/day
- Continued valproate 500 mg four times a day

Case Outcome: First Interim Followup, Week 4

- One month later, doing well except for occasional fatigue and occasional "down" feelings in terms of energy and mood
- Wife notes patient seems more tired
- Advised no change in medication for another month

Case Outcome: Second Interim Followup, Week 8

- The month passes, and patient still feels a bit tired but not depressed
- Decided to discontinue bupropion SR and reduce valproate from 500 mg four times a day to 500 mg three times a day
- Outpatient contingency plan for the next month:
  - Given extra valproate to reload himself in case of recurrent mania
  - Instructed to take clonazepam 0.5 mg to 2.0 mg per day in case of early signs of mania
  - Instructed to take risperidone 1–2 mg in case of moderate signs of emerging mania and prepare for hospitalization

Case Outcome: Third and Fourth Interim Followup, Weeks 12 and 16 Followup Visits

- One month later, doing well
- Reduced valproate from 500 mg three times a day to 500 mg twice a day
- Another month later, mood stable, no more daytime napping and wife agrees he appears less lethargic; no signs of mania or depression
- Instructed to continue off bupropion, and to taper divalproex to 500 mg at night, and if stable, to decrease to 250 at night in 2 to 4 weeks, and if stable, discontinue completely
- Given instructions for oral loading dose of valproate if moderate mania re-emerges, and contingency plan for clonazepam, risperidone and/or rehospitalization depending upon outcome
- Given instructions to restart bupropion if he becomes depressed

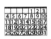

Case Outcome: Fifth Interim Followup, Weeks 24 to 52 Followup Visits

- Two months later:
  - Lost 20 pounds of weight
  - BMI now 29, no longer obese
  - Has better glucose control
  - Exercising
  - Mind clearer
  - Not sedated
  - No naps
  - Stable mood
  - Has insomnia; no initial insomnia, but trouble falling asleep after getting up his usual 1–3x nightly with nocturia
  - Insomnia not responsive to eszopiclone 3 mg at night, to zolpidem 10 mg at night, or to the combination of eszopiclone 3 mg plus clonzazepam 1 mg at night
- Insomnia finally responds to 20 mg zolpidem at night

- Continues hypnotic but no other medication for another six months
- Doing well in terms of mood
- Continued to lose weight
- No more "drugged" feeling for past six months
- "Doctor, this was a life altering process to come off drugs"
- Lost 40 pounds
- Feels like himself again
- Taking golf lessons
- Maybe some irritability
- Nocturia and middle insomnia continue intermittently

Attending Physician's Mental Notes: Fifth Interim Followup, Weeks 24 to 52

So Far So Good?

- Seems like the decision to taper the mood stabilizer was a good one so far
- Does he live happily ever after?
- He does if the case stops here, however:
- The case continues. . . .

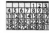

Case Outcome: Sixth Interim Followup, Week 60

- Maintains the hypnotic zolpidem at 20 mg at night, but no other medication for another six months
- Doing well in terms of mood
- Continues to lose weight
- However, wife asks to see attending physician alone
- States her husband seems happy, grilling/BBQ-ing, more interest in sex
- However, this past month, he rented a $2000 per month apartment in another state in a city where his mother lives and they visit frequently
- Bought a late model used car there for him to use when visiting there
- Did this all without consulting his wife
- Also, has bought computers, cameras, golf shoes, everyday something else and is giving these types of items as inappropriately expensive gifts to friends and those not really close to them
- According to the patient, "I am extremely well"
- Losing weight, seems relaxed, no pressured speech
- Denies racing thoughts
- No signs whatsoever of hypomania at the time of the interview
- Wife asks me to call their daughter while they are there and ask her about the prior weekend
- Daughter states by phone and patient agrees that last weekend the daughter told him to "dial it down" meaning less talking which was too much and a bit intrusive and argumentative at times

- Daughter agrees with the wife and thinks some of the recent gifts are inappropriate
- No other signs of hypomania or irritability and the patient actually seems pleasant and relaxed
- Patient also states his wife is unsophisticated about money and was traumatized by their loss of money in the stock market and now doesn't want to spend anything
- He states he has always had money and by contrast knows how to handle the ups and downs
- Told me to ignore her perspective on finances and gifts
- Found out also has had two speeding tickets in the past year, none in the past 6 weeks

What is going on here?
- An exuberant and talented man freed from restrictive side effects
- Domestic/marital conflict
- Irritability but not hypomania, as the patient reverts to his personality traits of 7 years ago prior to taking valproate
- Hypomanic relapse
- Other

Attending Physician's Notes: Sixth Interim Followup, Week 60

- Patient and wife were informed that this is possible incipient mania and given a prescription for quetiapine 100 mg at night to increase to 300 mg at night as tolerated over the next week
- Husband said this is domestic conflict, not hypomania and that if anything they need marriage therapy but he is not interested at the present time
- Asked them to bring daughter to the next appointment if possible
- Asked them all to observe for signs of escalating hypomania and to go to the emergency room if the situation worsens
- Patient says he is insulted

Case Outcome: Seventh Interim Followup, Week 64

- Patient seen with wife and daughter, 4 weeks later, as the holidays are about to start, on the day prior to their planned trip to another state to see family
- Patient refused to start quetiapine that was prescribed the last time
- "I can assure you this is not mania"
- "Sandy (his wife) is traumatized for the past 10 years because of our financial losses in the stock market"
- "She cried all the way over here"
- "I am not bipolar; she needs therapy"

- "I am exhausted"
- Seems slightly irritable and also tired
- No pressured speech, relaxed in the office, seems calm
- No signs of mania/hypomania and patient denies symptoms of hypomania

So far, can you diagnose hypomania on the basis of the information provided by the patient?

- – Yes
- – No

Attending Physician's Notes: Seventh Interim Followup, Week 64

- If the patient's presentation of the history is not sufficient for a diagnosis of hypomania, the interim history according to the wife and confirmed by the daughter provides important additional information
- Patient has had 19 new credit card charges in the past month to the computer store for computers, parts, supplies and gifts
- The patient opened a new $64,000 line of credit "for his business" but has not charged anything against it yet, and did this on his own, informing his wife after the fact
- The patient was asked if he would agree to a voluntary hospitalization rather than go on his trip
- Patient refuses, seems angry at the suggestion, and clinical assessment shows he is not sufficiently impaired to be involuntarily hospitalized and to do so would also compromise rapport and therapeutic alliance with him
- Alternative plan for the holidays:
  - – Agrees not to spend more than $200 per week without consulting his wife
  - – Wife agrees to give him $200 cash per week and he surrenders his credit cards to her in the office
  - – Told he is hypomanic and must take medications
  - – Given 100 mg sample of quetiapine which he was observed to take while in the office, and additional samples
  - – Instructed to take 200 mg quetiapine tomorrow and then increase dose to at least 300 mg and not more than 600 mg as needed and as tolerated over the holidays
  - – Instructed to start valproate 500 mg twice a day building up to 500 mg four times a day
  - – Instructed to return for an appointment as soon as he gets back from his trip in 2 weeks
  - – Not to depart for the trip tomorrow if wife feels he should not go

- To go to the local emergency room in the city he is visiting if condition escalates
- Wife and daughter agree to the plan

Case Outcome: Eighth Interim Followup, Weeks 64 Through 68

- The next day
  - Wife calls the next day
  - Quetiapine "knocked him out" and he went to sleep shortly after taking the pill in the office the previous day
  - Was unable to get up today to catch the airplane this morning, because the patient was still too sedated from the quetiapine 100 mg taken in the office yesterday
  - Advised to try another 100 mg tonight and not increase the dose if 100 mg still too sedating
- Patient and wife actually return for a followup visit 4 weeks later
  - They waited until after the holidays and then travelled to the other state to see family. Patient is going to set up a business and look for employment there and hopefully relocate there from California
  - The patient rented an office there and looked at condos but did not buy one
  - Wife says this is far in excess of what the circumstances warrant and what they can afford
  - Patient states he did not fill the prescriptions for either quetiapine or for valproate
  - "Immediately after our last appointment it settled everything down."
  - The patient states that the trip out of state one week ago was "a quantum leap forward" whatever that means
  - "I am totally positive because the medication is continuing to leave my system"
  - "This wasn't mania"
  - Bought a second late model used car, this time for his mother to use in the other city
  - "I am back to my normal self, active, engaged and everything else"
  - Asked why he needs an office in the other city before he has a business running there and he states "To get away from my wife's yelling and screaming"

Attending Physician's Mental Notes: Eighth Interim Followup, Weeks 64 Through 68

- This is getting very uncomfortable for all parties
- The patient is clearly hypomanic
- I wonder if I can convince him to go into the hospital
- I must convince him to take medication
- I fear disaster looms but so far he is clearly too rational to be

hospitalized against his will and any assessment in the emergency room will readily reverse any involuntary hospitalization

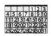

Case Outcome: Eighth Interim Followup, Weeks 64 Through 68, Continued

- Getting further history from the wife on this visit makes the situation go from bad to worse
- Wife says "tell him about the trip to Switzerland"
  - Patient states that it is not relevant
  - Wife claims the patient has now run up $85,000 of credit card debt
  - Charged $8000 of this for first class tickets to Zurich because he told her they need to go there "to open a lockbox there because this is where Jews put their money to avoid Naziism"
  - Patient admits to buying the tickets and laughs at the lockbox statement, denying ever saying it
  - Offers to return the tickets and cancel the trip
- Seems irritable, hypomanic, refusing medications
- Not psychotic
- Patient still refuses to take the quetiapine samples or to fill the quetiapine prescription or the valproate prescription
- Given another prescription and samples of aripiprazole
- Strongly encouraged him to be hospitalized, and patient refuses, and does not yet reach the threshold for involuntary hospitalization
- States he will never come back to the attending psychiatrist if the psychiatrist keeps insisting on medications and hospitalization and he will get a lawyer to reverse any involuntary hospitalization attempted
- Asked wife whether we should try to call the police to come to the office to restrain him and hospitalize him, and it is clear that this is not agreed
- Wife and daughter do not want to make a scene and agree to one last attempt at outpatient medication management
- Patient informed that if he does not improve in the next few days, that he will either agree to voluntary hospitalization or the attending physician will have to resign from the case and send him to another psychiatrist
- Patient given the names and numbers of three other psychiatrists and the number and location of the psychiatric emergency room

Case Outcome: Ninth Interim Followup, Week 74

- Misses next appointment, comes in 6 weeks later
- Seems contrite, says he has looked over his behavior the past 4 months and believes he did become irritable and hypomanic
- Now, however, he is worried about his finances, going back to work, and the future
- Admits he is not "over" his illness

- Wife observes that he has become placid and quiet and agrees he needs to get a job
- Seems less irritable, more tired and now depressed
- Suggested we add the aripiprazole he has refused to take to date
- Patient agrees and aripiprazole 5 mg prescribed along with continuation of zolpidem for sleep
- However, he has not followed through on taking medications other than zolpidem for months, so not clear what action he will take

What is Going On Here?

- He finally has some insight into the fact that he has become hypomanic
- Since he seems to be getting better without mood stabilizers or atypical antipsychotics means he was never hypomanic in the first place
- He is switching from hypomanic to depressed
- Other

Case Outcome: Tenth Interim Followup, Week 76

- 2 weeks later, too agitated by aripiprazole so stopped it
- Seems more depressed, irritable and possibly mixed but not pure hypomania
- Very anxious, depressed, now problems concentrating
- Agrees to take olanzapine 2.5 mg and to start lamotrigine
- Olanzapine to be increased to 5.0 mg then to 10 mg if necessary over the next several days to relieve symptoms

Case Outcome: Eleventh Interim Followup, Week 78

- 2 weeks later, bouts of crying, depression
- Fighting with wife about finances
- Olanzapine seems to help his irritability, his anxiety and his desperation, but still quite desperate and depressed
- Now gaining weight on Zyprexa but beginning to respond to it
- Increase olanzapine to 20 mg
- Continue lamotrigine and zolpidem
- Restrict calories

Case Outcome: Twelth Interim Followup, Week 80

- "Miserable"
- Taking olanzapine 15 mg at night and takes another 5 mg in the morning and then 5 mg in the afternoon because very anxious and agitated, total of 25 mg/day
- Agree to increase dose to 30 mg olanzapine

What is happening now?

- Remorse from bad financial decisions
- Continuing marital conflict
- Switch to bipolar depressive episode
- Switch to bipolar mixed episode
- Other

Case Outcome: Thirteenth Interim Followup, Week 84

- "Worst 3 months of my life"
- No longer depressed
- Looking to buy cars again
- Did buy a rifle
- Agrees not to pick it up
- Denies suicidality or plan but is has lost his credibility in terms of his lack of insight and being honest and forthright in reporting his symptoms
- Wife says he screams lately
- Mood on this visit actually seems a bit high
- Agrees to surrender his credit cards to his wife and to cancel sale of gun
- Has gained 20 pounds
- Impression is that the patient first became hypomanic off valproate, then without treatment spontaneously cycled into a depressed state, now cycling into hypomania again with lots of mixed symptoms over the past several weeks
- "I will take anything but valproate again"

How would you treat him?

- Continue his olanzapine, lamotrigine and zolpidem
- Stop one or more of these
- Switch to another antipsychotic
- Increase his olanzapine
- Add fluoxetine
- Add benzodiazepine
- Other

Case Outcome: Fourteenth and Subsequent Interim Followup, Weeks 88 to 104

- Patient subsequently cycled down into depression with waxing and waning mixed states for the next few months
- Eventually stabilized on:
  - Olanzapine 30 mg
  - Fluoxetine 20 mg
  - Lamotrigine 200 mg

– Clonazepam 1 mg twice a day and 1 mg as needed for anxiety/
      agitation/hypomania
    – Zolpidem 20 mg at night

Case Debrief

- It is an exhausting ride just reading this case
- In retrospect, he has some form of bipolar disorder, probably bipolar II disorder, with periods of euphoric hypomania, irritable hypomania, depression and mixed depression/irritable hypomanic
- In retrospect, it was not worth the risk of discontinuing his medications
- Brings up the issue of whether all cases of antidepressant-induced mania require lifetime mood stabilizers
- Once a bipolar, always a bipolar, even if substance-induced mood disorder?

Take-Home Points

- Bipolar disorder can be devastating when not stable and this risk must be seriously weighed against the risk of side effects of mood stabilizers, including sedation, weight gain, diabetes, cardiovascular events and potentially premature death
- The benefits of stable mood usually will outweigh not only the risks of mood stabilizing/atypical antipsychotic medication, but also the risks of the natural history of the untreated disorder since this illness when out of control recently has caused this patient and his family much suffering and financial hardship that lasted over a year after having been stabilized for more than 7 years on treatment
- These risk benefit calculations must be made on a case by case basis and repeated over time for each individual case
- Substance-induced mood disorder may be more appropriately reserved for patients taking drugs of abuse than for patients taking antidepressants, and antidepressant-induced mania/hypomania may need to be considered a form of bipolar disorder and treated as such until proven otherwise
- Using antidepressants in bipolar disorder remains controversial, and guidelines for treating antidepressant-induced mania in patients with no prior spontaneous mania, especially duration of treatment, remain unclear
- It is now a "no brainer" that mood stabilizers cannot be stopped again in this patient, a lesson learned

Performance in Practice: Confessions of a Psychopharmacologist

- What could have been done better here?
  - One wonders whether the attending psychiatrist should have agreed to supervise a trial off valproate in this patient with substance-induced mood disorder
  - One wonders whether a forced hospitalization at the risk of compromising therapeutic alliance would have prevented some of the complications and shortened the period of hypomania
  - Should the need for very high doses of hypnotics for insomnia have been a clue that the patient may have had some residual subsyndromal hypomania, even when mood was apparently stable following valproate and bupropion withdrawal?
- Possible action item for improvement in practice
  - Try harder to convince patients with just a substance-induced mood disorder not to attempt a trial of medication discontinuation
  - Get better history, because it seems possible that in retrospect there could have been some missed symptoms of bipolar disorder that could have predated his substance-induced mood disorder and hospitalization and could have tipped the balance in favor of not stopping mood stabilizers
  - It is also possible that the patient with unacceptable side effects can be convinced to try different mood stabilizers/atypical antipsychotics rather than just stop them

Tips and Pearls

- When mood stabilizers are discontinued, perhaps especially lithium, they need to be tapered very slowly
- Treatment criteria for substance induced mood disorder, especially for long term treatment, are not clear

Two-Minute Tute: A brief lesson and psychopharmacology tutorial (tute) with relevant background material for this case – Issues and Questions in Managing Bipolar Disorder

- Despite DSM IV, is Substance-Induced Mood Disorder a form of bipolar disorder that should be treated as such?
  - Do patients who get manic on drugs such as antidepressants or stimulants have a predisposition for mania?
  - Is drug induced mania actually a form of mania requiring life long treatment?
- Diagnostic criteria require that the patient experiences an elevated, expansive or irritable mood in which evidence from the history, physical exam and lab findings reflects that the mood disturbance

developed during or within a month of substance intoxication/
withdrawal
- Is use of an antidepressant "intoxication"?
- Medication use is etiologically related to the mood disturbance

Posttest Self Assessment Question: Answer

*Precipitous discontinuation of mood stabilizers has been reported
to induce manic relapse, so discontinuation of mood stabilizer when
indicated should be tapered over several months.*

A. True
B. False

Answer: A

References

1. Stahl SM, Mood Disorders, in Stahl's Essential
   Psychopharmacology, 3rd edition, Cambridge University Press, New
   York, 2008, pp 453–510
2. Stahl SM, Antidepressants, in Stahl's Essential
   Psychopharmacology, 3rd edition, Cambridge University Press, New
   York, 2008, pp 511–666
3. Stahl SM, Mood stabilizers, in Stahl's Essential
   Psychopharmacology, 3rd edition, Cambridge University Press, New
   York, 2008, pp 667–720
4. Stahl SM, Valproate, in Stahl's Essential Psychopharmacology The
   Prescriber's Guide, 3rd edition, Cambridge University Press, New
   York, 2009, pp 569–74
5. Stahl SM, Olanzapine, in Stahl's Essential Psychopharmacology The
   Prescriber's Guide, 3rd edition, Cambridge University Press, New
   York, 2009, pp 497–502
6. Stahl SM, Lamotrigine, in Stahl's Essential Psychopharmacology
   The Prescriber's Guide, 3rd edition, Cambridge University Press,
   New York, 2009, pp 259–66
7. Stahl SM, Zolpidem, in Stahl's Essential Psychopharmacology The
   Prescriber's Guide, 3rd edition, Cambridge University Press, New
   York, 2009, pp 595–8

The Case: Suck it up, soldier and quit whining

The Question: What is wrong with a soldier returning from his deployment in Afghanistan?

The Dilemma: Is it traumatic brain injury, PTSD or post-concussive syndrome, and how do you treat him?

Pretest Self Assessment Question (answer at the end of the case)

Which symptom(s) below distinguish PTSD from persistent post concussive syndrome following a mild traumatic brain injury?

A. Problems with concentration/attention

B. Depression

C. Irritability/anger

D. Fatigue

E. Hyperarousal

F. Apathy

G. Emotional lability

H. None of the above

Patient Intake

- 27-year-old corporal
- Returns from Afghanistan after a Humvee accident in which he suffered a head injury
- Upon his return to the US one week later, experiences tremors and heart palpitations and feels that his surroundings are unreal

Psychiatric History

- Toward the end of his tour in Afghanistan, had a Humvee accident in which the vehicle flipped and he hit his head and lost consciousness momentarily
- Afterwards he was "stunned", upset but remembered the accident
- He denies that it frightened him in any way
- Upon return to the US he saw his primary care provider on the military base for his symptoms

Social and Personal History

- Has been in the army for 6 years
- Married 4 years, 2 young children
- One week ago finished his first 15-month deployment to Iraq
- Has been exposed to combat
- Smokes one to two packs of cigarettes per day
- No drinking or alcohol in Iraq
- Binge drinker on weekends at home in the US

Medical History

- None
- BP normal
- BMI normal
- Normal blood tests

Family History

- Father: alcohol abuse

Treatment History

- Given a few zolpidem for sleep and a few lorazepam for anxiety by a medic in the field before departing Iraq
- None since returning home last week

Attending Physician's Mental Notes: Initial Psychiatric Evaluation

- Because of complaints of tremors and heart palpitations and a sense of unreality, the army primary care provider back on base in the US thinks this is mostly a normal stress reaction and a soldier decompressing from a combat experience
- Suspects also that the soldier might also be having some panic attacks
- Prescribes duloxetine and told the patient that his symptoms are probably to be expected given the circumstances of decompressing from a war zone and that he doubts whether any damage was done by the head injury
- The patient is reassured that his symptoms are common in soldiers when they first come back from combat, and that he mostly just needs a few weeks of down time
- Also told that if he "sucks it up" he will get over it but if he complains and whines to others in his unit, he could lose respect

Case Outcome: First Interim Followup, Week 1

- Patient not improving
- Now tells the army primary care provider something that he did not mention last week
- The patient says he constantly hears a buzzing sound and has done so ever since the Humvee accident
- "It is like a swarm of bees are buzzing right into my ear"
- The patient also appears insensitive to external stimuli, doesn't react to sounds or voices
- He is also sweating constantly which he attributes to the fact that he feels extremely nauseated

- Fearing a psychotic event, but not wanting to put that in the patient's chart or to prescribe an antipsychotic, both of which could end the patient's military career, the primary care provider prescribes a high dose of lorazepam 1 or 2 mg three or four times a day
- The primary care provider tells the patient it is probably just a normal stress reaction that most soldiers get when they return home and that it will go away soon but if it gets worse, to go to the mental health clinic
- Meanwhile, an appointment is made for one week back in primary care
- The next day, however, the patient comes back exhibiting loss of balance, having to hold onto chairs while walking
- Also exhibits odd rapid eye movements
- Army primary care provider decides to admit the patient to the hospital on base for a medical evaluation
- Also checks blood alcohol level (which was zero)
- Primary care provider calls the patient's wife and asks about the patient's drinking but she says he is not drinking and is mostly just complaining about the buzzing in his ear and the increasing loss of balance, which got worse yesterday

Based on just what you have been told so far about this patient's history and recurrent episodes of depression, do you think is going on with him?

- Acute stress disorder
- Post traumatic stress disorder
- Panic disorder
- Psychotic reaction
- Mild traumatic brain injury
- Persistent Post Concussive Syndrome
- Reaction and side effects from benzodiazepines
- Drug abuse
- Other

Case Outcome: First Interim Followup, Week 1, Continued

- Psychiatry was not consulted in the hospital so that the patient would not think he was crazy and to keep mental health notes out of his medical records
- ENT(ear nose and throat specialist) was consulted who felt that there might have been some mild vestibular damage from the Humvee accident but that it would likely resolve
- ENT also tells the primary care manager that vestibular dysfunction may cause anxiety and thinks maybe the patient is freaking out from his vestibular symptoms and is developing panic attacks

- The patient is told that once his vestibular symptoms resolve, any mental health issues should also be resolved
- Meanwhile the patient continued his duloxetine 60 mg/day and lowered his lorazepam to 0.5 mg as needed

Case Debrief

- Lots of information is missing here
- Need more details of the patient's symptoms following the head injury
- Did he really lose consciousness or was he just dazed, confused or seeing stars (the latter appears more likely here since he remembered the accident)
- Was he really not frightened by the Humvee accident?
- Any delusions or hallucinations? (doubt that they are present)
- Is his lack of reaction to external events accompanied by a subjective sense of numbing, detachment or absence of emotional responsiveness and if so
  - Does he seem to be in a daze?
  - Does he experience depersonalization or derealization?
  - Does he have any dissociative amnesia for events in Iraq?
  - Nightmares?
  - Flashbacks?
- Is his problem with balance episodic, coming in attacks that might represent panic and is it accompanied by tremors and palpitations?
- Are his balance symptoms entirely due to the high dose lorazepam or were these symptoms present previously and worsened by lorazepam?
- Much more will be clear in a month, in which case persisting symptoms probably represent something more serious
- Hopefully, all symptoms resolved and if so, it is likely this soldier was sent back for another combat tour in Iraq but further followup is not available

Two-Minute Tute: A brief lesson and psychopharmacology tutorial (tute) with relevant background material for this case – Differential Diagnosis of PTSD, acute stress and traumatic brain injury

Table 1: What is an Acute Stress Disorder and How Does It Differ from PTSD?

- Anxiety, dissociative symptoms within a month after exposure to an extreme traumatic stressor
- Requires the same exposure to a traumatic event as required for the diagnosis of PTSD, namely:
  - The person experienced, witnessed or was confronted with an event or events that involved actual or threatened death or serious injury, or threat to the physical integrity of self or others, and the person's response was intense fear, helplessness or horror
- Has dissociative symptoms of numbing, reduced awareness of surrounds, derealization, depersonalization or dissociative amnesia
- Reexperiencing, avoidance and hyperarousal occurs and causes distress or impairment
- Lasts 2 days and a maximum of 4 weeks
- If it lasts longer, it is considered PTSD
- How common is acute stress disorder in returning combat troops?
- Is this a "normal" reaction to deployment in war?
- PTSD does seem to occur in 10–20% of combat troops
- Acute stress reactions that do not go on to become PTSD resolve within a month by definition

Table 2: What is TBI (Traumatic Brain Injury)?

- A physical or mechanical brain injury causing temporary or permanent impairment of brain function
- Can be open (foreign object penetrating the brain) or closed (blunt force, acceleration/deceleration)
- Mild TBI
- Alteration in level of consciousness or loss of consciousness lasting up to 30 minutes
- Normal CT and/or MRI scans
- Glasgow Coma Scale score of 13–15
- TBIs are the most frequent physical injury among personnel serving in the Iraq and Afghanistan wars, sometimes called the "signature wound" of these conflicts and are typically closed, resulting from explosion or blast injury

Table 3: Glasgow Coma Scale

Points	Eye Opening Response	Verbal Response	Motor Response
6			Obeys commands for movement
5		Oriented	Purposeful movement to painful stimulus
4	Spontaneous – open with blinking at baseline	Confused conversation, but able to answer questions	Withdraws in response to pain
3	To verbal stimuli, command, speech	Inappropriate words	Flexion in response to pain (decorticate posturing)
2	To pain only (not applied to face)	Incomprehensible speech	Extension response in response to pain (decerebrate posturing)
1	No response	No response	No response

Table 4: Can TBI and PTSD Co-occur?

- Controversy over whether it is possible for both PTSD and TBI to result from the same trauma
- Many soldiers would rather call their injury TBI than PTSD, one denoting heroic injury, and the other, weakness
- The "signature wound" of the Iraq/Afghanistan conflict may be PTSD rather than TBI, or maybe both
- How can you tell the difference between mild TBI and PTSD?
- How can they co occur if TBI generally involves amnesia of the traumatic injury while PTSD presumably requires recollection of the traumatic event?
- Large scale population studies suggest that TBI and PTSD can co-occur, with severe TBI actually protective against PTSD whereas mild TBI may increase risk for PTSD, perhaps because resulting cognitive deficits impair the ability to process emotional information related to the trauma

Table 5: What is PPCS (Persistent Post Concussive Syndrome?

- The majority of individuals who suffer a mild TBI (traumatic brain injury) experience acutely:
  - Disorientation
  - Confusion
  - Agitation
- Many also experience
  - Fatigue
  - Headaches
  - Dizziness
  - Sleep disturbances
  - Seizures
  - Irritability/anger
- Symptoms usually resolve over several days to weeks
- A significant minority may experience persistent symptoms that comprise PPCS
- All of the above symptoms plus additional cognitive impairments:
  - Memory
  - Attention
  - Concentration
  - Executive function
  - Plus additional emotional symptoms
  - Apathy
  - Emotional lability
  - Disinhibition

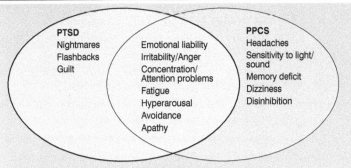

Figure 1: PPCS and PTSD: Symptom Overlap

Posttest Self Assessment Question: Answer

Which symptom(s) below distinguish PTSD from persistent post concussive syndrome (PPCS) following a mild traumatic brain injury (TBI)?

A. Problems with concentration/attention

B. Depression

C. Irritability/anger

D. Fatigue

E. Hyperarousal

F. Apathy

G. Emotional lability

H. None of the above

Answer: H – none of the above, meaning that any of the symptoms listed can by common to both PTSD and PPCS. Distinguishing symptoms that occur in PTSD but not PPCS include nightmares, flashbacks and guilt. Distinguishing symptoms that occur in PPCS but not PTSD include headaches, sensitivity to light and sound, memory deficit, dizziness and disinhibition.

References

1. Kaplan GB, Vasterling JJ, and Vedak PC. Brain-derived neurotrophic factor in traumatic brain injury, post-traumatic stress disorder and their comorbid conditions: role in pathogenesis and treatment. Behav Pharmacol 2010; 21(506): 427–37

2. Sayer NA, Rettmann NA, Carlson KF et al. Veterans with history of mild traumatic brain injury and posttraumatic stress disorder: challenges from provider perspective. J Rehabil Res Dev 2009; 46(6): 703–16

3. Vanderploeg RD, Belanger HG, and Curtiss G. Mild traumatic brain injury and posttraumatic stress disorder and their associations with health symptoms. Arch Phys Med Rehabil 2009; 90(7): 1084–93

4. Hill JJ 3rd, Mobo BH Jr, and Cullen MR. Separating deployment-related traumatic brain injury and posttraumatic stress disorder in veterans: preliminary findings from the Veterans Affairs traumatic brain injury screening program. Am J Phys Med Rehabil 2009; 88(8): 605–14

5. Pietrzak RH, Johnson DC, Goldstein MB et al. Posttraumatic stress disorder mediates the relationship between mild traumatic brain injury and health and psychosocial functioning in veterans of Operations Enduring Freedom and Iraqi Freedom. J Nerve Ment Dis 2009; 197(10): 748–53

6. Hoge CW, Wilk JE, and Herrell R. Methodological issues in mild traumatic brain injury research. Arch Phys Med Rehabil 2010; 91(6): 963

7. Hoge CW, McGurk D, Thomas JL et al. Mild traumatic brain injury in U.S. soldiers returning from Iraq. N Engl J Med 2008; 358(5): 453–63

8. Hoge CW, Goldberg HM, Castro CA, Care of war veterans with mild traumatic brain injury – flawed perspectives, New Eng J Med 2009 360: 1588–91

9. Stahl SM, Anxiety Disorders and Anxiolytics, in Stahl's Essential Psychopharmacology, 3rd edition, Cambridge University Press, New York, 2008, pp 721–72

10. Stahl SM, Duloxetine, in Stahl's Essential Psychopharmacology The Prescriber's Guide, 3rd edition, Cambridge University Press, New York, 2009, pp 165–70

11. Stahl SM, Lorazepam, in Stahl's Essential Psychopharmacology The Prescriber's Guide, 3rd edition, Cambridge University Press, New York, 2009, pp 295–9

12. Stahl SM, Stahl's Illustrated Anxiety, Stress and PTSD, Cambridge University Press, New York, 2010

The Case: The young man who is failing to launch

The Question: What is the underlying illness and when can you make a long term diagnosis?

The Dilemma: What can you do for a young adult on a tragic downhill course of social and cognitive decline?

Pretest Self Assessment Question (answer at the end of the case)

Individuals who ultimately develop schizophrenia typically exhibit what pattern of cognitive functioning prior to disorder onset?

A. Normal cognitive functioning during premorbid and prodromal phases
B. Impaired cognitive functioning that is stable across premorbid and prodromal phases
C. Impaired cognitive functioning premorbidly with further decline during the prodromal phase
D. Progressive decline of cognitive functioning across premorbid and prodromal phases

Patient Intake

- 21-year-old man who states he has no chief complaint but is here because his parents made him come
- The chief complaint of the parents is that their son is not transitioning successfully into independent adult life (i.e., failure to launch)

Early Psychiatric History: Childhood and Adolescence

- Obtained from the parents and from medical and school records
- The patient has been aloof and a loner with strange ideas and behaviors since childhood
- Somewhat rigid and obsessive; needs to follow a strict order when doing things
- Language development in grade school appeared normal, but had difficulty reading and was considered learning disabled by third grade
- Was considered to have possibly a form of ADHD and thus given methylphenidate (Ritalin) as a child without clear therapeutic effects
- Was then considered to have possibly a form of OCD and thus given trials of fluvoxamine (Luvox, Faverin) and venlafaxine (Effexor XR) as an adolescent to treat some obsessive compulsive tendencies but without clear therapeutic effects

Recent Psychiatric History

Late Adolescence and Early Adulthood

- After graduation from high school, went on a two year mission for his church
- On his mission, he was picked on, as his peers considered him slow and dumb
- Upon his return, his family immediately noted a dramatic change in function and behavior
- He seemed disorganized and confused, had strange behavioral changes and displayed noticeable deterioration in his handwriting, reading, and communicating including using simple language
- Did not complete sentences, had long delays in conversation in order to organize his thoughts, was not engaging in conversations, and let his conversations trail off
- There was a noticeable change in his voice quality and he had inappropriate facial grimaces
- He has been losing things, including pay checks; doesn't seem to know how to use an ATM (Automated Teller Machine at the bank) or fill out deposit slips
- Does not groom or change his clothes unless prompted by his mother
- Appears immature and childlike and seems to have difficulty understanding nuances and complex language, both written and spoken
- Some are wondering whether he had exposure to meningitis while on his mission, but no accurate diagnosis appears in his mission chart
- Patient was recently prescribed atomoxetine (Strattera) with no clear response

Social and Personal History

- Non smoker
- No past or current history of drug abuse, including alcohol and marijuana
- Few friends, no dating
- Has not attended college since graduating high school
- Has been living at home for a year since returning from his mission

Family History

- Father: history of learning disabilities, but is a successful small businessman now
- Sister: ADHD and learning disabilities
- Two maternal uncles: depression
- Paternal cousin: diagnosed with Landau Kleffner syndrome

(a rare disorder of childhood with aphasia and an abnormal EEG, sometimes confused with or misdiagnosed as autism, Aspberger's Syndrome, pervasive developmental disorder, hearing impairment, learning disability, auditory/verbal processing disorder, ADHD, mental retardation, childhood schizophrenia or emotional/behavioral problems)

Attending Physician's Mental Notes: Initial Psychiatric Evaluation

- This started out looking like a case of ADHD or some sort of minor learning disability, possibly morphing into OCD in adolescence, but then something horrible seems to have happened during his mission
- Does he have a condition related to what his cousin has (Landau Kleffner syndrome)?
- Although this could be a schizophrenic prodrome, could it also be an organic brain disorder from infection, chronic subdural hematoma, brain tumor, or seizure disorder?

Medical History

- Normal BMI, BP
- Routine blood tests normal
- Normal physical and neurological exams

Further Investigation:

Is there anything else you would like to know about this patient?
  – What about a detailed neurological evaluation and neuropsychological testing?
- Neurological Evaluation
  – Possible diagnosis of previous developmental learning difficulties in grade school
  – In retrospect, had a period of severe somnolence during a bad respiratory infection while on his mission, so considered the possiblility of a missed diagnosis of previous meningitis
  – MRI several months after this episode of somnolence and respiratory infection is negative except for a few non-specific bilateral frontal lobe white matter high-signal foci
  – EEG is within normal limits
- Neuropsychological Testing
  – Neuropsychological testing shows problems with executive functioning, organization, and suggestion of schizoid personality disorder or schizophrenia
  – Has a documented decline in IQ

Score in 9th grade:
- – Verbal IQ of 107
- – Performance IQ of 113
- – Full Scale IQ of 111

Score now:
- – Verbal IQ of 89
- – Performance IQ of 85
- – Full Scale IQ of 87

Patient Intake

- First time patient is seen, he is accompanied by his father and mother
- Patient is awkward, detached, aloof, and seems anxious and withdrawn
- He is able to relate tentatively to physician and to speak with a reserved and simple language processing style
- He is able to understand and relate to simple questions, but seems to get lost when the pace of the conversation between physician and parents accelerates and becomes more complex and subtle
- Second time patient is seen, he is accompanied by his mother only
- He is more socially engaged and relaxed, has better eye contact and shows humor
- At times, he is even poignant in his relationship with his mother: when she discusses his qualities of having empathy and tenderness his mother becomes tearful and the patient is able to connect with her in way that shows he is clearly able to track the nature of the conversation
- His memory appears to be intact
- Has good judgment
- Uses only simple language but is not bizarre and has no delusions or hallucinations
- There is evidence of slow cognition and executive dysfunction but no actual problems with short term memory
- Has some insights into his condition
- Wishes to have a job where he could work by himself, i.e., as a truck driver, and live in the mountains
- Is willing to go to school and live at home for a while, but would like to live independently

PATIENT FILE

Attending Physician's Mental Notes: Initial Psychiatric Evaluation

- It appears as though organic causes of this patient's symptoms have been ruled out
- However, prodromal symptoms of schizophrenia overlap with normal behaviors and also with behaviors of numerous other more benign psychiatric disorders and cannot be considered diagnostic: superstitiousness, irritability, distractibitiliy, anxiety, social withdrawal
- The parents want to know if there are genetic tests or biological markers yet available to help make the diagnosis of eventual schizophrenia or if they must simply wait for the next shoe to drop, namely a first break episode of psychosis

What would you do?

- Tell them that there are no genetic tests for schizophrenia
- Tell them that there is no way to prevent schizophrenia
- Refer them to an academic medical center for research
- Refer them to the internet

Case Outcome: First Interim Followup

- At this point, the family was informed that genetic or biological predictors of schizophrenia remain research tools, although many lines of evidence converge upon abnormalities of the NMDA (N-methyl-d-aspartate) glutamate receptor and glutamate synapses in schizophrenia
- A potential referral was discussed with the family to a schizophrenia genetics research center, for potential genotyping of affected and unaffected family members, particularly on the father's side, including the cousin with Landau Kleffner syndrome
- However, the family was cautioned that this information would not have immediate value in informing the family about the diagnosis of this patient, but might help future family members or others with similar symptoms
- Besides glutamate genes, the research center could evaluate genetic variants of both the dopamine metabolizing enzyme COMT (catechol-O-methyl transferase) and the L-methyl folate forming enzyme MTHFR (methylene tetrahydrofolate reductase), since variants of these enzymes interact to enhance the chances of cognitive dysfunction in schizophrenia
- However, these studies are "ahead of the curve" for clinical practice and would not be covered by insurance and it is not yet possible to use this strategy to predict the outcome of this patient, even though such a possibility may be introduced into clinical practice soon

From the information given, what do you think is his most likely diagnosis?
- Asperger's Syndrome
- Prodrome of schizophrenia
- Schizophrenia
- Schizoid personality disorder
- Severe form of social anxiety with underlying developmental delays

Attending Physician's Mental Notes: First Interim Followup

- Patient possibly meets diagnostic criteria for Asperger's Syndrome at the present time, although the disorder and its symptoms are not stable and continue to evolve:
  - Pervasive developmental disorder characterized predominantly by impairment in social interaction without profound delay in language
- Recent step off in his function may be categorized as prodrome of schizophrenia
  - Diagnosis of schizophrenia is not currently possible, but social oddities and cognitive disturbances, predominantly of an executive dysfunctioning, is quite typical of a schizophrenic prodrome
- Severe form of social anxiety superimposed upon developmental delays and/or schizoid personality may be considered but is less probable
- The patient is provisionally diagnosed as pervasive developmental disorder of the Asperger's type, but is monitored for the possible progression of further symptoms of schizophrenia
- No diagnosis of schizophrenia made at this point
- One new concept that could fit this patient is "ultra high risk for developing psychosis," as he meets the criteria of state and trait risk factors (i.e., has a first degree relative with a psychotic disorder plus he has experienced a significant decrease in functioning)
- Now the family wants to know if there is any treatment for their son, to reduce his symptoms or to prevent the onset of schizophrenia

What would you do?
- Tell the patient and his family that there is no approved treatment for the schizophrenia prodrome
- Tell them that there is no known treatment that can prevent progression of a prodrome to schizophrenia and that not all patients with a prodrome progress to schizophrenia anyway
- Tell them that treatments for schizophrenia have considerable expense and risks, including diabetes, weight gain, dyslipidemia, sedation, and tardive dyskinesia and that the risk:benefit calculation is in favor of observation without treatment

- Tell them that symptomatic treatments with anxiolytics, antidepressants, omega-3 fatty acids, or antipsychotics may be justified but are "off label" and unapproved

Attending Physician's Mental Notes: First Interim Followup, Continued

- No approved treatment for schizophrenia prodrome
- Many studies of atypical second generation antipsychotics, antidepressants, omega-3 fatty acids and anxiolytics in patients at high risk for developing psychosis have some encouraging results in reducing current symptoms but not necessarily delaying onset of first episode psychosis
- Should one err on the side of overtreatment or undertreatment?
- On balance, it was decided to treat the patient psychopharmacologically

Of the following choices, how would you treat this patient?
- Continue atomoxetine
- Stop atomoxetine and start an anxiolytic drug
- Stop atomoxetine and start an antidepressant
- Stop atomoxetine and start an atypical antipsychotic

Attending Physician's Mental Notes: First Interim Followup, Continued

- Discontinued atomoxetine
- A trial of an atypical antipsychotic may be indicated, at least to treat current symptoms, as some studies have shown symptomatic relief but not convincing prophylactic measures against progression to psychosis, nor improvement in current functional disability
  - Might be beneficial to help the patient interact socially and reduce his anxiety as well as improve cognitive functioning, although the latter is the least likely effect of antipsychotic treatment
  - In order to justify short term trials of antipsychotics, criteria will be established to determine whether continuing treatment is indicated
  - Specifically, over the next 6 months look to see if the following three items improve in order to define a positive outcome from medication treatment:
    - More flexibility
    - Less anxiety in social settings
    - More organizing skills
- Atypical antipsychotics may also be useful in treating certain symptoms associated with pervasive developmental disorder, but this is also an "off label" use of antipsychotics

- Started aripiprazole (Abilify) (can have less weight gain and sedation than some other choices, but actually not as well studied in the schizophrenia prodrome as other choices), dosed at 2.5 mg per day for 3–4 days, increasing then to 5 mg per day for several days to reach to a maximum of 10 mg per day
- The risks, benefits, and alternatives were explained to the patient and his parents and they consented to this treatment plan
- Patient is also advised to continue rehabilitative efforts:
  - Mathematics classes at a community college to supplement his training
  - Social skills settings to improve his interaction with peers

Case Outcome: Second and Subsequent Interim Followup, Over the Next 3 Months

- Minor improvements, no notable side effects
- Sertraline (Zoloft) added for social anxiety and apathy
- No dramatic changes, and no onset of psychosis (yet)

Case Debrief

- Asperger's syndrome or pervasive developmental disorder is a subset of the broader autism phenotype
- Many children, especially those with Asperger's syndrome, are initially misdiagnosed with ADHD
- Unlike Asperger's syndrome, schizoid personality disorder does not involve an impairment in non-verbal communication (i.e., lack of eye-contact) or a pattern of restricted interests or repetitive behaviors
- Prodrome refers to an early set of symptoms, and in schizophrenia has been characterized as the period of decreased functioning that precedes the onset of psychotic symptoms
- This patient did exhibit lack of non-verbal communication at one appointment but not at the second one; he may not fit neatly into the diagnostic criteria of any specific disorder which makes this case interesting
- Only the future will tell. . . .

Take-Home Points

- It is not possible to predict with great accuracy who will get schizophrenia, but certain symptoms such as social withdrawal and cognitive decline can identify teenagers and young adults at high risk
- Genetic and neuroimaging tests of high risk individuals seek to predict who will get schizophrenia, but these remain research tools
- To treat or not to treat: that is the question

- No drug is approved for the social withdrawal and cognitive decline in the schizophrenia prodrome, but numerous studies of antipsychotics, antidepressants, anxiolytics and omega 3 fatty acids suggest that some patients can attain symptomatic relief and may even delay the onset of first episode psychosis, but there is little evidence of disease modification by these medications such that schizophrenia can be prevented
- Nevertheless, it may be justified in some cases to treat symptomatically if risks are outweighed by the potential benefits, in recognizing that such use of these medications is not approved

Performance in Practice: Confessions of a Psychopharmacologist

- What could have been done better here?
  - Is false hope being raised by referral for genetic testing?
  - Is the possibility of an unproven therapeutic benefit short term justified by the costs and risks of psychotropic medications?
  - Is watchful waiting without treatment therapeutic nihilism or the correct approach?
- Possible action item for improvement in practice
  - Have available written materials for the patient and parents to read about genetic testing and prodromal treatment studies in schizophrenia
  - Utilize more aggressive approaches to psychotherapy and rehabilitation

Tips and Pearls

- Children with ever-changing psychiatric symptoms and diagnoses without robust treatment responses should be monitored carefully for progression of symptoms
- Clinicians must decide whether to err on the side of undertreatment (error of omission) or on the side of overtreatment (error of commission) since prodromal cases have unpredictable outcomes
- Genetic testing and biological markers are poised to enter clinical practice but are not understood well enough for routine clinical use
- Schizophenia, is well known for its positive symptoms of delusions and hallucinations, which in turn are proven to improve with antipsychotic medications; however it is actually a disease beginning with cognitive and negative symptoms, erupting into positive symptoms later, but with functional outcome more clearly linked to severity of cognitive and negative symptoms than to positive symptoms

Two-Minute Tute: A brief lesson and psychopharmacology tutorial (tute) with relevant background material for this case
– Clinical and genetic predictions of schizophrenia
– Genetic influences on cognition in schizophrenia

Table 1. Criteria for Ultra High Risk of Psychosis (One or More of the Following)

1. Attenuated psychotic symptoms, having experienced sub-threshhold attenuated psychotic symptoms during the past year
2. Brief limited intermittent psychotic symptoms, having experienced episodes of frank psychotic symptoms that have not lasted longer than a week and have been spontaneously abated
3. State and trait risk factors, having schizotypal personality disorder or a first-degree relative with a psychotic disorder and have experienced a significant decrease in functioning during the previous year

Table 2. Susceptibility Genes for Schizophrenia
Genes for

- Dysbindin (dystrobrevin binding protein1 or DTNBP1)
- Neuregulin (NRG1)
- DISC-1 (disrupted in schizophrenia 1)
- DAOA (d-amino acid oxidase activator;G27/G30)
- DAO (d-amino acid oxidase)
- RGS4 (regulator of G protein signaling 4)
- COMT (catechol-0-methyl transferase)
- CHRNA7 (alpha-7 nicotinic cholinergenic receptor)
- GAD1 (glutamic acid decarboxylase 1)
- GRM3 (mGluR3)
- PPP3CC

- PRODH2
- AKT1
- ERBB4
- FEZ1
- MUTED
- MRDS1 (OFCC1)
- BDNF (brain-derived neurotrophic factor)
- Nur77
- MAO-A (monoamine oxidase A)
- Spinophylin
- Calcyon
- Tyrosine hydroxylase
- Dopamine D2 receptor (D2R)
- Dopamine D3 receptor (D3R)

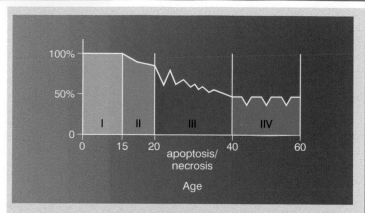

Figure 1: Clinical Course of Schizophrenia
The stage of schizophrenia are shown here over a lifetime. The progressive nature of schizophrenia supports a **neurodegenerative** basis for the disorder.

Stage I: The patient has full (100%) functioning early in life and is virtually asymptomatic.

Stage II: During a prodromal phase that starts in the teens, there may be odd behaviors and subtle negative symptoms.

Stage III: The acute phase of the illness usually announces itself fairly dramatically in the twenties with positive symptoms, remissions, and relapses. But the patient never quite returns to previous levels of functioning. This is often a chaotic stage of illness with a progressive downhill course.

Stage IV: The final phase of the illness may begin in the forties or later, with prominent negative and cognitive symptoms. Although there is some waxing and waning, this is often more of a "burnout" stage of continuing disability. The illness may not necessarily take a continual and relentless downhill course, but the patient may become progressively resistant to treatment with antipsychotic medications during this stage.

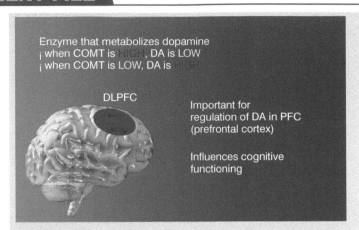

Figure 2: COMT
Genetic influence on circuits that regulate executive functioning can be
demonstrated by comparing functional neuroimaging date from individuals
with different variants of the catechol-O-methyl transferase (COMT)
gene while they are performing the n-back test. COMT is an enzyme that
metabolizes dopamine. Although COMT is active at all DA synapses, it is
most important for regulating DA levels in brain areas that are relatively
lacking in DA transporters, such as the PFC (prefrontal cortex).

Thus, when COMT activity is **high**, dopamine levels are **low**. Since
dopamine profoundly affects the information processing of pyramidal
neurons in the PFC, it also profoundly influences cognitive functioning.

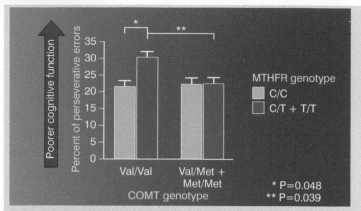

Figure 3: Interactive Effects of MTHFR (methylene-tetra-hydro-folate-reductase) and COMT (catechol-O-methyltransferase) on Executive Functioning in Schizophrenia

Roffman and colleagues (2008) investigated the interactive effects of MTHFR and COMT genetic polymorphisms on Wisconsin Card Sorting Task (WCST) performance in 185 outpatients with schizophrenia. This figure shows the differences in perseverative errors, a WCST measure consistently associated with schizophrenia. Individuals homozygous for the COMT Val allele (i.e., those with high COMT activity and low prefrontal dopamine) who also carried at least one copy of the MTHFR T allele (i.e., those with low formation of the methyl donor L-methylfolate and presumably less methylation of the COMT promoter with thus more synthesis of COMT and even lower prefrontal dopamine) exhibited a significantly higher percentage of perseverative errors than patients in the other genotype groups. Thus, these two genotypes interact, hypothetically at the level of dopamine in prefrontal cortex, to worsen cognitive functioning in those schizophrenic patients with these genetic variants. Prodromal patients with these same genotypes could theoretically be at greater risk for progressing to schizophrenia, but this is yet unproven.

Posttest Self Assessment Question: Answer

Individuals who ultimately develop schizophrenia typically exhibit what patter of cognitive functioning prior to disorder onset?

A. Normal cognitive functioning during premorbid and prodromal phases
B. Impaired cognitive functioning that is stable across premorbid and prodromal phases
C. Impaired cognitive functioning premorbidly with further decline during the prodromal phase
D. Progressive decline of cognitive functioning across premorbid and prodromal phases

Answer: C

References

1. Stahl SM, Psychosis and Schizophrenia, in Stahl's Essential Psychopharmacology, 3rd edition, Cambridge University Press, New York, 2008, pp 247–326
2. Stahl SM, Antipsychotic Agents, in Stahl's Essential Psychopharmacology, Cambridge University Press, New York, 2008, pp 327–452
3. Roffman JL, Weiss AP, Deckersback T et al. Interactive effects of COMT Val108/158Met and MTHFR C677T on executive function in schizophrenia. Am J Med Genetics part B (Neuropsychiatric Genetics) 2008; 147B: 990–5
4. Coyle JT, Glutamate and schizophrenia: beyond the dopamine hypothesis. Cellular and Mol Neurobiol 2006; 26: 365–84
5. Stahl SM, Methylated spirits: epigenetic hypotheses of psychiatric disorders. CNS Spectrums 2010; 15: 220–30
6. deKoning MB, Bloemen OJN, va Amelsvoort TAMH et al. Early intervention in patients at ultra high risk of psychosis: benefits and risks. Acta Psychiatrica Scand 2009; 119: 426–42
7. Stahl SM, Prophylactic antipsychotics: do they keep you from catching schizophrenia? J Clin Psychiat 2004; 65: 1445–6
8. McGorry PD, Nelson B, Amminger GP et al. Intervention in individuals at ultra high risk for psychosis: a review and future directions. J Clin Psychiatry 2009; 70: 1206–12
9. Cornblatt BA, Lencz T, Smith CW et al. Can antidepressants be used to treat the schizophrenia prodrome? Results of a prospective-naturalistic treatment study of adolescents. J Clin Psychiatry 2007; 68: 546–57
10. McGlashan TH, Zipursky RB, Perkins D et al. Randomized, double-blind trial of olanzapine versus placebo in patients prodromally symptomatic for psychosis. Am J Psychiatry 2006; 163: 790–9
11. Seidman LJ, Guiliano AJ, Meyer EC et al. Neuropsychology of the prodrome to psychosis in the NAPLS consortium. Arch Gen Psychiatr 2010; 67: 578–88
12. Lencz T, Smith CW, McLaughlin D et al. Generalized and specific neurocognitive deficits in prodromal schizophrenia. Biol Psychiatr 2006; 59: 863–71
13. Howes OK, Montgomery AJ, Asselin MC et al. Elevated striatal dopamine function linked to prodromal signs of schizophrenia. Arch Gen Psychiat 2009; 66: 13–20
14. Amminger GP, Shafer, MR, Papageorgiou K, et al. Long chain omega-3 fatty acids for indicated prevention of psychotic disorders. Arch Gen Psychiat 2010; 67: 146–54

The Case: The young cancer survivor with panic

The Question: Why is this patient resistant to medication treatments?

The Dilemma: How aggressive should psychopharmacological treatment be in terms of dosing and duration of drug treatment for panic?

Pretest Self Assessment Question (answer at the end of the case)

Which of the following is true regarding dosing of duloxetine (Cymbalta) for depression?

A. Efficacy is dose-dependent, with greater response typically seen above 60 mg/day

B. There is no evidence of increased efficacy above 60 mg/day, though some patients may benefit from it

C. The maximum dose is 60 mg/day due to a significant increase in side effects at higher doses

Patient Intake

- 30-year-old man with a chief complaint of anxiety and depression

Psychiatric History

- Onset of panic attacks was approximately nine years ago
- He has also suffered from moderate depression for several years
- He has been treated with every selective serotonin reuptake inhibitor (SSRI) and several different benzodiazepines without good response
- Some medications, specifically sertraline and paroxetine, seemed to worsen his sweating and fatigue
- He has never taken venlafaxine XR, desvenlafaxine, buspirone, or chlordiazepoxide
- Three years ago, he was diagnosed with non-Hodgkin's lymphoma, which complicated treatment of his anxiety disorder
- Specifically, there was confusion regarding the side effects of psychotropic medications, the recurrence of his tumor, and the side effects of chemotherapy, so anxiety treatment was suspended
- He is now in complete remission from his cancer and is assumed cured; he stopped chemotherapy two years ago
- His anxiety and depression, however, have continued unabated

Social and Personal History

- Single, never married, no children
- Non smoker
- No drug or alcohol abuse
- College educated
- Works in software but feels under employed

Medical History

- Status post non-Hodgkin's lymphoma, treated and presumably cured 2 years ago
- BP normal
- BMI normal
- Other lab tests normal

Family History

- Father: depression and panic disorder
- Paternal grandfather: committed suicide
- Aunt: anxiety disorder

Current medications

- Duloxetine 60 mg in the morning
- Clonazepam 2 mg in the morning

Patient Intake

- He has six to seven panic attacks a day, including some night panic
- His attacks are characterized by sweating and a "toxic feeling," and they make it difficult for him to interact with people
- He feels that duloxetine has helped his mood, but not his panic attacks, and that clonazepam has helped his daytime panic attacks
- However, he feels some resurgence of his depression in the evenings, and he continues to experience multiple panic attacks each day
- He is distressed and concerned about his symptoms, and he feels that they are preventing him from living a "normal life," having social relationships, and pursuing fulfilling employment

Considering this patient's partial response, which of the following medication adjustments would you most likely make?

- None, maintain his current medications
- Increase the doses of his current medications
- Switch duloxetine to a different antidepressant
- Switch clonazepam to a different anxiolytic
- Switch both duloxetine and clonazepam to a different treatment regimen

Attending Physician's Mental Notes, Initial Psychiatric Evaluation

- Although the patient continues to have several panic attacks a day, he has experienced some reduction in his anxiety since starting clonazepam

- Similarly, although he has residual depressive symptoms, he has experienced improvement while on duloxetine
- Considering his history of nonresponse with other medications, it may be more prudent to increase the dose of one or both medications than to switch

Which of the following dose adjustments would you most likely make for this patient?

- Increase duloxetine dose only
- Increase clonazepam dose only
- Increase duloxetine dose, then increase clonazepam dose
- Increase clonazepam dose, then increase duloxetine dose
- Increase duloxetine and clonazepam doses simultaneously

Attending Physician's Mental Notes: Initial Psychiatric Evaluation, Continued

- Although 60 mg/day is the usual dose for duloxetine when treating depression and anxiety, it is frequently prescribed at doses up to 120 mg/day
- Studies have not generally demonstrated increased efficacy beyond 60 mg/day; however, in relapse prevention studies in depression, a significant percentage of patients who relapsed on 60 mg/day responded and remitted when the dose was increased to 120 mg/day
- For clonazepam, the usual dose in panic disorder is 0.5 to 2 mg/day; the maximum recommended dose is 4 mg/day
- It is usually preferable to use the lowest possible effective dose of benzodiazepines because the risk of dependence may increase with higher doses
- Thus, the decision is made to increase the dose of duloxetine up to 120 mg/day
- Duloxetine is increased to 60 mg in the morning and 30 mg at night

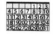

Case Outcome: First and Second Interim Followup, Weeks 2 and 4

- After two weeks, the patient reports no improvement; the dose is thus increased to 60 mg twice per day
- After another two weeks, he reports that his mood is improved and that on most days he does not feel increasing depressed as the evening approaches
- However, he has not experienced any reduction in his panic attacks, and he continues to be disabled by them
- Asked whether he would be willing to try cognitive behavioral

therapy for his panic attacks since they have been so resistant to medications, but he wants to try higher doses of clonazepam first
- Because the patient's panic has not improved adequately, the dose of clonazepam is increased by adding a 4 p.m. dose of 1 mg

Case Outcome: Third Interim Followup, Week 8
- The patient experiences partial improvement at this dose; the dose is thus increased to 2 mg twice per day

Case Outcome: Fourth Interim Followup, Week 12
- The patient experiences only one panic attack a week and thus is advised to continue clozazepam at 2 mg twice a day

Case Outcome: Fifth Interim Followup, Week 16
- The patient experiences only one panic attack a week and thus is advised to continue clozazepam at 2 mg twice a day

How long would you continue this regimen, which includes high-dose benzodiazepine therapy?
- Until his symptoms are suppressed
- For one year following remission of his symptoms
- Indefinitely

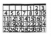

Attending Physician's Mental Notes: Fifth Interim Followup, 16 Weeks
- Although it is somewhat controversial to give a young person long-term, high-dose benzodiazepine therapy, there are unique considerations in this case that justify it
- First, the patient has just conquered cancer, but despite this triumph he is having serious residual disability from ongoing depression and anxiety
- Thus, the risk of creating additional dependence with benzodiazepine exposure may be trivial compared to the upside of helping him get his life back together now that he is healthy
- To maximize the chances of a successful outcome, it may be best to continue his treatment for one year after his symptoms are completely suppressed
- If successful, one could consider at that point a slow taper of some of his medication to see if he could be maintained in the long run with lower doses
- During the next year he will be encouraged to reconsider trying CBT since there is evidence that CBT may be more effective in keeping panic attacks In remission after stopping this therapy than after stopping benzodiazepine treatment

- If he wants to have symptom-free remission without medications, his best bet might be to try CBT
- Some argue that CBT is not as beneficial when giving benzodiazepines or when symptoms are in remission, so a good time to consider this is if he experiences breakthrough symptoms on his current medications, to initiate CBT rather than raise the dose of clonazepam further

Case Debrief

- This patient had prominent panic disorder with secondary depression, and was not very responsive to treatment with moderate doses of SSRIs, SNRIs or benzodiazepines and never had CBT
- After surviving a bout with non-Hodgkin's lymphoma, wanted to get life on track and become better controlled in terms of panic attacks
- Prudent, stepwise increase of duloxetine and clonazepam doses to the top of their therapeutic ranges but not in heroic doses was successful in suppressing most panic attacks and improving depression

Take-Home Points

- When using benzodiazepines to treat anxiety disorders, it is generally advisable to use the lowest possible effective dose for the shortest possible period of time (benzodiazepine sparing strategy) because the risk of dependence increases with dose and duration
- In particular, it is somewhat controversial to use long-term, high-dose benzodiazepine therapy
- Nonetheless, there may be some patients for whom such treatment is warranted

Performance in Practice: Confessions of a Psychopharmacologist

- What could have been done better here?
  - Higher doses of clonazepam would probably have been effective if given earlier, including during his convalescence from treatment for non-Hodgkin's lymphoma
  - CBT could have been effective if given earlier
- Possible action item for improvement in practice
  - Provide more written information about dosing of psychotropic drugs and about CBT for panic disorder to patients

Tips and Pearls

- Duloxetine is not specifically approved for treating panic disorder, but like other SSRIs and SNRIs, there are data suggesting that all agents in this class are effective not only for major depression and generalized anxiety disorder, but also for panic disorder and other anxiety disorders
- The duloxetine may have contributed to therapeutic actions in this patient's panic disorder, with a delayed onset of action

Two-Minute Tute: A brief lesson and psychopharmacology tutorial (tute) with relevant background material for this case – Benzodiazepines and panic

Table 1: Benzodiazepines in Panic Disorder

- Alprazolam and clonazepam best studied
- Rapid onset of action
- Can be used short term to boost efficacy of SSRIs/SNRIs, and also to block some of the anxiogenic actions of SSRIs/SNRIs, and then often can be tapered without loss of efficacy a few months later
- Alprazolam dosing in panic is 0.5 mg three or four times a day and can be increased 1 mg/day until a maximum dose of 10 mg is reached
- Alprazolam is dosed about twice that of clonazepam
- Thus, clonazepam dose is 0.5 mg twice a day, increasing by 0.5 mg per day until a maximum usually of 4–5 mg/day for panic
- Treatment for over 4 months may require slow taper to avoid withdrawal effects
- Generally benzodiazepines should not be given to substance abusers or to those who continually escalate their dose without supervision

Posttest Self Assessment Question: Answer

Which of the following is true regarding dosing of duloxetine for depression?

A. Efficacy is dose-dependent, with greater response typically seen above 60 mg/day
B. There is no evidence of increased efficacy above 60 mg/day, though some patients may benefit from it
C. The maximum dose is 60 mg/day due to a significant increase in side effects at higher doses

Answer: B

References

1. Nardi AE and Perna G. Clonazepam in the treatment of psychiatric disorders: an update. Int Clin Psychopharmacol 2006; 21(3): 131–42
2. Rosenbaum JF. The development of clonazepam ass a psychotropic: the Massachusetts General Hospital Experience. J Clin Psychiatry 2004; 65(suppl5): 3–6
3. Rosenblaum JF, Moroz G, and Bowden CL. Clonazepam in the treatment of panic disorder with or without agoraphobia: a dose-response study of efficacy, safety, and discontinuance. Clonazepam Panic Disorder Dose-Response Study Group. J Clin Psychopharmacol 1997; 17(5): 390–400
4. Susman J and Klee B. The role of high-potency benzodiazepines in the treatment of panic diosorder. Prim Care Companion J Clin Psychiatry 2005; 7(1): 5–11
5. Pollack MH, Otto MW, Tesar GE et al. Long-term outcome after acute treatment with alprazolam or clonazepam for panic disorder. J Clin Psychopharmacol 1993; 13(4): 257–63
6. Stahl SM, Mood Disorders, in Stahl's Essential Psychopharmacology, 3rd edition, Cambridge University Press, New York, 2008, pp 453–510
7. Stahl SM, Antidepressants, in Stahl's Essential Psychopharmacology, 3rd edition, Cambridge University Press, New York, 2008, pp 511–666
8. Stahl SM, Anxiety Disorders and Anxiolytics, in Stahl's Essential Psychopharmacology, 3rd edition, Cambridge University Press, New York, 2008, pp 721–72
9. Stahl SM, Stahl's Illustrated Anxiety, Stress and PTSD, Cambridge University Press, New York, 2010
10. Stahl SM, clonazepam, in Stahl's Essential Psychopharmacology The Prescriber's Guide, 3rd edition, Cambridge University Press, New York, 2009, pp 97–101
11. Stahl SM, duloxetine, in Stahl's Essential Psychopharmacology The Prescriber's Guide, 3rd edition, Cambridge University Press, New York, 2009, pp 165–70

The Case: The man whose antipsychotic almost killed him

The Question: How closely should you monitor atypical antipsychotic augmentation in a Type 2 diabetic with treatment resistant depression?

The Dilemma: Can you rechallenge a patient with an atypical antipsychotic for his highly resistant depression when he developed hyperglycemic hyperosmotic syndrome on the medicine the last time he took it?

Pretest Self Assessment Question (answer at the end of the case)

The presence of diabetes is a contraindication to treatment with atypical antipsychotics, especially high risk agents such as olanzapine or clozapine

A. True
B. False

Patient Intake

- 56-year-old man
- Chief complaint of unremitting depression, unresponsive to treatments

Psychiatric History Prior to Diagnosis

- Although he has only been treated for the past 10 years, in retrospect, has always had mood fluctuations and other psychiatric comorbidities
- As a child, adolescent and young adult, always a loner, few friends, chronic low grade depression
- In teens and adulthood, always shy, inappropriate in social settings
- Developed first major depressive episode 10 years ago after retiring as a firefighter and losing his routine, and this also occurred shortly after his third divorce

Social and Personal History

- Alcohol helped his social discomfort, so abused it until 1 year ago
- Joined AA (Alcoholics Anonymous) and has been sober since
- Abused LSD several years ago
- Abused marijuana until one year ago, now only uses occasionally
- Has used crack cocaine for a six month period of time approximately two years ago
- "Made me feel great" and in fact possibly induced mania transiently
- Married 3 times; 2 children from first marriage, one from the second, none from the third
- Non smoker
- Some college now retired after a long career as firefighter

Family History

- Mother: alcoholic
- No first degree relatives with depression or bipolar disorder known

Medical History

- Thin, normal BP
- Type II diabetes, good control on oral hypoglycemics

Medications One Year Following the First Episode of Depression

- Glucotrol
- Glucophage
- Levothyroxine
- Prilosec
- Lithium
- Clomipramine

Psychiatric History

Treatment of Mood Disorder, Past 10 years

- Treated with SSRIs, venlafaxine, then hospitalized and received ECT
- Transient improvement on ECT, relapsed on venlafaxine, tricyclic antidepressants
- Rehospitalized, received ECT again, transient response again
- Relapsed again despite treatment with MAO inhibitor phenelzene, and then augmentation of SSRIs with bupropion, lithium, valproate, lamotrigine, mirtazapine, stimulants, modafinil, then trials of protriptyline, and clomipramine plus lithium, all without effect

Patient Intake

- The patient was soft spoken, withdrawn, flat, monotone affect
- Rates himself as 9 out of 10 on a 10 point scale of severity (10 worst)
- Clearly suicidal; has thoughts of taking a garden hose and duct tapking it to his car exhaust to kill himself with carbon monoxide
- States he does not do it because he still has some hope that he might get better and is also concerned that he does not want to hurt his children
- Agrees to no harm verbally and wishes to try several treatment options and does not want to be hospitalized at the present time
- Patient does not want ECT again as it causes memory problems

Attending Physician's Mental Notes: Initial Psychiatric Evaluation

- The patient clearly has had long standing social anxiety disorder with superimposed drug and alcohol abuse, the latter recently in remission

- He has a recurrent depressive disorder, but unclear whether any of his hypomania was spontaneous or only cocaine-induced
- Clearly is treatment-resistant
- Has not tried an atypical antipsychotic

Based on just what you have been told so far about this patient's history and recurrent episodes of depression, how would you treat him?

- Refer for another neurostimulation treatment (VNS, TMS, DBS)
- Treat with an atypical antipsychotic
- Check therapeutic blood levels of his antidepressants to see if nonabsorption/rapid metabolism
- Other

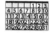

Case Outcome: First and Second Interim Followup, Weeks 1–4

- The patient was given olanzapine 5 mg added to his regimen of lithium and clomipramine
- He had an almost immediate response within about 3 days
- Doing much better with renewed interest in life, resolution of suicidal thoughts and increased energy levels
- Bought a puppy
- No hypomania
- About a month later, lost much of the effect, and increased olanzapine to 7.5 mg, and responded again, relapsed again in another month, increased olanzapine to 10 mg and responded again
- However, got a call from the emergency room, patient presented with dehydration, confusion, obtundation and fever, with blood glucose over 600 but no ketosis or acidosis
- Was diagnosed as HHS (hyperglycemic hyperosmotic syndrome), treated briefly with insulin and discharged off olanzapine

What do you think?

- In retrospect, should olanzapine not have been given to this patient?
- If given, should olanzapine treatment have been closely monitored with frequent blood glucose measurements?
- Should diabetics avoid atypical antipsychotics?
- Should a different atypical antipsychotic have been given?

Attending Physician's Mental Notes: First and Second Interim Followup, Weeks 1 and 4

- The patient, a known type II diabetic, developed a complication of atypical antipsychotic use
- At the time of this evaluation, olanzapine had just been reported to be effective in treatment-resistant depression by the attending

physician and colleagues, and there were no warnings yet about the risk for sudden DKA (diabetic ketoacidosis) or HHS (hyperglycemic hyperosmotic syndrome) in the literature or in FDA labels

- The patient had stable glucose measurements for years, well controlled on oral hypoglycemics, the patient's internist was aware of the treatment with olanzapine, but there was no specific monitoring of blood glucose levels in this patient following administration of olanzapine
- The standard has now evolved so that warnings about acute and chronic complications of atypical antipsychotics should be given, and those risks weighed against the potential benefits of treatment
- Also, some antipsychotics like olanzapine are considered higher risk for metabolic complications than other antipsychotics like ziprasidone or aripiprazole, but all agents have a class warning about metabolic complications

Case Outcome: Third Interim Followup

- As might be expected, discontinuation of the olanzapine led to relapse and recurrence of suicidal ideation
- Now the patient feels desperate and without options
- Referred for VNS which was available at the time (TMS not available then)
- Received VNS and had an excellent response to it
- Even experienced some hypomania on it
- Because of some nausea during stimulation, the patient's VNS stimulator was turned off for a while, and the patient relapsed, then responded again when stimulation began again
- After about a year, the VNS was no longer effective and the patient fell back into a deep depression
- Augmentation with quetiapine, aripiprazole and ziprasidone all ineffective once the VNS no longer worked
- Felt forced to undergo ECT again, and this third set of treatments worked transiently, and fell back into deep depression despite maintenance ECT

Would you rechallenge this patient with olanzapine or prescribe a trial of clozapine?

- Yes
- No

Case Outcome: Third Interim Followup, Continued

- The patient was advised of the risks and benefits of another trial of olanzapine, and with the input of his internist and close metabolic monitoring, olanzapine was given again
- The patient responded again but without any metabolic complications this time
- However, the response was not sustained despite augmentation with lithium and the patient yet again relapsed into deep depression with recurrent suicidal ideation
- The patient has not had therapeutic drug monitoring, or genetic testing
- Considering now DBS and, despite the possible metabolic risks, clozapine
- The case goes on. . . .

Case Debrief

- Despite life threatening complications from olanzapine, the patient was given a second olanzapine trial because the risks of his depression were thought to outweigh even the risks of olanzapine to him
- Now, he may even be a candidate for clozapine, perhaps the antipsychotic with the greatest metabolic risk, even though the patient is a diabetic and has experienced HHS on olanzapine
- Therapeutic decisions in cases like this can be quite difficult but risks can be justified if taken prudently to attempt to save the life of a patient like this

Two-Minute Tute: A brief lesson and psychopharmacology tutorial (tute) with relevant background material for this case – Hyperglycemic hyperosmotic syndrome

Table 1: Hyperglycemic Hyperosmotic Syndrome (HHS) Warning Signs and Symptoms to Know and to Tell the Patient

- Dry, parched mouth
- Extreme thirst (although this may gradually disappear)
- Warm, dry skin that does not sweat
- High fever (over 101 degrees Fahrenheit, for example)
- Sleepiness or confusion
- Loss of vision, speech impairment
- Hallucinations (seeing or hearing things that are not there)
- Weakness on one side of the body
- Blood sugar level over 600 mg/dl
- Coma
- Convulsions
- Nausea
- Weight loss
- Increased heart rate with low blood pressure
- Increased serum osmolality
- High BUN (Blood Urea Nitrogen) and creatinine
- Only mild or absent ketosis
- Get to a doctor or emergency room
- Rehydration with fluids
- Potassium
- Insulin
- Death rate may be as high as 40%
- Circulatory collapse (shock)
- Stroke
- Cerebral edema
- Differs from diabetic ketoacidosis which Is the combination of hyperglycemia with both ketosis and acidosis, absent from HHS
- DKA (Diabetic Ketoacidosis) even more dangerous and life threatening than HHS
- HHS is much more common than DKA in type II diabetes

Posttest Self Assessment Question: Answer

The presence of diabetes is a contraindication to treatment with atypical antipsychotics, especially high risk agents such as olanzapine or clozapine

A. True

B. False

Answer: B

Although closer monitoring would be necessary if a patient has diabetes, it is not a contraindication to give a diabetic patient an atypical antipsychotic. There are far too many patients with diabetes to exclude them from antipsychotic treatment, and no antipsychotic is without risk. The point is to calculate a risk: benefit ratio for an individual patient, inform them, monitor them and get their consent. Taking risks can yield therapeutic rewards, but does not always turn out well.

References

1. Stahl SM, Mood Disorders, in Stahl's Essential Psychopharmacology, 3rd edition, Cambridge University Press, New York, 2008, pp 453–510
2. Stahl SM, Antidepressants, in Stahl's Essential Psychopharmacology, 3rd edition, Cambridge University Press, New York, 2008, pp 511–666
3. Stahl SM, Mood Stabilizers, in Stahl's Essential Psychopharmacology, 3rd edition, Cambridge University Press, New York, 2008, pp 667–720
4. Stahl SM, olanzapine, in Stahl's Essential Psychopharmacology The Prescriber's Guide, 3rd edition, Cambridge University Press, New York, 2009, pp 387–92
5. Shelton RC, Tollefson GD, Tohen M et al. A novel augmentation strategy for treatment-resistant major depression. Am J Psychiatry 2001; 158: 131–4
6. Marangell LB, Martinez M, Jurdi RA et al. Neurostimulation therapies. Acta Psychiatrica Scandinavica 2007; 116: 174–81
7. Henderson DC, Cagliero E, Copeland PM et al. Elevated hemoglobin A1c as a possible indicator of diabetes mellitus and diabetic ketoacidosis in schizophrenia patients receiving atypical antipsychotics. J Clin Psychiatry 2007; 68; 533–41
8. Jin H, Meyer JM, Jeste DV. Phenomenology of and risk factors for new-onset diabetes mellitus and diabetic ketoacidosis associated with atypical antipsychotics: an analysis of 45 published cases. Ann Clin Psychiatry 2002; 14: 59–64

9. Gouni-Berthold I, Krone W. Diabetic ketoacidosis and hyperosmolar hyperglycemic state. Med Klin (Munich) 2006; 101(Suppl 1): 100–5

10. Johnson DE, Yamazaki H, Ward KM et al. Inhibitory effects of antipsychotics on carbachol-enhanced insulin secretion from perifused rat islets: role of muscarinic antagonism in antipsychotic-induced diabetes and hyperglycemia. Diabetes 2005; 54: 1552–8

11. Jindal RD, Keshavan MS. Critical role of M3 muscarinic receptor in insulin secretion: Implications for psychopharmacology. J Clin Psychopharmacol 2006; 26(5): 449–50

12. Gautam D, Han SJ, Hamdan FF et al. A critical role for beta cell M3 muscarinic acetylcholine receptors in regulating insulin release and blood glucose homeostasis in vivo. Cell Metab 2006; 3: 449–61

13. Gautam D, Han SJ, Duttaroy A et al. Role of M3 muscarinic acetylcholine receptor in beta-cell function and glucose homeostasis. Diabetes Obes Metab 2007; 9(Suppl 2): 158–62

14. Houseknecht KL, Robertson AS, Zavadoski W et al. Acute effects of atypical antipsychotics on whole-body insulin resistance in rats: implications for adverse metabolic effects. Neuropsychopharmacology 2007; 32: 289–97

15. Vestri HS, Maianu L, Moellering DR et al. Atypical antipsychotic drugs directly impair insulin action in adipocytes: effects on glucose transport, lipogenesis, and antilipolysis. Neuropsychopharmacology 2007; 32: 765–72

16. Stahl SM, Mignon L and Meyer JM. What comes first: atypical antipsychotics or the metabolic syndrome? Acta Psychiatrica Scand 2209; 119: 171–9

17. Meyer JM and Stahl SM. The metabolic syndrome and schizophrenia. Acta Psychiatrica Scand 2009; 119: 4–14

The Case: The painful man who soaked up his opiates like a sponge

The Question: What do you do for a complex chronic pain patient whose symptoms progress despite treatment?

The Dilemma: How far can medications go to treat chronic pain?

Pretest Self Assessment Question (answer at the end of the case)

Various theories propose which of the following as hypothetical causes of chronic pain?

A. Nerve damage
B. Central sensitization of brain and spinal cord pain circuits
C. Psychological factors
D. A plea for help and attention and a desire to be cared for
E. Somatic expression of psychological conflict

Patient Intake

- 58-year-old man with a history of chronic pain
- Referred to you by his primary care physician who also specializes in chronic pain, for new ideas regarding psychopharmacologic pain management for this patient

Psychiatric and Pain History

- Relatively well until 6 years ago when he developed painful tinnitus in his right ear
- ENT (ear nose and throat) evaluation did not reveal any diagnosable problem
- The patient found that hydrocodone worked for approximately three to four years at 15 mg per day and then required 30 mg per day until last year at which time that dose stopped working
- For the past several years has been diagnosed as having Dercum's Disease (adiposis dolorosa, multiple painful subcutaneous lipomas) and since then has had over 50 lipomas surgically resected from areas all over his body, particularly his trunk
- About a year ago also began having difficulties with pain in his lower legs and had to increase his opiate use to 60 to 80 mg/day of hydrocodone.
- The patient states that the pain in his lower legs is "hard to explain" and feels as though someone is "pumping them up with fluid"
- In the past 4 to 5 months he has now developed low back pain
- Orthopedic evaluations suggest that he has degenerative disc disease and may at some point require back surgery
- In an attempt to avoid this, the patient has escalated his opiate use

to 80 to 120 mg of hydrocodone per day and has also had epidural blocks

- The epidural blocks were helpful for his low back pain for a short period of time but actually, if anything, made the pain in his legs worse
- The hydrocodone is now sedating and interferes with his ability to concentrate and makes him too sedated to do creative or consulting work during the day; however, if he lowers the dose of hydrocodone below 80 mg/day, he is in too much pain to work anyway
- His pain is distressing to him and interferes with his ability to function as a self employed entrepreneur, inventor and consultant, but does not really make him feel sad, hopeless, apathetic, loss of interest, or in the midst of a major depressive episode now or in the past
- Over the past few years has had an extensive history of psychotropic drug utilization and has had numerous agents which caused unusual or difficult side effects
  - Numerous TCAs not tolerated (urinary retention, constipation, sedation) and did not work on his pain
  - Gabapentin, far too sedating but also seemed to cause a withdrawal reaction with increased tinnitus, paresthesias and gastrointestinal pain when he stopped it
  - Numerous SSRIs not effective, caused burning sensation in upper and lower distal extremities
  - Quetiapine very sedating even at low doses
- A few years back when he was living in another city, a US physician prescribed low dose sulpiride for him for an unknown reason which he had shipped to him from France and which helped his pain
- When the patient ran out of medication and moved, he stopped the sulpiride

Social and Personal History

- Married 9 years
- One daughter 8 years old
- Non smoker
- No illicit drug or alcohol abuse
- Graduate of an elite engineering school
- Successful patent holder and entrepreneur until 2 years ago when he could no longer work full time, but only consult and not invent

Medical History

- Hypercholesterolemia
- BMI 29
- Obstructive sleep apnea

- Dercum's disease
- Sinus surgery several years ago

Family History

- Father: chronic pain and anxiety

Current Medications

- Synthroid 75 mcg
- Duloxetine (Cymbalta) 60 mg
- Atomoxetine (Strattera) 40 mg
- Hydrocodone up to 120 mg/day
- Zolpidem 10 mg for sleep
- Zetia for hypercholesterolemia
- Uses CPAP (continuous positive airway pressure) machine most nights for obstructive sleep apnea

Based on just what you have been told so far about this patient's history and various pain conditions, what do you think is his diagnosis?

- Pain secondary to Dercum's Disease plus degenerative lumbar disc disease
- Pain Disorder, somatoform
- Somatization disorder
- Depression
- Fibromyalgia
- Other

Attending Physician's Mental Notes, Initial Psychiatric Evaluation

- There are no obvious psychosocial stressors that come out of his history on the initial evaluation, but it is difficult to assess psychological factors on only one visit
- His multiple and vague pain complaints involving many parts of his body without an obvious medical explanation seem excessive
  - Painful tinnitus
  - Painful lumps all over his body
  - Painful lower legs
  - Painful lower back
- Dercum's Disease is a rare and controversial condition and many people have lipomas that are not painful
- It seems possible that his "pain all over" is fibromyalgia instead but his referring physician is not clear about that
- Orthopedic reports do not suggest that degenerative disc disease is very severe or advanced nor that it will imminently need surgery

- The patient is escalating his opiate use in a somewhat concerning matter
- It may be useful to explore psychological factors in followup visits and even to get personality testing
- For now, a working diagnosis could be one of the somatoform disorders, namely pain disorder, with pain in multiple anatomical sites of severity to warrant medical attention and which impair functioning
- There is as yet the unconfirmed suspicion that psychological factors may play an important role in the onset, severity, exacerbation or maintenance of the pain and this must be investigated further
- He does not appear to have somatization disorder because his complaints did not start before age 30, and he has only pain symptoms and not other somatic symptoms
- He does not seem excessively depressed

How would you treat him?

- Increase duloxetine dose
- Increase atomoxetine dose
- Suggest reduction in opiate dose, maybe switching to long acting formulations but lower total daily dose
- Referral to insight oriented psychotherapy
- Referral to biofeedback
- Referral to CBT
- Other

Attending Physician's Notes: Initial Psychiatric Evaluation, Continued

- Advised to increase duloxetine to 120 mg/day
- Suggested simultaneously discontinuing atomoxetine
- Suggested low dose pregabalin since it is less sedating than the gabapentin he did not tolerate previously
- If duloxetine and pregabalin are somewhat effective, advised to attempt to lower hydrocodone dose
- Consider mofafinil augmentation both for opiate induced impairment in concentration/sedation and sleepiness/executive dysfunction that may result from his obstructive sleep apnea

Case Outcome: First Interim Followup, Month 6

- Seen again in consultation 6 months later
- Patient sent back to inquire about use of sodium oxybate/gamma hydroxybutyrate (Xyrem) for his pain, but strongly advised against it while taking sedative hypnotics and opiates
- Has not reduced his total daily opiate dose, but now taking as a

sustained release oxycodone in the form of Oxycontin 40 mg three times a day!
- Patient feels he needs opiates for:
  - Painful tinnitus which continues
  - Pain all over, either from his Dercum's lipomas or fibromyalgia
  - Lumbosacral pain radiating into his legs
- Also, taking zolpidem 10 mg plus eszopiclone 6 mg to get a good night's sleep now
- Thus, sodium oxybate, approved for fibromyalgia, would be off label for his pain condition and potentially dangerous to mix with his other medications
- Patient taking only 40–60 mg per day of duloxetine because higher doses increased his blood pressure
- Modafinil has been very helpful for concentration and especially for fatigue
- Trial of 25 mg of pregabalin is helpful for pain
- Had a brief trial of mexiletine, an antiarrhythmic used off label for pain, but ineffective
- However, he feels his pain is now well controlled
- Recent resection of 4 more painful lipomas
- No more epidural injections
- Suggested trial of venlafaxine (Effexor XR) rather than duloxetine (Cymbalta) if he cannot tolerate an increase in duloxetine dose
- Mentioned that at the time another SNRI, milnacipran in clinical testing and may become available
- Could increase pregabalin dose
- Should consider reducing hypnotic dose and opiate dose
- Patient states that it will be up to his other physician, and that he does not see any problem with his current opiates as the alternatives are not acceptable as it will be too much pain

Case Outcome: Second Interim Followup, Month 24

- Seen again in consultation 18 months later, 2 years from the time of the original appointment
- Patient wants to know if there is anything new in terms of nonopiates for him because his pain condition has worsened and he is taking high doses of opiates but nothing else works
- Patient now has new bilateral wrist pain which is worse than his tinnitus or back pain
- States he has developed seronegative rheumatoid arthritis but was unable to tolerate methotrexate or azulfidine
- Also has been diagnosed with a small pituitary adenoma with decreased growth hormone and decreased testosterone and getting testosterone replacement cream

- Gained 30 pounds, no exercise
- Working very little
- Now taking Oxycontin 120 mg three times a day!
- Supplements this with hydrocodone 7.5 mg plus ibuprofen 200 mg or with hydrocodone 10 mg plus acetaminophen 500 up to 8 tablets a day (i.e., another 60 to 80 mg of hydrocodone a day on top of the oxycodone)!
- Taking duloxetine 120 mg/day unless his blood pressure raises and then he holds the dose
- Modafinil 400 mg in the morning and 200 mg in the afternoon
- Takes pregabalin as needed, 50 mg four times a day, perhaps three days in a row but he develops clumsiness, atoxia and a withdrawal syndrome so he does not continue pregabalin more than 3 days in a row
- Still taking zolpidem 10 mg plus eszopiclone 6 mg for sleep

What would you do?

- Trial of trazodone to reduce sedative hypnotics
- Trial of quetiapine again to reduce sedative hypnotics
- Referral to opiate detoxification program in a pain specialty clinic
- Insist on a psychotherapy evaluation
- Psychological/personality testing
- Report the referring physician to the medical board
- Resign from the case
- Other

Attending Physician's Mental Notes: Second Interim Followup, Month 24

- Obviously the patient is now opiate dependent and reaching a dangerous ceiling on dosing, particularly with his concomitant medications and his history of obstructive sleep apnea
- The patient should be warned about potential overdose implications of continuing his opiates at these doses and the possibility of respiratory depression or respiratory arrest
- He is actually not abusing the opiates in the sense that he is taking more than prescribed, and is not having daytime sedation by history, nor by examination at the followup appointment
- This may be as much a problem of a compassionate but enabling opiate prescribing physician sliding down the slippery slope of opiate dependence as it is opiate dependence on the patient's part
- Medications are not the way out of this dilemma, and the patient should be told that
- Strongly advised to decrease opiate dose and the danger of his current treatment program

- Suggested he consider referral to a new pain center for reduction but not elimination of his opiates
- Patient is not interested in that as he believes it would be disloyal to his current physician upon whom he depends for opiate prescriptions
- Strongly suggested scheduling more time to explore psychological dimensions to his condition
- Has poor insurance coverage and not working much at all any more, so income is low, and can only come back every 3 months
- Referred him to a psychotherapist anyway
- Advised him to try trazodone as a way to decrease his zolpidem and/or his eszopiclone

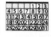

Case Outcome: Third Interim Followup, Month 27

- Seen again in consultation 3 months later, 27 months from the time of the original appointment
- Now told by specialists that his bone scan was positive in his wrists and that a form of rheumatoid arthritis may be causing wrist pain
- Considering anti-TNF (tumor necrosis factor) drugs such as etanercept (Embrel), adalimumab (Humira), and infliximab (Remicaid), but insurance will not cover these extremely expensive agents that cost thousands of dollars a month, as he does not have a classical case of rheumatoid arthritis
- Wife asked for a divorce a few months ago
- Now feeling depressed
- Thinks relationship might be salvageable
- According to the patient, his wife thinks he is too preoccupied with his pain and takes too many drugs
- Patient was advised that it was urgent to see a psychotherapist for himself, a couples therapist with his wife, and to try to reduce opiates
- No other suggestions given for psychotropic drugs and the patient was told that psychopharmacology was not the answer to his problems
- Patient was further told that he should take a non-medication approach such as psychotherapeutic and behavioral approach to this situation
- Patient said he will think about it

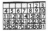

Case Outcome: Fourth Interim Followup, Month 30

- Three months later, seen again
- "Things are complicated"
- Still looks like his wife wants a divorce but they are living together although not talking about it
- He has "attacks" of pain now, with burning in his joints diffusely
- Feels he is deteriorating
- Was given a trial of an immunosuppressant, leflunomide for his possible rheumatoid arthritis, which caused anxiety, itching, infections and rebound of his arthritic pain in his wrists and the burning in all his other joints after discontinuing it
- Current medications:
  - Oxycodone sustained release (Oxycontin) 80 mg, 3–4/day (240–320 mg/day)
  - Oxycodone immediate release 30 mg 4 times a day (120 mg/day)
  - Hydrocodone/ibuprofen 7.5mg/200 mg, 2 per day
  - Extra ibuprofen, 200 mg as needed
  - Now taking clonazepam 1 mg three times a day
  - Duloxetine 120 mg/day
  - Herbs for sleep
  - Zolpidem 10 mg plus eszopiclone 6 mg for sleep
  - Thyroid
  - Modafinil 200 mg in the morning and 100 mg in the afternoon
  - Testosterone cream
  - Nutritional supplements
- Did not followup on opiate reduction program
- Did not followup on psychotherapy program
- However, wants to know the attending physician's opinion on following the teachings of George Gurdjieff and "consciousness" as a way of dealing with the pain
  - Gurdjieff is a late 19th century/early 20th century "mystic" and spiritual teacher sometimes described as teaching esoteric Christianity
  - The idea is to gain self awareness in one's daily life and in humanity's place in the universe
  - The patient agrees with Gurdjieff's apparent claim that people cannot perceive reality in their current state because they do not possess "consciousness" but rather live in a state of a hypnotic waking sleep
  - "Man lives his life in sleep and in sleep he dies"
  - Patient has been reading about Gurdjieff on his own and agrees with his ideas
- Patient asked if he felt suicidal but he denies this

- Patient advised that perhaps a better strategy would be meditation and that a better source of information might be Jon Kabatt-Zinn who has specifically applied meditation practices to the treatment of pain
- Patient states he will explore this direction

Case Outcome: Fifth Interim Followup, Month 34

- Seen again in consultation 4 months later, almost 3 years since the original psychiatric evaluation
- Wants attending physician's advice on some disability litigation in which the patient has been involved regarding his painful conditions
- Had a private disability policy for his consulting practice and self employment and now cannot work because of pain
- Insurance company is disputing his disability as being "real" and also thinks his major problem is drug addiction which they do not cover
- The patient has been in litigation for over a year, with independent medical examinations both by the insurance company and through his own lawyer
- Patient feels he can no longer work, and fears losing his wife's income from her job once she divorces him
- Advised him that his pain condition even if a somatoform disorder, can be disabling and his drug condition is secondary to the pain disorder
- Insurance company argues that his condition is a pre-existing psychological disorder with which he was able to work for many years and now that he is 61 he should retire, and does not merit disability payments
- It is common for patients with somatoform disorders to be involved in litigation and often they do not prevail nor receive good financial settlements
- Current medications:
  - Long acting oxycodone (Oxycontin) 80 mg three or four a day (240–320 mg/day)
  - Oxycodone immediate release 15 mg, 6–8 per day (90–120 mg/day)
  - Hydrocodone/ibuprofen, 7.5/200 mg, 2–4/day
  - Pregabalin 100 mg/day most days
  - Thyroid
  - Modafinil 200 mg in the morning, 100 mg in the afternoon
  - Duloxetine 120 mg/day
  - Clonazepam 1 mg two or three times a day
  - Alprazolam 1 mg 0 to 2 a day
  - Zolpidem 20–30 mg at night for sleep
- Discussed his litigation documents
- Pressed him on reducing his opiates and getting nonmedication treatment

- Patient wants sulpiride
- Attending physician unwilling to prescribe an unapproved agent from Europe unless patient makes a serious attempt to reduce opiates and get nonmedication treatments

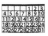

Case Outcome: Sixth Interim Followup, Month 37

- Seen again in consultation 3 months later
- Wife and daughter moved out
- Wife will not let him see his daughter
- Wife has taken daughter to a therapist
- Patient getting some support from family by phone from out of state but still no psychotherapy
- Patient trying to run his consulting business a few hours a day as he is in dire financial condition
- Still fighting with disability insurance company for a settlement
- Now he has to hire someone to clean house and do laundry
- Denies suicidal ideation
- Denies alcohol
- Has stopped the hydrocodone although continues to take his oxycodone at huge doses
- Other medications unchanged
- States that "pain varies from awful to unbelievable" with lots of day to day variation
- Asked why he comes back every few months if he does not take attending physician's advice
- States "I respect you."

Case Outcome: Seventh Interim Followup, Month 41

- Seen 4 months later
- "I have come through a lot"
- Still awaiting results of disability law suit
- Sees daughter once or twice a week
- Brings new article on Dercum's Disease
- Has finally begun seeing a psychotherapist weekly
- Has not pursued biofeedback or meditation which he was again encouraged to do
- Medications unchanged

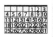

Case Outcome: Eighth Interim Followup, Month 45

- Seen for the last time 4 months later, almost 4 years following initial psychiatric evalutation
- Took a trip to New York and found a physician who will prescribe sulpiride again

- Got it in the mail, started 50 mg at night
- Decreased duloxetine to 60 mg/day
- Started "feeling better" and more energetic
- Other medications remain unchanged
- Except has tried some "medical marijuana" and some oral THC (tetrahydrocannabinol) which reduces the pain, but makes him feel quite "stoned" and intoxicated so only takes it once in a while
- Less pain, better sense of well being
- Still seeing his regular prescribing physician
- His therapist agrees with attending physician that patient is addicted to pain meds and also wants him to enroll in a detoxification program
- Plan is 6 to 8 months of psychotherapy, then enter detoxification, then another 6 to 12 months of psychotherapy
- Patient says he cannot afford it
- Wants to try milnacipran now

Case Debrief

- This man has a mixture of many painful conditions, the sum of which cause him great misery and disability
- Avoidant of psychological issues, psychotherapy or psychological interpretations of pain
- Always chasing a solution in another drug
- At high risk for premature death from accidental overdose or deliberate overdose
- High risk of suicide
- Poor outcome is likely
- Part of the problem is his physician prescribing the opiates
- Psychological factors are likely to have had an important role in this patient's pain
    - Concern about his waning influence in his field as his honors, recognition, patents, inventions and substantial financial rewards were on the wane and had mostly occurred several years before the onset of his tinnitus
    - Likely domestic conflict with his wife and his increasing dependency on her as his career waned was another likely factor in maintaining his pain

Take-Home Points

- It can be difficult to understand the causes of chronic pain in any given patient
- When a patient has an ever-escalating consumption of opiates, the result is not good

- Sometimes, opiates and psychopharmacologic agents allow a pain patient to avoid dealing with the real issues that cause the pain and the disability and the distress in their lives

Performance in Practice: Confessions of a Psychopharmacologist

- What could have been done better here?
  - It is possible that a more direct intervention with the opiate prescribing physician could have been done and done early to prevent the high dosing and the dependence that resulted
  - Perhaps the attending physician should have resigned from the case or used this as leverage to change behavior as the patient seemed to respect the attending physician and came back for more than 4 years
- Possible action item for improvement in practice
  - Make a concerted effort to get the patient involved in meditation programs, psychotherapy programs, or specialty pain centers
  - Find low cost psychotherapy options, including access to trainees in mental health training programs that may be available for psychotherapy at reduced cost

Tips and Pearls

- Once you go opiate, you never go back
- It is dangerous to begin opiates for chronic and vague pain conditions, particularly somatoform disorders that are likely to be lifelong because as in this case, it is the first step down a slippery slope to high dosing and dependence
- Patients with somatoform disorders may not get better but may be able to learn to live with their condition and still have a productive life

Two-Minute Tute: A brief lesson and psychopharmacology tutorial (tute) with relevant background material for this case – Differential diagnosis of chronic pain disorders in psychiatry

Table 1: What Are Somatoform Disorders?

- Names change over the years
- Body dysmorphic disorder
- Conversion disorder
- Hypochondriasis
- Pain Disorder
- Somatoform pain disorder
- Psychogenic pain disorder
- Somatization disorder
- Undifferentiated somatoform disorder

Table 2: Pain Disorder (Somatoform)

- Pain in one of more anatomical sites is the main complaint and is of sufficient severity to warrant clinical attention
- Pain causes clinically significant distress or impairment in social, occupational functioning
- Psychological factors are judged to have an important role in the onset, severity, exacerbation or maintenance of the pain
- Pain is not feigned
- Pain is not better accounted for by another disorder
- Symptoms can be a plea for help
- Symptoms may be a somatic expression of psychological conflict
- Often involved in litigation
- Often become opiate dependent
- Outcomes often poor

Table 3: Somatization Disorder

- Many physical complaints beginning before age 30 over many years and many types of treatment sought or significant functional impairments caused
- Needs 4 pain symptoms, 2 gastrointestnal symptoms, one sexual symptom, one pseudoneurological symptom
- Not caused by a medical condition or substance, and complaints out of proportion to medical findings
- Not feigned
- Symptoms can be a plea for help
- Symptoms may be a somatic expression of psychological conflict

Table 4: Dercum's Disease "Adiposis Dolorosa"

- Extremely rare disorder
- Multiple painful growths consisting of fatty tissue (lipomas)
- Mainly on the trunk, upper arms, upper legs, and found subcutaneously
- Pain possibly caused by growths pressing on nearby nerves
- Might be mistaken for fibromyalgia or it might be fibromyalgia

Table 5: Does Chronic Pain Change the Brain?

- Neuronal reorganization may occur in the grey matter of brain structures in the pain pathway and cause them to shrink
- Has been seen in structural brain scans of chronic pain patients
- Prefrontal cortex atrophy can occur in chronic pain states and has been linked to cognitive dysfunction in such patients
- Other areas where grey matter shrinkage has been reported include the brainstem and thalamus, in many chronic pain conditions

Posttest Self Assessment Question: Answer

Various theories propose which of the following as hypothetical causes of chronic pain?

A. Nerve damage
B. Central sensitization of brain and spinal cord pain circuits
C. Psychological factors
D. A plea for help and attention and a desire to be cared for
E. Somatic expression of psychological conflict

Answer: All of the above are proposed as theories for chronic pain causation.

References

1. Stahl SM, Pain and the Treatment of Fibromyalgia and Functional Somatic Syndromes, in Stahl's Essential Psychopharmacology, 3rd edition, Cambridge University Press, New York, 2008, pp 773–814
2. Stahl SM, Antidepressants, in Stahl's Essential Psychopharmacology, 3rd edition, Cambridge University Press, New York, 2008, pp 511–666
3. Stahl SM, Mood Stabilizers, in Stahl's Essential Psychopharmacology The Prescriber's Guide, 3rd edition, Cambridge University Press, New York, 2009, pp 667–720
4. Stahl SM, Stahl's Illustrated Chronic Pain and Fibromyalgia, Cambridge University Press, New York, 2009
5. Stahl SM, Sulpiride, in Stahl's Essential Psychopharmacology The Prescriber's Guide, 3rd edition, Cambridge University Press, New York, 2009, pp 503–7
6. Stahl SM, Duloxetine, in Stahl's Essential Psychopharmacology The Prescriber's Guide, 3rd edition, Cambridge University Press, New York, 2009, pp 165–70
7. Silberstein SD, Marmua MJ, Stahl SM (Ed), Mexiletine in Essential Neuropharmacology, The Prescriber's Guide, Cambridge University Press, 2010, pp 218–20
8. Kroenke K, Rosmalen JG. Symptoms, syndromes, and the value of psychiatric diagnostics in patients who have functional somatic disorders. Med Clin North Am 2006; 90: 603–26
9. Kroenke K, Spitzer RL, deGruy FV et al. Multisomatoform disorder: an alternative to undifferentiated somatoform disorder for the somatizing patient in primary care. Arch Gen Psychiatry 1997; 54: 352–8
10. de Waal MW, Arnold IA, Eekhof JA et al. Somatoform disorders in general practice: prevalence, functional impairment and comorbidity with anxiety and depressive disorders. Br J Psychiatry 2004; 184: 470–6
11. Barsky AJ, Orav EJ, Bates DW. Somatization increases medical utilization and costs independent of psychiatric and medical comorbidity. Arch Gen Psychiatry 2005; 62: 903–10
12. Hahn SR, Thompson KS, Wills TA et al. The difficult doctor-patient relationship: somatization, personality and psychopathology. J Clin Epidemiol 1994; 47: 647–57
13. Hahn SR, Kroenke K, Spitzer RL et al. The difficult patient: prevalence, psychopathology, and functional impairment. J Gen Intern Med 1996; 11: 1–8

14. Jackson JL, Kroenke K. Difficult patient encounters in the ambulatory clinic: clinical predictors and outcomes. Arch Intern Med 1999; 159: 1069–75

15. O'Malley PG, Jackson JL, Santoro J et al. Antidepressant therapy for unexplained symptoms and symptom syndromes. J Fam Pract 1999; 48: 980–90

16. Kroenke K, Swindle R. Cognitive-behavioral therapy for somatization and symptom syndromes: a critical review of controlled clinical trials. Psychother Psychosom 2000; 69: 205–15

17. Jackson JL, O'Malley PG, Kroenke K. Antidepressants and cognitive-behavioral therapy for symptom syndromes. CNS Spectr 2006; 11: 212–22

18. Allen LA, Escobar JI, Lehrer PM et al. Psychosocial treatments for multiple unexplained physical symptoms: a review of the literature. Psychosom Med 2002; 64: 939–50

19. Raine R, Haines A, Sensky T et al. Systematic review of mental health interventions for patients with common somatic symptoms: can research evidence from secondary care be extrapolated to primary care? BMJ 2002; 325: 1082

20. Mayou R, Bass C, Sharpe M, editors. Treatment of Functional Somatic Symptoms. Oxford: Oxford University Press; 1995

21. Looper KJ, Kirmayer LJ. Behavioral medicine approaches to somatoform disorders. J Consult Clin Psychol 2002; 70: 810–27

22. Smith GR, Monson RA, Ray DC. Psychiatric consultation in somatization disorder: a randomized, controlled study. N Engl J Med 1986; 314: 1407–13

23. Rost K, Kashner TM, Smith GR. Effectiveness of psychiatric intervention with somatization disorder patients: improved outcomes at reduced costs. Gen Hosp Psychiatry 1994; 16: 381–7

24. Kashner TM, Rost K, Cohen B et al. Enhancing the health of somatization disorder patients. Effectiveness of short-term group therapy. Psychosomatics 1995; 36: 462–70

25. Allen LA, Woolfolk RL, Escobar JI et al. Cognitive-behavioral therapy for somatization disorder: a randomized controlled trial. Arch Intern Med 2006; 166: 1512–8

26. Smith GR, Rost K, Kashner TM. A trial of the effect of a standardized psychiatric consultation on health outcomes and costs in somatizing patients. Arch Gen Psychiatry 1995; 52: 238–43

27. Sumathipala A, Hewege S, Hanwella R et al. Randomized controlled trial of cognitive behaviour therapy for repeated consultations for medically unexplained complaints: a feasibility study in Sri Lanka. P. Psychol Med 2000; 30: 747–57

28. Schilte AF, Portegijs PJ, Blankenstein AH et al. Randomised controlled trial of disclosure of emotionally important events in somatisation in primary care. BMJ 2001; 323: 86

29. Larisch A, Schweickhardt A, Wirsching M et al. Psychosocial interventions for somatizing patients by the general practitioner: a randomized controlled trial. J Psychosom Res 2004; 57: 507–14

30. Dickinson WP, Dickinson LM, deGruy FV, Main DS, Candib LM, Rost K. A randomized clinical trial of a care recommendation letter intervention for somatization in primary care. Ann Fam Med 2003; 1: 228–35

31. Kroenke K, Messina N, III, Benattia I et al. Venlafaxine extended release in the short-term treatment of depressed and anxious primary care patients with multisomatoform disorder. J Clin Psychiatry 2006; 67: 72–80

32. Volz HP, Moller HJ, Reimann I et al. Opipramol for the treatment of somatoform disorders results from a placebo-controlled trial. Eur Neuropsychopharmacol 2000; 10: 211–7

33. Volz HP, Murck H, Kasper S et al. St John's wort extract (LI 160) in somatoform disorders: results of a placebo-controlled trial. Psychopharmacology (Berl) 2002; 164: 294–300

34. Muller T, Mannel M, Murck H et al. Treatment of somatoform disorders with St. John's wort: a randomized, double-blind and placebo-controlled trial. Psychosom Med 2004; 66: 538–47

35. Hellman CJC, Budd M, Borysenko J et al. A study of the effectiveness of two group behavioral medicine interventions for patients with psychosomatic complaints. Behav Med 1990; 16: 165–73

36. Speckens AEM, van Hemert AM, Spinhoven P, et al. Cognitive behavioural therapy for medically unexplained physical symptoms: a randomized controlled trial. BMJ 1995; 311: 1328–32

37. Lidbeck J. Group therapy for somatization disorders in general practice: effectiveness of a short cognitive-behavioural treatment model. Acta Psychiatr Scand 1997; 96: 14–24

38. McLeod CC, Budd MA, McClelland DC. Treatment of somatization in primary care. Gen Hosp Psychiatry 1997; 19: 251–8

39. Peters S, Stanley I, Rose M et al. Randomized controlled trial of group aerobic exercise in primary care patients with persistent, unexplained physical symptoms. Fam Pract 2002; 19: 665–74

40. Kolk AM, Schagen S, Hanewald GJ. Multiple medically unexplained physical symptoms and health care utilization: outcome of psychological intervention and patient-related predictors of change. J Psychosom Res 2004; 57: 379–89

41. Smith, RC, Lyles JS, Gardiner JC et al. Primary care clinicians treat patients with medically unexplained symptoms: a randomized controlled trial. JGIM 2006; 21: 671–7

42. Rosendal M, Olesen F, Fink P et al. Randomized controlled trial of brief training in the assessment and treatment of somatization in primary care: effects on patient outcome. Gen Hosp Psychiatry 2007; 29: 364–73

43. Rief W, Martin A, Rauh E. Evaluation of general practitioners' training: how to manage patients with unexplained physical symptoms. Psychosomatics 2006; 47: 304–11

44. Martin A, Fichter MM, Rauh, E et al. A one-session treatment for patients suffering from medically unexplained symptoms in primary care: a randomized clinical trial. Psychosomatics 2007; 48: 294–303

45. Warwick HM, Clark DM, Cobb AM et al. A controlled trial of cognitive-behavioural treatment of hypochondriasis. Br J Psychiatry 1996; 169: 189–95

46. Clark DM, Salkovskis PM, Hackmann A et al. Two psychological treatments for hypochondriasis. A randomised controlled trial. Br J Psychiatry 1998; 173: 218–25

47. Fava GA, Grandi S, Rafanelli C et al. Explanatory therapy in hypochondriasis. J Clin Psychiatry 2000; 61: 317–22

48. Visser S, Bouman TK. The treatment of hypochondriasis: exposure plus response prevention vs cognitive therapy. Behav Res Ther 2001; 39: 423–42

49. Barsky AJ, Ahern DK. Cognitive behavior therapy for hypochondriasis: a randomized controlled trial. JAMA 2004; 291: 1464–70

50. Moene FC, Spinhoven P, Hoogduin KA et al. A randomised controlled clinical trial on the additional effect of hypnosis in a comprehensive treatment programme for in-patients with conversion disorder of the motor type. Psychother Psychosom 2002; 71: 66–76

51. Moene FC, Spinhoven P, Hoogduin KA et al. A randomized controlled clinical trial of a hypnosis-based treatment for patients with conversion disorder, motor type. Int J Clin Exp Hypn 2003; 51: 29–50

52. Ataoglu A, Ozcetin A, Icmeli C et al. Paradoxical therapy in conversion reaction. J Korean Med Sci 2003; 18: 581–4

53. Rosen JC, Reiter J, Orosan P. Cognitive-behavioral body image therapy for body dysmorphic disorder. J Consult Clin Psychol 1995; 63: 263–9

54. Veale D, Gournay K, Dryden W et al. Body dysmorphic disorder: a cognitive behavioural model and pilot randomised controlled trial. Behav Res Ther 1996; 34: 717–29

55. Phillips KA, Albertini RS, Rasmussen SA. A randomized placebo-controlled trial of fluoxetine in body dysmorphic disorder. Arch Gen Psychiatry 2002; 59: 381–8

56. Mayou R, Kirmayer LJ, Simon G et al. Somatoform disorders: time for a new approach in DSM-V. Am J Psychiatry 2005; 162: 847–55

57. Henningsen P, Zimmermann T, Sattel H. Medically unexplained physical symptoms, anxiety, and depression: a meta-analytic review. Psychosom Med 2003; 65: 528–33

58. Nezu AM, Nezu CM, Lombardo ER. Cognitive-behavior therapy for medically unexplained symptoms: a critical review of the treatment literature. Behav Ther 2001; 32: 537–83

59. Kroenke K. Patients presenting with somatic complaints: epidemiology, psychiatric comorbidity and management. Int J Methods Psychiatr Res 2003; 12: 34–43

60. Greco T, Eckert G, Kroenke K. The outcome of physical symptoms with treatment of depression. J Gen Intern Med 2004; 19: 813–8

61. Lin EH, Katon W, Von Korff M et al. Effect of improving depression care on pain and functional outcomes among older adults with arthritis: a randomized controlled trial. JAMA 2003; 290: 2428–9

62. Williams J, Hadjistavropoulos T, Sharpe D. A meta-analysis of psychological and pharmacological treatments for Body Dysmorphic Disorder. Behav Res Ther 2006; 44: 99–111

63. Kazis LE, Anderson JJ, Meenan RF. Effect sizes for interpreting changes in health status. Med Care 1989; 27: S178–S189

64. Ruddy R, House A. Psychosocial interventions for conversion disorder. Cochrane Database Syst Rev 2005; (4): CD005331.

65. Hahn SR. Physical symptoms and physician-experienced difficulty in the physician-patient relationship. Ann Intern Med 2001; 134: 897–904

66. Kroenke K, Sharpe M, Sykes R. Revising the classification of somatoform disorders: key questions and preliminary recommendations. Psychosomatics 2007; 48: 277–85

The Case: The woman with an ever fluctuating mood

The Question: Where does her personality disorder end and where does her mood disorder begin?

The Dilemma: Can medication work for mood instability of a personality disorder?

Pretest

When a patient has mood symptoms resulting from a personality disorder, medication treatment by itself is not likely to provide substantial benefit.

A. True
B. False

Patient Intake

- 27-year-old woman with a chief complaint of depression

Psychiatric History

- According to the patient's report, she has been depressed since age 5, with suicidal thoughts that began at age 7
- She began to have dissociative experiences of being outside of her body at age 8
- She also has an ambiguous memory about whether she was abused as a child (her half sister was sexually abused as a child)
- She began cutting herself at age 15
- She had some boyfriends in high school but was very socially anxious, though this has gotten better in recent years
- She graduated from high school and has worked several minimum wage or low-skill jobs during the nine years since graduation; the longest job held was for two years
- Other than working, she would mostly lie in bed all day watching television
- She says that she has been employed about 80% of the time but is not employed now; instead, she lies in bed all day with no motivation
- She picks at herself a great deal, and has muscle tension and leg shaking
- She also smokes marijuana daily and states that "it is the only thing that works for [her] agitation"
- Until one year ago, she lived independently; now she is on social security and disability, and her older sister frequently takes care of her
- She wants to go back to work, specifically to train dogs ("It helps put me back into my body"), but she is beginning to think that she will never recover sufficiently to do that

Treatment

- She first saw a psychiatrist at age 16; the psychiatrist started her on paroxetine (Paxil, Seroxat) and referred her back to her primary care physician
- She took paroxetine for three months, but it had no effect and she discontinued it
- After graduating from high school, she went into a residential treatment program for 45 days because of her cutting behavior
- She tried fluoxetine (Prozac) and then paroxetine, which "worked really good" and "gave [her] optimism"
- She stopped it after less than a year because she lost her insurance coverage; she relapsed within one month but did not restart medication for at least two years
- During this time, she had a boyfriend, got pregnant, and had an abortion
- She continued to be depressed and at age 20, restarted paroxetine, but discontinued it quickly because of side effects
- At age 21, she again saw a psychiatrist, who diagnosed major depression and gave her paroxetine, on which she partially improved
- Over the next two years, she took a long series of medications in an effort to achieve greater improvement
- She had side effects with most of these and was not very patient about trying them for a long enough period of time
- Because of lack of response, she had an endocrine evaluation and was told that she had low estrogen, for which she was given birth control pills
- She briefly tried lamotrigine (Lamictal) but discontinued it because she said it caused weight gain
- At age 25, while on birth control pills alone, she had a four-month period of complete remission
- She then stopped her birth control pills, relapsed into depression, and reinstated her birth control pills; however, this did not reverse her depression
- She restarted paroxetine and then several other medications, with no effect
- She developed more and more picking behavior of her fingers, scalp, and face
- Approximately one year ago, at age 26, she was hospitalized for suicidal ideation
- She was given lithium, which she did not like because it made her feel tired and groggy; she stopped it after six weeks
- At that time, she had a repeat hormone test and was told that her estrogen was normal

- She says does not remember much of the details of her outpatient psychotropic drug treatment for the past year, mostly because she has been noncompliant
- She states that since she was discharged from the hospital, she has been unmotivated, depressed, tearful, emotional, and negative, but not suicidal
- She does recall being retried on paroxetine, as well as on divalproex and other treatments, without benefit

Current Medications

- Paroxetine 30 mg/day
- Quetiapine 50 mg/day
- Thyroid
- Modafinil
- Zolpidem
- Birth control

Social and Personal History

- Never married
- Smokes cigarettes
- Smokes marijuana daily

Medical History

- BP normal
- BMI normal
- Normal routine blood tests except lightly hypothyroid

Family History

- Half sister: anxiety disorder
- Mother and maternal grandparents: alcoholism

Patient Intake

- She states that she is agitated, picks at herself, and occasionally has a surge of energy and feels like crawling outside of her body
- She also has superficial self-mutilation/cutting behavior every few days during the past month
- There is no suicidal ideation at present time, but she wishes that she were dead
- Abuses marijuana
- During the interview, she displays inappropriate affect, smiling when talking about her disability and seeming nervous and fidgety
- She often has awkward positioning of her head and posturing of her extremities and hands
- She is an excellent historian but has very little insight

PATIENT FILE

Based on just what has been presented so far, what do you think is this patient's diagnosis?

- Cluster B personality disorder?
  - Antisocial
  - Borderline
  - Histrionic
  - Narcissistic
- Cluster C personality disorder?
  - Avoidant
  - Dependent
  - Obsessive compulsive
- Social anxiety disorder
- Obsessive compulsive disorder
- Recurrent major depressive disorder
- Bipolar spectrum disorder, bipolar NOS
- Other

Whatever her diagnosis, do you think that this patient will likely recover fully and resume employment?

- **Yes**, with the right treatment
- No, but with the right treatment, partial improvement may be possible
- No, she is unlikely to recover

Attending Physician's Mental Notes, Initial Psychiatric Evaluation

- This patient has a complex situation
- She likely has a polymorphic mixed personality disorder with borderline, histrionic and dependent features that will take more time and possibly psychological testing to sort out
- Her personality disorder is also characterized by cutting behavior, dissociative states, inappropriate affect, and dependency
- She also has signs of compulsive picking behavior and social anxiety, and avoidance
- She also has a highly unstable mood
  - Unclear, however, if this is the unstable mood of a personality disorder, or the unstable mood of a unipolar depressive disorder, or of a bipolar spectrum disorder order since she has never been manic and it is unclear whether any of her other episodes in the past represent unequivocal hypomania
  - She clearly has had depressive episodes in the past and seems to describe mixed states as well, though there is no unequivocal hypomania

- It is possible that antidepressants have sometimes activated her
- Seems as though her treatment so far has been to chase a psychopharmacologic solution for her symptoms, so far unsuccessfully for over 10 years
- Not clear that she has ever had substantial psychotherapy in the 20 years since symptoms began
- Medication stabilization is not likely to be as robust a treatment for this patient as it would be for someone without her complex personality features, particularly if her mood instability is due to her personality disorder and not to a mood disorder
- Has not taken medication reliably enough and does not take it long enough to clearly see the effectiveness of past psychopharmacologic interventions
- She definitely needs psychotherapy
- The prognosis for a patient with a complex mixture of personality disorder features as well as mood disorder features can be quite challenging to try to stabilize with the combination of both psychotherapy and medications, and often is not successful as her history over the past 20 years already suggests
- Nonetheless, consistent and aggressive psychopharmacological management may have a role here and is worth a try in the hopes that it may help, along with psychotherapy, to recompensate this patient sufficiently so that she can attain a much higher level of functioning
- Psychopharmacologic management now, however, should not distract from now attempting to deal with her problems through psychotherapy

How confident are you that medication treatment for this case will be effective in improving functioning for this patient?

- She is unlikely to experience improvement with medication treatment
- She could experience some improvement with medication treatment, though it may not be robust
- She should be able to experience substantial improvement with the right medication combination

What type(s) of medication might be most beneficial for this patient?

- Antidepressant
- Mood-stabilizing anticonvulsant
- Atypical antipsychotic
- Antidepressant plus mood-stabilizing anticonvulsant
- Antidepressant plus atypical antipsychotic

- Lithium
- Other

Would you be more likely to switch her current medications or adjust the doses of her current medications?

- Switch
- Adjust doses

Attending Physician's Mental Notes: Initial Psychiatric Evaluation, Continued

- It may be useful to exploit her current medication portfolio by increasing the doses
- Specifically, quetiapine is currently at a low dose (50 mg/day), but the therapeutic dose for bipolar depression is often 300 mg/day
- The dose of paroxetine could also be increased to 40 mg/day
- Medications such as lamotrigine or lithium could be beneficial; however, she has already tried both
  - She believes that lamotrigine caused her weight gain (though this is not typically a side effect of lamotrigine), and she did not tolerate lithium well; thus, she is unlikely to be willing to try either option again
- Some patients with treatment-resistant bipolar disorder have responded to novel treatments, including riluzole, memantine, and pramipexole
  - Although these are low-yield possibilities and may have their own side effects, they could be worth a try
- Memantine in particular is noted for not having side effects
- However, in a case like this, psychotherapy may be the cornerstone of any improvement in function, and keeping medications stable for a longer period of time, no matter what combination is chosen, may be more important than constantly looking for a solution in a better medication combination, distracting therapeutic interventions away from psychotherapy

Case Debrief

- This is a complex patient with multiple problems, including adult development issues, personality disorder, and unstable mood of a non-classic, bipolar condition
- She may not benefit much from medication treatment because of her personality disorder, but it is still worth pursuing to try to maximize any improvement in functioning that she may be able to achieve
- If she would be willing and able to adhere to it, the best medication treatment option may be to combine an atypical antipsychotic and an antidepressant

- Other options may include a mood stabilizing anticonvulsant or even novel treatment with riluzole, memantine, or pramipexole
- Regardless of the medication strategy, she should pursue psychotherapy

Take-Home Points

- Medication is not the solution for all cases of mood instability
- Prognosis for mood fluctuations and other symptoms due to comorbid mood disorder with personality disorder is not necessarily very good, especially after 20 years of unresolved symptoms and after functional disability has set in
- Stability of therapist, prescribing psychopharmacologist, psychotherapy and medications without constant switching and changing is indicated so as not to contribute to the chaos and instability of her long term clinical course

Performance in Practice: Confessions of a Psychopharmacologist

- What could have been done better here?
  - Earlier psychotherapeutic intervention
  - Keeping the same therapist and prescribing psychopharmacologist
  - Trying treatments over longer periods of time
  - More attempts to have her stop daily marijuana use
  - Have the sister come to the office with the patient to get another perspective
  - Being realistic about long term outcomes
- Possible action item for improvement in practice
  - Being careful not to overpromise on the potential effectiveness of psychopharmacology interventions in a case like this
  - Transferring the psychopharmacologic management to a psychotherapist who can also manage the medications or who has close collaboration with a prescriber as coordination between psychopharmacology and psychotherapy for a case like this is essential

Tips and Pearls

- Try to reduce wild mood fluctuations and prevent overt mania and deep unremitting depressions with medications
- Do not attempt to control the rapid and short duration mood swings of a personality disorder with medications, but with psychotherapy

Two-Minute Tute: A brief lesson and psychopharmacology tutorial (tute) with relevant background material for this case
– Types of bipolar disorders
– Bipolar disorder vs personality disorder

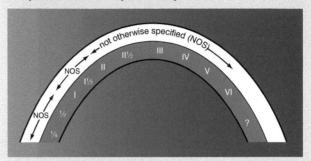

Figure 1: The Bipolar Spectrum
The only formal unique bipolar diagnoses identified in the Diagnostic and Statistical Manual of Mental Disorders, fourth edition (DSM-IV) are bipolar I, bipolar II, and cyclothymic disorder, with all other presentations that include mood symptoms above the normal range lumped together in a single category called "not otherwise specified (NOS)." However, there is a huge variation in the presentation of patients within this bipolar NOS category. It may be more useful instead to think of these patients as belonging to a bipolar spectrum and to identify subcategories of presentations, as has been done by Akiskal and other experts and illustrated in the next several figures.

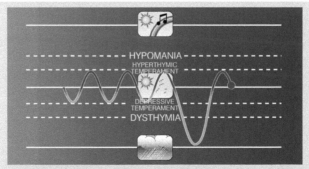

Figure 2: Cyclothymic with Major Depression
Patients such as the one discussed here may present with a major depressive episode in the context of cyclothymic temperament, which is characterized by oscillations between hyperthymic or hypomanic states (above normal) and depressive or dysthymic states (below normal) upon which a major depressive episode intrudes (bipolar II½). Individuals with cyclothymic temperament who are treated for the major depressive episodes may be at increased risk for antidepressant-induced mood cycling.

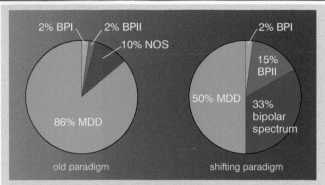

Figure 3: Prevalence of Mood Disorders.
In recent years there has been a paradigm shift in terms of recognition and diagnosis of patients with mood disorders. That is, many patients once considered to have major depressive disorder (MDD; old paradigm, left) are now recognized as having bipolar II disorder or another form of bipolar illness within the bipolar spectrum (shifting paradigm, right).

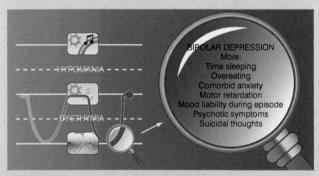

Figure 4: Bipolar Depression Symptoms.
Although all symptoms of a major depressive episode can occur in either unipolar or bipolar depression, some symptoms may present more often in bipolar vs. unipolar depression, providing hints if not diagnostic certainty that the patient has a bipolar spectrum disorder. These symptoms include increased time sleeping, overeating, comorbid anxiety, psychomotor retardation, mood lability during episode, psychotic symptoms, and suicidal thoughts.

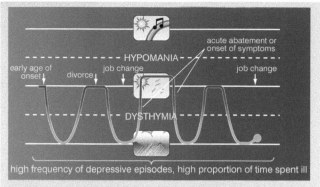

Figure 5: Identifying Bipolar Depression: History.
Even in the absence of any previous (hypo)manic episodes, there are often specific hints in the untreated course of illness that suggest depression is part of the bipolar spectrum. These include early age of onset, high frequency of depressive episodes, high proportion of time spent ill, acute onset or abatement of symptoms, and behavioral symptoms such as frequent job or relationship changes.

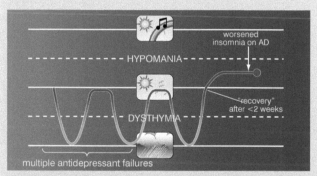

Figure 6: Identifying Bipolar Depression: Response to Antidepressants.
Treatment-response history, particularly prior response to antidepressants, may provide insight into whether depression is unipolar or bipolar. Prior responses that suggest bipolar depression may include multiple antidepressant failures, rapid response to an antidepressant, and activating side effects such as insomnia, agitation, and anxiety.

Table 1: Is It a Personality Disorder or a Mood Disorder?

- No foolproof way to tell
- No genetic test yet
- No reliable neuroimaging test yet
- General symptoms of personality disorders can greatly overlap with symptoms of a bipolar spectrum disorder
  - Frequent mood swings
  - Unstable mood
  - Excessively emotional
  - Suicidal behavior
  - Stormy, volatile relationships
  - Angry outbursts
  - Poor impulse control
  - A need for instant gratification
  - Constantly seeking attention
  - Suspicion or mistrust of others
  - Social isolation
  - Difficulty making friends
  - Alcohol or substance abuse
- Onset in childhood, poor response to antidepressants and mood stabilizers should increase the suspicion of a personality disorder, either as the sole cause of these symptoms, or as a comorbid cause of these symptoms with a concomitant mood disorder
- The problem with treatment of a patient with a mood disorder comorbid with a personality disorder is that a patient may oscillate from the symptoms of a mood disorder when that is out of control, to the symptoms of a personality disorder when the mood disorder is in control, never appearing to reach stability or a symptom free state

Posttest Self Assessment Question: Answer

When a patient has mood symptoms resulting from a personality disorder, medication treatment by itself is not likely to provide substantial benefit.

A. True
B. False
Answer: A

References

1. Stahl SM, Mood Disorders, in Stahl's Essential Psychopharmacology, 3rd edition, Cambridge University Press, New York, 2008, pp 453–510

2. Stahl SM, Antidepressants, in Stahl's Essential Psychopharmacology, 3rd edition, Cambridge University Press, New York, 2008, pp 511–666

3. Stahl SM, Mood stabilizers, in Stahl's Essential Psychopharmacology, 3rd edition, Cambridge University Press, New York, 2008, pp 667–720

4. Stahl SM, Quetiapine, in Stahl's Essential Psychopharmacology The Prescriber's Guide, 3rd edition, Cambridge University Press, New York, 2009, pp 459–64

5. Stahl SM, Paroxetine, in Stahl's Essential Psychopharmacology The Prescriber's Guide, 3rd edition, Cambridge University Press, New York, 2009, pp 409–15

6. Judd LL, Akiskal HS, Maser JD et al. Major depressive disorder: a prospective study of residual subthreshold depressive symptoms as predictor of rapid relapse. J Affect Disord 1998; 50(2–3): 97–108

7. Kendler, KS, Thornton, LM, Gardner, CO. Stressful life events and previous episodes in the etiology of major depression in women: an evaluation of the "kindling" hypothesis. Am J Psychiatry 2000; 157: 1243–51

8. Angst J. The Bipolar Spectrum. British Journal of Psychiatry 2007; 190: 189–191

9. Judd LL, Akiskal HS, Schettler PJ et al. A prospective investigation of the natural history of the long term weekly symptomatic status of bipolar II disorder. Arch Gen Psychiatry 2003; 60: 261–269

10. Merikangas KR, Akiskal HS, Angst J et al. Lifetime and 12-month prevalence of bipolar spectrum disorder in the national Comorbidity Survey replication. Arch Gen Psychiatry 2007; 64(5): 543–52

11. Benazzi F and Akiskal HS. How best to identify bipolar-related subtype among major depressive patients without spontaneous hypomania: superiority of age at onset. J Affect Disord 2008; 107(1–3): 77–88

12. Ng B, Camacho A, Lara DR et al. A case series on the hypothesized connection between dementia and bipolar spectrum disorders: bipolar type VI? J Affect Disord 2008; 107(1–3): 307–15

13. Akiskal HS and Benazzi F. Continuous distribution of atypical depressive symptoms between major depressive and bipolar II disorder: dose-response relationship with bipolar family history. Psychopathology 2008; 41(1): 39–42

14. Vázquez GH, Kahn C, Schiavo CE et al. Bipolar disorders and affective temperaments: a national family study testing the "endophenotype" and "subaffective" theses using the TEMPS-A Buenos Aires. J Affect Disord 2008; 108(1–2): 25–32

15. Oedegaard KJ, Neckelmann D, Benazzi F et al. Dissociative experiences differentiate bipolar-II from unipolar depressed patients: the mediating role of cyclothymia and the Type A behavior speed and impatience subscale. J Affect Disord 2008; 108(3): 207–16

16. Savitz J, van der Merwe L and Ramesar R. Dysthymic and anxiety-related personality trait in bipolar illness. J Affect Disord 2008; 109(3): 305–11

17. Correa R, Akiskal H, Gilmer W et al. Is unrecognized bipolar disorder a frequent contributor to apparent treatment resistant depression? J Affect Disord 2010; 127(1–3): 10–8

Lightning Round

The Case: The psychotic sex offender with grandiosity and mania

The Question: How to stabilize an assaultive patient with deviant sexual fantasies not responsive to standard doses of antipsychotics and mood stabilizers?

The Dilemma: Should heroic doses of quetiapine be tried when standard doses give only a partial response?

Pretest Self Assessment Question (answer at the end of the case)

Which of the following is a reasonable approach to treatment resistant psychosis when clozapine is not an option?

A. Dose olanzapine (Zyprexa) >40 mg/day to attain plasma drug levels >120 ng/ml but lower than 700–800 ng/ml which are associated with QTc prolongation
B. Dose quetiapine (Seroquel) up to 1200 mg/day
C. Dose quetiapine up to 1800 mg/day
D. Use olanzapine plus quetiapine
E. Use risperidone (Risperdal) with quetiapine
F. Augment with lamotrigine (Lamictal)
G. Augment with high dose benzodiazepines
H. Use nonpharmacologic interventions

Patient Intake

- 33-year-old man diagnosed with schizoaffective disorder, bipolar type, polysubstance abuse in remission in a controlled environment and antisocial personality disorder
- Diagnosed as conduct disorder prior to age 18 with criminal activity, then after age 18 as a psychotic and mood disorder for the past 15 years, with intermittent assaultive behavior, grandiose and grossly disorganized thinking and behavior
- Truancy, fighting, abuse of alcohol, methamphetamine and other drugs, continuing minor criminal activity
- Dropped out of college age at 21 when drinking heavily and initially diagnosed as bipolar disorder and treated with lithium and carbamazepine (Tegretol); also later diagnosed as schizoaffective
- Developed deviant sexual fantasies involving coerced sexual activity with adult women linked to grandiose delusions associated with hypersexuality in the context of mania but also without empathy or remorse
- Then became intoxicated and joined a group in a park which raped and sodomized a woman; following arrest his charges were reduced to assault with a deadly weapon

- Was convicted of this charge, sentenced to state prison, but required psychiatric treatment so that at the time of parole he was declared to be a mentally disordered offender and hospitalized in a forensic facility

Psychiatric History

- Despite treatment with standard doses of multiple different antipsychotics, continues to exhibit signs and symptoms of irritability, hostility towards women, loosening of associations, persecutory ideation, grandiose ideation, and auditory and visual hallucinations
- Patient has low frustration tolerance and bizarre, violent, and sexual delusions, plus rape fantasies with the belief that by excessively washing his hands he can cleanse himself of sexually deviant thoughts
- Continues to make verbal threats and engages in overt physical confrontations with staff and other patients and also exposes himself to other patients
- He also has a low grade and intermittent leucopenia that medical consultants have not diagnosed but are reluctant to approve the patient for clozapine treatment

Treatment History

- Inadequate responses to standard doses of risperidone, haloperidol and olanzapine, plus lithium, carbamazepine, lamotrigine and valproate (Depakote)
- Currently taking quetiapine 400 mg twice a day plus topiramate (Topamax) 200 mg twice a day

Of the following choices, what would you do?
- Increase the quetiapine dose
- Add a second antipsychotic
- Add a benzodiazepine
- Stop the topiramate

Case Outcome: First Interim Followup, Week 8

- Recommended increasing the dose of quetiapine by 100 mg/wk to 1200 mg/day
- No response in 8 weeks but tolerating it well
- Some weight gain, little sedation
- Is obese and has dyslipidemia

Of the following choices, what would you do?
- Keep increasing the quetiapine dose
- Add a second antipsychotic
- Add a benzodiazepine
- Stop the topiramate

Case Outcome: Second Interim Followup, Week 14

- Recommended increase the dose of quetiapine by 100 mg/wk to 1400 mg/day
- No response in 6 weeks; still tolerating it well
- Recommended increasing the dose to 1800 mg/day
- At 1800 mg/day, patient did remarkably well
- Decline in auditory hallucinations, improvement in irritability, no further violent sexual fantasies and excessive handwashing declined

Case Debrief

- It appears as though this patient has some sort of mixed psychotic and mood disorder. During development, the patient showed signs of conduct disorder and later antisocial personality disorder without regard for his victims
- He may also have a sexual disorder or paraphilia, as well as having conscious criminal intent, refusing to show remorse for his victims, and also refusing to pursue conditional outpatient treatment as he does not believe he should be required to participate in a criminal sex offender treatment program, this despite continuing to expose himself
- It is not clear whether antipsychotic treatments can target all of his behavioral symptoms, and thus whether his treatment resistance is due to comorbid personality and sexual disorders or to treatment resistant psychosis
- Nevertheless, given the severity of his condition, and few other options since many antipsychotics have failed, the cautious step-wise increase of quetiapine doses to heroic levels seems to have been empirically effective
- Whether he is failing to absorb the drug, or is having therapeutic effects from actions of quetiapine other than blocking D2 dopamine receptors is not clear
- Whether he could benefit from more standard doses of clozapine is not clear, but an intermittent and undiagnosed leucopenia makes medical consultants hesitant to approve him for clozapine treatment
- There is almost no written documentation in the literature for treating cases at these doses of quetiapine, with the literature that does exist suggesting that 1200 mg/day is no more effective than 600 mg/day

- The dilemma is whether to risk the danger to the staff and to the patient by treating with ineffective but evidence based doses of quetiapine, or to risk medical complications of heroic (or desperate) off-label use
- A treatment committee with a patient advocate reluctantly approved this treatment approach, with quarterly reviews and the patient agreed to this plan

Posttest Self Assessment Question: Answer

Which of the following is a reasonable approach to treatment resistant psychosis when clozapine is not an option?

A. Dose olanzapine >40 mg/day to attain plasma drug levels >120 ng/ml but lower than 700–800 ng/ml which are associated with QTc prolongation
   - This appears to be a prudent choice with cautious monitoring
B. Dose quetiapine up to 1200 md/day
   - Data suggest that this dose may have more side effects but not be more effective than 600 mg/day; however, anecdotes suggest that some patients respond to such high doses
C. Dose quetiapine up to 1800 mg/day
   - Almost no significant experience with this dose, and only in institutional settings with extraordinary cases and extraordinary monitoring; like this case, some anecdotes suggest that only doses this high help some patients
D. Use olanzapine plus quetiapine
   - Antipsychotic polypharmacy is not well studied but may be justified when all monotherapies fail
E. Use risperidone with quetiapine
   - Antipsychotic polypharmacy is not well studied but may be justified when all monotherapies fail
F. Augment with lamotrigine
   - This is a standard recommendation with a bit of data to support it
G. Augment with high dose benzodiazepines
   - Can help some patients but improvement may be proportional to sedation
H. Use nonpharmacologic interventions
   - This is obvious, but seclusion, restraint, isolation or disciplinary housing are not long term options and often are instituted after an assault, and may not prevent assaults to others or self harm

Answer: All of the above in selected cases under unusual circumstances only.

References

1. Stahl SM, Lamotrigine, in Stahl's Essential Psychopharmacology The Prescriber's Guide, 3rd edition, Cambridge University Press, New York, 2009, pp 259–65
2. Stahl SM, Clozapine, in Stahl's Essential Psychopharmacology The Prescriber's Guide, 3rd edition, Cambridge University Press, New York, 2009, pp 113–8
3. Stahl SM, Risperidone, in Stahl's Essential Psychopharmacology The Prescriber's Guide, 3rd edition, Cambridge University Press, New York, 2009, pp 475–81
4. Stahl SM, Olanzapine, in Stahl's Essential Psychopharmacology The Prescriber's Guide, 3rd edition, Cambridge University Press, New York, 2009, pp 387–92
5. Citrome L, Kantrowitz JT, Olanzapine dosing above the licensed range is more efficacious than lower doses: fact or fiction? Expert Reviews Neurother 2009; 9: 1045–58
5. Citrome L, Quetiapine: dose response relationship to schizophrenia. CNS Drugs 2008; 22: 69–72
7. Lindenmayer J-P, Citrome L, Khan A, Kaushik S, A randomized double-blind, parallel-grou, fixed dose, clinical trial of quetiapine 600 mg/day vs 1200 mb/day for patients with treatment-resistant schizophrenia or schizoaffective disorder. Abstracts of the Society for Biological Psychiatry, 2010, New Orleans Louisiana
8. Stahl SM, Antipsychotics, in Stahl's Essential Psychopharmacology, 3rd edition, Cambridge University Press, New York, 2008, pp 327–452
9. Goff DC, Keefe R, Citrome L, Davy K, Krystal JH, Large C, Ghompson TR, Volavka J, Webster E, Lamotrigine as add-on therapy in schizophrenia. J Clin Psychopharmacol 2007; 27: 582–9
10. Stahl SM, Grady MM. A critical review of atypical antipsychotic utilization: Comparing monotherapy with polypharmacy and augmentation. Cur Med Chem 11, 313–26

Lightning Round

The Case: The elderly man with schizophrenia and Alzheimer's disease

The Question: How do you treat a patient with schizophrenia who is poorly responsive to antipsychotics and then develops Alzheimer's dementia?

The Dilemma: Can you give an antipsychotic for one disorder when this is relatively contraindicated for another disorder in the same patient at the same time?

Pretest Self Assessment Question (answer at the end of the case)

Which of the following is a reasonable approach to treating an aging patient with schizophrenia who then develops Alzheimer's dementia?

A. Risk of cardiovascular events and death associated with the diagnosis of Alzheimer disease generally mean that antipsychotics should not be given even though the patient has long standing schizophrenia

B. Generally the needs for treating schizophrenia and the benefits of antipsychotic treatment of this condition outweigh the risks associated with antipsychotics when given in the presence of the additional condition of Alzheimer's disease

C. Cholinesterase inhibitors can be combined with antipsychotics

D. Best to treat a patient like this with cholinesterase inhibitors alone

Patient Intake

- 65-year-old man with a psychotic disorder since age 26 currently diagnosed as paranoid schizophrenia, with multiple hospitalizations for auditory hallucinations, ideas of reference, persecutory delusions, disorganization of thinking and aggressive behavior
- He has exhibited episodes of psychomotor agitation and aggressive behavior but has never met full criteria for either mania or major depression, but has carried the diagnosis of schizoaffective disorder at times in the past
- About 18 years ago stabbed the manager of his board and residential care facility during an argument and was convicted of attempted murder but found not criminally responsible by reason of insanity and admitted to a forensic facility
- Now developing deficits in cognition and short term memory consistent with early Alzheimer's disease and confirmed on neuropsychological testing

Psychiatric History

- Currently, his psychosis is out of control plus he now has worsening cognitive symptoms superimposed

- He was previously controlled on olanzapine (Zyprexa) 40 mg/day prior to the onset of progressive cognitive decline over the past year
- He refused medication for about a week recently, and his mental status declined with increasing confusion, more difficult to direct and more threatening
- Involuntary medication administration procedures were approved and the patient has been doing better, but still perseverates and seems confused with poor short term memory
- Also taking valproate (Depakote) 1000 mg in the morning and 1250mg at night
- Not only is there a question as to whether olanzapine can be given to a patient with Alzheimer's disease due to the black box warning for increased risk of cardiovascular events and death in elderly dementia patients, but there is even the consideration that his olanzapine dose may need to be increased beyond what even younger psychotic patients without Alzheimer's disease normally take in order to gain behavioral control

Of the following choices, what would you do?
- Taper his valproate
- Taper his olanzapine
- Increase olanzapine dose (after obtaining plasma drug levels)
- Start a cholinesterase inhibitor

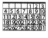

Case Outcome

- Plasma drug levels were measured and proved to be in the low to normal range despite the high dose of olanzapine 40 mg/day
- Olanzapine dose was thus increased slowly to 20 mg in the morning and 40 mg at night with good response
- IM olanzapine was given prn a few times during the tapering up to manage behavioral disturbances
- A good response was seen to his uncooperativeness and threatening behaviors, but he still perseverates and seems confused
- Donepezil (Aricept) 5 mg was started with perhaps a slight improvement in cognition
- If this does not work, the plan is either to increase the donepezil dose or try a cautious lowering of his valproate dose

Case Debrief

- It appears as though this patient has a long-standing psychotic illness now complicated by Alzheimer's disease, with somewhat mutually contradictory treatment requirements

- The patient cannot even withstand a few days discontinuation of his antipsychotic without behavioral decompensation, and standard to high doses of olanzapine are only partially effective
- Despite his age and the controversy of giving very high antipsychotic doses and the added controversy of administering antipsychotics to an Alzheimer's patient, the risks, and benefits were weighed and found in favor of trying very high olanzapine doses with good results, at least short-term
- Given the severity of his long standing psychotic condition, which is still the most disabling condition for him, and few other options since many antipsychotics have failed, the cautious step wise increase of olanzapine doses to heroic levels seems to have been empirically effective
- He may be partially noncompliant or partially failing to absorb his drug, thus necessitating higher than normal oral doses
- There is almost no written documentation in the literature for treating cases at these doses of olanzapine, especially at his age and, in particular, in the presence of comorbid Alzheimer's disease
- The dilemma is whether to risk cardiovascular events and premature death in order to control psychosis
- A treatment committee with a patient advocate reluctantly approved this treatment approach, with quarterly reviews, and the patient agreed to this treatment plan

Posttest Self Assessment Question: Answer

Which of the following is a reasonable approach to treating an aging patient with schizophrenia who then develops Alzheimer's dementia?

A. Risks of cardiovascular events and death associated with the diagnosis of Alzheimer disease generally mean that antipsychotics should not be given even though the patient has long standing schizophrenia
   - Such risks are low and generally documented in patients with Alzheimer disease alone and not in elderly schizophrenics, for whom antipsychotics are still indicated
B. Generally the needs for treating schizophrenia and the benefits of antipsychotic treatment of this condition outweigh the risks associated with antipsychotics when given in the presence of the additional condition of Alzheimer's disease
   - Although this is an individual determination, this is generally true for patients with continuing active symptoms of psychosis convincingly improved by antipsychotics
C. Cholinesterase inhibitors can be combined with antipsychotics
   - This is true and may even improve the cognitive symptoms

associated with schizophrenia as well as the cognitive symptoms
associated with Alzheimer's disease

D. Best to treat a patient like this with cholinesterase inhibitors alone
   – This approach is not likely to be successful as it will leave
     psychosis untreated

Answer: B and C

References

1. Stahl SM, Olanzapine, in Stahl's Essential Psychopharmacology The
   Prescriber's Guide, 3rd edition, Cambridge University Press, New
   York, 2009, pp 387–92
2. Stahl SM, Donepezil, in Stahl's Essential Psychopharmacology The
   Prescriber's Guide, 3rd edition, Cambridge University Press, New
   York, 2009, pp 145–9
3. Citrome L, Kantrowitz JT, Olanzapine dosing above the licensed
   range is more efficacious than lower doses: fact or fiction? Expert
   Reviews Neurother 2009; 9: 1045–58
4. Stahl SM, Antipsychotics, in Stahl's Essential Psychopharmacology,
   3rd edition, Cambridge University Press, New York, 2008, pp
   327–452
5. Stahl SM, Dementia and its Treatment, in Stahl's Essential
   Psychopharmacology, 3rd edition, Cambridge University Press, New
   York, 2008, pp 899–1012

Index of Drug Names

Note: page numbers in *italics* refer to figures and tables

Index of Case Studies